Long Term Safety of Assisted Reproduction

Long Term Safety of Assisted Reproduction

Edited by

Arianna D'Angelo, MD, Associate MRCOG
Clinical Lead and Consultant in Reproductive Medicine
Wales Fertility Institute, Swansea Bay University Health Board
Senior Clinical Lecturer in Obstetrics and Gynaecology
Cardiff University
Cardiff, UK

Kenny A. Rodriguez-Wallberg, MD, PhD
Professor and Clinical Head, Programme for Fertility Preservation
Department of Oncology-Pathology, Karolinska Institutet
Laboratory of Translational Fertility Preservation, BioClinicum
Head of the Subspecialist Training Program in Reproductive Medicine
Karolinska University Hospital
Stockholm, Sweden

Daniela Nogueira, PhD
Scientific Director, Groupe Inovie Fertilité
Co-Head, Institut de Fertilité La Croix du Sud
Toulouse, France

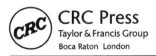

CRC Press is an imprint of the
Taylor & Francis Group, an **informa** business

First edition published 2022
by CRC Press
6000 Broken Sound Parkway NW, Suite 300, Boca Raton, FL 33487–2742

and by CRC Press
2 Park Square, Milton Park, Abingdon, Oxon, OX14 4RN

© 2022 Taylor & Francis Group, LLC

CRC Press is an imprint of Taylor & Francis Group, LLC

This book contains information obtained from authentic and highly regarded sources. While all reasonable efforts have been made to publish reliable data and information, neither the author[s] nor the publisher can accept any legal responsibility or liability for any errors or omissions that may be made. The publishers wish to make clear that any views or opinions expressed in this book by individual editors, authors or contributors are personal to them and do not necessarily reflect the views/opinions of the publishers. The information or guidance contained in this book is intended for use by medical, scientific or health-care professionals and is provided strictly as a supplement to the medical or other professional's own judgement, their knowledge of the patient's medical history, relevant manufacturer's instructions and the appropriate best practice guidelines. Because of the rapid advances in medical science, any information or advice on dosages, procedures or diagnoses should be independently verified. The reader is strongly urged to consult the relevant national drug formulary and the drug companies' and device or material manufacturers' printed instructions, and their websites, before administering or utilizing any of the drugs, devices or materials mentioned in this book. This book does not indicate whether a particular treatment is appropriate or suitable for a particular individual. Ultimately it is the sole responsibility of the medical professional to make his or her own professional judgements, so as to advise and treat patients appropriately. The authors and publishers have also attempted to trace the copyright holders of all material reproduced in this publication and apologize to copyright holders if permission to publish in this form has not been obtained. If any copyright material has not been acknowledged please write and let us know so we may rectify in any future reprint.

Except as permitted under U.S. Copyright Law, no part of this book may be reprinted, reproduced, transmitted, or utilized in any form by any electronic, mechanical, or other means, now known or hereafter invented, including photocopying, microfilming, and recording, or in any information storage or retrieval system, without written permission from the publishers.

For permission to photocopy or use material electronically from this work, access www.copyright.com or contact the Copyright Clearance Center, Inc. (CCC), 222 Rosewood Drive, Danvers, MA 01923, 978–750–8400. For works that are not available on CCC please contact mpkbookspermissions@tandf.co.uk

Trademark notice: Product or corporate names may be trademarks or registered trademarks and are used only for identification and explanation without intent to infringe.

Library of Congress Cataloging-in-Publication Data
Names: D'Angelo, Arianna, editor. | Rodriguez-Wallberg, Kenny A., editor. | Nogueira, Daniela, editor.
Title: Long term safety of assisted reproduction / edited by Arianna D'Angelo, Kenny A. Rodriguez-Wallberg, Daniela Nogueira.
Description: First edition. | Boca Raton : CRC Press, [2022] | Includes bibliographical references and
 index. | Summary: "A much needed overview of the available information now accumulating to indicate that Assisted Reproductive Technologies are generally safe for both babies and mothers. However, the literature abounds with reports of a higher risk of obstetrical and perinatal complications; regarding the long-term outcomes for both women and children, the data are still scarce. The chapters summarized in this book review the current knowledge on long-term safety of assisted reproduction and indicate the need for continued research to cover the lack of data in some specific patient groups and for recently developed treatments that only have a short period of follow-up"—Provided by publisher.
Identifiers: LCCN 2021043781 (print) | LCCN 2021043782 (ebook) | ISBN 9780367511234 (hardback) |
 ISBN 9780367511203 (paperback) | ISBN 9781003052524 (ebook)
Subjects: MESH: Reproductive Techniques, Assisted | Outcome Assessment, Health Care—methods | Safety
 Management—trends
Classification: LCC RG135 (print) | LCC RG135 (ebook) | NLM WQ 208 | DDC 618.1/7806—dc23
LC record available at https://lccn.loc.gov/2021043781
LC ebook record available at https://lccn.loc.gov/2021043782

ISBN: 978-0-367-51123-4 (hbk)
ISBN: 978-0-367-51120-3 (pbk)
ISBN: 978-1-003-05252-4 (ebk)

DOI: 10.1201/9781003052524

Typeset in Times
by Apex CoVantage, LLC

Contents

Acknowledgments vii
Contributors viii

1   The effect of ovarian stimulation on short term maternal outcomes 1
     Carol Coughlan, Barbara Lawrenz, and Human Fatemi

2   Evidence of the long term safety of ART and fertility drugs regarding cancer risk 8
     Frida E. Lundberg

3   Maternal and obstetric outcomes after IVF indicated by a male factor 20
     Begoña Prieto and Maria Diaz-Nuñez

4   The long term outcomes of children conceived through ART 28
     Kenny A. Rodriguez-Wallberg and Panagiotis Tsiartas

5   Maternal and obstetric outcomes after transfer of cryopreserved embryos 42
     Anne Lærke Spangmose, Anna-Karina Aaris Henningsen, and Anja Pinborg

6   Safety of assisted reproduction and fertility preservation in women with
     Turner syndrome 61
     Kenny A. Rodriguez-Wallberg

7   Maternal and obstetric outcomes after oocyte cryopreservation 68
     Alessandra Alteri and Valerio Pisaturo

8   Perinatal complications in pregnancies achieved using donor oocytes 73
     Roberto Matorras, Héctor Sainz, and Ana Matorras

9   Obstetric risks and pregnancy outcomes specific to patients with very
     advanced maternal age (over 45) 86
     Filipa Rafael, Marta Carvalho, and Samuel Santos-Ribeiro

10 Obstetric, perinatal, and postnatal outcomes after PGT 98
     Danilo Cimadomo, Letizia Papini, Nicoletta Barnocchi, Laura Rienzi,
     and Filippo Maria Ubaldi

11 Multiple birth outcomes: A minimizing strategy for elective single embryo transfer 108
     Zdravka Veleva

12 Obstetric outcomes after cancer treatment with or without assisted
     reproductive technologies 117
     Giulia Maria Cillo and Arianna D'Angelo

13 An overview of ART and the risks of childhood cancer 132
     Julian Gardiner and Alastair Sutcliffe

14 **Obstetric and perinatal outcomes using a gestational carrier** 141
   Marieke O. Verhoeven, Henrike E. Peters, and Cornelis B. Lambalk

15 **Birth outcomes of children born after treatments still considered innovative:
   In vitro oocyte maturation** 148
   Julie Labrosse, Daniela Nogueira, and Christophe Sifer

16 **An overview on the clinical outcomes from ovarian tissue cryopreservation** 156
   Daniela Nogueira and Isabelle Demeestere

17 **In vitro embryo development: Implications for epigenetic regulation** 161
   Giovanni Coticchio and Andrea Borini

18 **Psychosocial effects of undergoing assisted reproductive technologies** 169
   Sofia Gameiro and Bethan Rowbottom

19 **Psychosocial adjustment in offspring conceived through assisted reproductive
   technologies: Childhood, adolescence, and young adulthood** 182
   Catherine McMahon and Caitlin Macmillan

20 **The long term safety of assisted reproductive technologies: Ethical aspects** 195
   Lucy Frith, Heidi Mertes, and Nicola Jane Williams

Index 205

Acknowledgments

The editors are very grateful for all the authors for their valuable contributions; without them this book would not have been possible. We would like to acknowledge the excellent work started by Bob Edwards and collaborators and continued by all of us working in the fertility field – in particular, to the scientists for their continued contribution to research.

We are also very grateful to our patients who trust science in the hope of fulfilling their parenting desire.

Finally, a big thank you goes to all our organizations, to the publishers for their continuous support, and to our families for their continuous patience and encouragement.

Arianna D'Angelo
Kenny A. Rodriguez-Wallberg
Daniela Nogueira

Contributors

Alessandra Alteri
Obstetrics and Gynecology Unit
IRCCS San Raffaele Scientific Institute
Milan, Italy

Nicoletta Barnocchi
G.e.n.e.r.a. Umbria
Genera Centers for Reproductive Medicine
Umbertide, Italy

Andrea Borini
Family and Fertility Center
Bologna, Italy

Marta Carvalho
Hospital Santa Maria
Lisbon, Portugal

Giulia Maria Cillo
Obstetrics and Gynaecology
Yorkshire and Humber HEE Deanery
UK

Danilo Cimadomo
G.e.n.e.r.a. Umbria
Genera Centers for Reproductive Medicine
Umbertide, Italy

Giovanni Coticchio
Family and Fertility Center
Bologna, Italy

Carol Coughlan
ART Fertility Clinics
Dubai and Abu Dhabi, UAE

Isabelle Demeestere
Research Laboratory on Human Reproduction and Fertility
Clinic Erasme–ULB
Bruxelles, Belgium

Maria Diaz-Nuñez
Human Reproduction Unit
Cruces University Hospital
Biocruces Bizkaia Health Research Institute
Barakaldo, Spain

Human Fatemi
ART Fertility Clinics
UAE and India

Lucy Frith
Bioethics and Social Science Philosophy
Institute of Population Health
University of Liverpool
Liverpool, UK

Sofia Gameiro
Cardiff Fertility Studies Group
School of Psychology
Cardiff University
Cardiff, Wales, UK

Julian Gardiner
Department of Education
University of Oxford
Oxford, UK

Anna-Karina Aaris Henningsen
Fertility Clinic
Copenhagen University Hospital
Rigshospitalet
Copenhagen, Denmark

Julie Labrosse
Department of Reproductive Medicine and Fertility Preservation
Hôpital Jean Verdier
Bondy, France

Cornelis B. Lambalk
Department of Obstetrics and Gynecology
Amsterdam University Medical Centers
Amsterdam, The Netherlands

Contributors

Barbara Lawrenz
ART Fertility Clinics
Abu Dhabi, UAE

Frida E. Lundberg
Department of Oncology-Pathology
Karolinska Institutet
Stockholm, Sweden

Caitlin Macmillan
Faculty of Health
School of Psychology
Deakin University
Burwood, Australia

Ana Matorras
Cruces University Hospital
Basque Country University
Instituto Valenciano de Infertilidad (IVI)
Bilbao, Spain

Roberto Matorras
Cruces University Hospital
Basque Country University and Instituto
  Valenciano de Infertilidad (IVI)
Bilbao, Spain

Catherine McMahon
Centre for Emotional Health
Psychology Department
Macquarie University
Sydney, Australia

Heidi Mertes
Philosophy and Moral Sciences
Department of Public Health and Primary Care
University of Ghent
Ghent, Belgium

Letizia Papini
G.e.n.e.r.a. Umbria
Genera Centers for Reproductive Medicine
Umbertide, Italy

Henrike E. Peters
Department of Obstetrics and Gynecology
Amsterdam University Medical Centers
Amsterdam, The Netherlands

Anja Pinborg
Fertility Clinic
Copenhagen University Hospital
Rigshospitalet
Copenhagen, Denmark

Valerio Pisaturo
Obstetrics and Gynaecology Department
Fondazione IRCCS Ca' Granda Ospedale
  Maggiore Policlinico
Milan, Italy

Begoña Prieto
Human Reproduction Unit
Cruces University Hospital
Barakaldo University of Medicine of
  the Basque Country
Biocruces Bizkaia Health Research Institute
Barakaldo Instituto Valenciano de Infertilidad
  (IVI) Bilbao
Lejona, Spain

Filipa Rafael
Faculdade de Medicina da Universidade do Porto
Portugal

Laura Rienzi
G.e.n.e.r.a. Umbria
Genera Centers for Reproductive Medicine
Umbertide, Italy

Bethan Rowbottom
Cardiff Fertility Studies Group
School of Psychology
Cardiff University
Cardiff, Wales, UK

Héctor Sainz
Cruces University Hospital
Basque Country University
Instituto Valenciano de Infertilidad (IVI)
Bilbao, Spain

Samuel Santos-Ribeiro
IVI-RMA Lisboa
Lisbon, Portugal

Christophe Sifer
Department of Cytogenetic and Reproductive
  Biology
Hôpital Jean Verdier
Bondy, France

Anne Lærke Spangmose
Fertility Clinic
Copenhagen University Hospital
Rigshospitalet
Copenhagen, Denmark

Alastair Sutcliffe
University College London and Great Ormond
    Street Institute of Child Health
London, UK

Panagiotis Tsiartas
Institute of Clinical Sciences
Department of Obstetrics and Gynecology,
    Sahlgrenska Academy
Section of Reproductive Medicine, Sahlgrenska
    University Hospital
Gothenburg, Sweden

Filippo Maria Ubaldi
G.e.n.e.r.a. Umbria
Genera Centers for Reproductive Medicine
Umbertide, Italy

Zdravka Veleva
Department of Obstetrics and Gynecology
Helsinki University
and
Helsinki University Central Hospital
Helsinki, Finland

Marieke O. Verhoeven
Department of Obstetrics and Gynecology
Amsterdam University Medical Centers
Amsterdam, The Netherlands

Nicola Jane Williams
Politics, Philosophy and Religion
Lancaster University
Lancaster, UK

1

The effect of ovarian stimulation on short term maternal outcomes

Carol Coughlan, Barbara Lawrenz, and Human Fatemi

Introduction

Ovarian hyperstimulation syndrome (OHSS) is an uncommon but serious complication associated with controlled ovarian stimulation (COS) during assisted reproductive technology (ART). Increasing evidence demonstrates that the number of oocytes retrieved after COS greatly influences the clinical outcome in terms of cumulative live birth per started cycle. For this reason, any COS should aim to optimize the number of oocytes according to the ovarian reserve of the patient. Although this strategy might improve reproductive outcome, there is a risk of iatrogenic occurrence of OHSS. This syndrome is clinically divided into three grades of severity: mild, moderate, and severe (Table 1.1). In a mild form, OHSS can occur in up to 40% of cycles during in vitro fertilization (IVF) (1). The incidence of moderate OHSS is 3%–6%, whereas that of severe OHSS is 0.1%–3% (2). However, the true incidence is difficult to delineate. The traditional description of this syndrome includes a number of findings such as ovarian enlargement, ascites, hemoconcentration, hypercoagulability, and electrolyte imbalance (3). Symptoms are frequently classified in accordance with severity (mild, moderate, or severe) and by the timing of onset (early or late) (Table 1.1) (3). There are two types of OHSS, the first of which is described as early onset, appearing <10 days after human chorionic gonadotropin (hCG) administration and is self-limiting when pregnancy does not occur, and the second is late onset, appearing ≥10 days after oocyte retrieval (4). Early-onset OHSS is associated with ovarian hyper-response to gonadotrophin stimulation in patients predominantly triggered with hCG, whereas late-onset OHSS is induced by hCG produced by the trophoblast of an implanting embryo (3). Most cases of OHSS are mild and self-limiting, but cases composed of early-onset followed by late-onset OHSS are often serious and prolonged (5).

Prediction of OHSS

Identification of women at high risk and appropriate intervention can reduce the incidence of OHSS without compromising treatment outcome.

Demographics

Individualizing patient care and pretreatment evaluation of each patient will allow the clinician to determine each patient's risk of developing OHSS and optimize the COS protocol. Factors associated with an increased risk of OHSS include young age (<30 years) (6), low body weight (7), and polycystic ovary syndrome (8). Ethnicity may also play a part in determining the risk of OHSS, as African American women undergoing IVF have been reported to be at greater risk of developing OHSS than Hispanic or Caucasian women (9).

DOI: 10.1201/9781003052524-1

TABLE 1.1

Classification of OHSS Symptoms

OHSS Stage	Clinical Features	Laboratory Features
Mild	Abdominal discomfort/distention Mild nausea/vomiting Mild dyspnea Diarrhea Enlarged ovaries	No important alterations
Moderate	Mild features as noted earlier Ultrasonographic evidence of ascites	Hemoconcentration (Hct >41%) Elevated WBCs (>15,000 mL)
Severe	Mild and moderate features Clinical evidence of ascites Hydrothorax Severe dyspnea Oliguria/anuria Intractable nausea/vomiting Low blood/central venous pressure Pleural effusion Rapid weight gain (>1 kg in 24 hours) Syncope Severe abdominal pain Venous thrombosis	Severe hemoconcentration (HCT >55%) WBC >25,000 mL CrCl <50 mL/min Cr >1.6 mg/dL Na$^+$ <135 mEq/L K$^+$ >5 mEq/L Elevated liver enzymes
Critical	Anuria/acute renal failure Arrhythmia Thromboembolism Pericardial effusion Massive hydrothorax Arterial thrombosis Adult respiratory distress syndrome Sepsis	Worsening of findings

Source: Practice Committee of the American Society for Reproductive Medicine. Prevention and treatment of moderate and severe OHSS. *Fertil Steril.* 2016.

Ovarian reserve

Markers of ovarian reserve, such as high anti-Müllerian hormone (AMH) concentrations (10) and high basal antral follicle count (AFC) (7, 8, 10), are widely used by clinicians when determining a patient's risk of developing OHSS. Despite the widespread use of these markers in quantifying the risk of OHSS, clear cut-off values of these markers have not been prospectively validated (11). While cut points require validation, AMH values >3.4 ng/mL, AFC >24, development of ≥25 follicles, estradiol values >3,500 pg/mL, or ≥24 oocytes retrieved are particularly associated with an increased risk of OHSS (Practice Committee of the American Society for Reproductive Medicine).

Ovarian response to stimulation

A patient who was previously diagnosed with OHSS will be at risk again in a subsequent stimulation cycle. During stimulation there are certain "red flags" that may alert a clinician to the risk of OHSS. Ovarian response to stimulation may facilitate the identification of patients at high risk during COS, enabling the clinician to modify the risk by altering the protocol or by deciding to proceed with an "elective freeze all". Possible indicators of an OHSS risk during stimulation include elevated or rapidly increasing serum estradiol levels (12) and the development of a large number of small follicles (8–12 mm) during ovarian stimulation (13). Development of multiple follicles (>20) and a high number of oocytes retrieved (>20) are positively related to OHSS (14). In order to reduce the risk of OHS clinicians should prescribe progesterone as opposed to hCG for luteal-phase support. Despite the clinician being alert to both patient characteristics and stimulation parameters in order to trigger preventative measures, a significant proportion of patients who develop OHSS are not recognized as being at risk of OHSS either prior to or during their treatment cycle (15). A particular problem is the inability to accurately predict late-onset OHSS, which is related to pregnancy occurring following a fresh embryo transfer (15). This clinical scenario is poorly predicted by ovarian response parameters (15).

Pathophysiology

Understanding the pathophysiology of this condition may help in identifying measures to prevent its development and treat associated symptoms. The pathophysiology of OHSS is characterized by enlarged ovaries and increased capillary permeability, resulting in leakage of fluid from intravascular to extravascular spaces (16, 17). This fluid shift results in a state of hypovolemic hyponatremia (3). Vascular endothelial growth factor (VEGF) appears to play an integral role in the development of this condition and has been shown to play a part in many processes, including follicular growth, corpus luteal function, angiogenesis, and vascular endothelial stimulation (18, 19, 20). Available evidence points towards VEGF as an important mediator of OHSS, and serum levels of VEGF have been shown to correlate with OHSS severity (18). In addition, hCG has been shown to increase VEGF expression in human granulosa cells, with related increases in VEGF concentration (20). Other mediators that have been implicated in the pathogenesis of OHSS include angiotensin II, insulin-like growth factor I, and interleukin-6 (3: The Practice Committee of ASRM, 2006).

Preventative measures

It is not possible to completely eliminate OHSS, but significant reductions in incidence can be achieved with early identification of risk factors and careful monitoring of patients undergoing ovarian stimulation. Primary measures to prevent OHSS focus on individualizing patient care by personalizing the stimulation protocol to an individual patient's risk factors for ovarian response. Gonadotrophin dose should be tailored according to AMH and AFC (10). Previous responses to ovarian stimulation with exogenous gonadotrophins should be taken into account when planning the forthcoming treatment cycle. Women with risk factors such as polycystic ovary syndrome (PCOS) or a previous history of OHSS should be identified prior to starting treatment and an appropriate treatment plan put in place. A variety of protocols can be employed such as low-dose step-up, mild stimulation, and the withholding of follicle-stimulating hormone (FSH) on the day of hCG trigger. Metformin is an insulin-sensitizing drug that is commonly used for treating type 2 diabetes and has been widely studied in patients with PCOS, particularly in relation to OHSS. Some studies suggest that metformin does not decrease OHSS risk in non-obese PCOS patients (21) or those with PCO morphology only (Figure 1.1) (22). However, on balance, there is good evidence that metformin decreases the risk of OHSS in PCOS patients (23, 24, 25).

There are multiple studies demonstrating that stimulation protocols utilizing gonadotropin- releasing hormone (GnRH) antagonists for ovulation suppression are associated with a lower incidence of OHSS compared with protocols that use a GnRH agonist (26, 27). A Cochrane review compiled data from 29 randomized controlled trials (RCTs) that evaluated live birth (45 studies total in Cochrane) and demonstrated a statistically significant lower incidence of OHSS in the GnRH antagonist group and no difference in live-birth rates compared with the GnRH agonist group (28).

Secondary measures aim to avoid OHSS in patients who have had an excessive response to ovarian stimulation. The most efficient secondary OHSS prevention strategy is GnRH agonist triggering of final oocyte maturation. This approach secures sufficient oocyte maturation and significantly reduces – and in the majority of cases eliminates – the risk of OHSS. However, the GnRH agonist trigger can only be applied to cycles co-treated with a GnRH antagonist (29). Another modification includes lowering the dose of hCG used for trigger, but this does not reduce the risk of late OHSS (10).

Kisspeptin is a hormone that offers a novel approach to triggering oocyte maturation in women undergoing IVF treatment at high risk of developing OHSS. It stimulates the release of endogenous

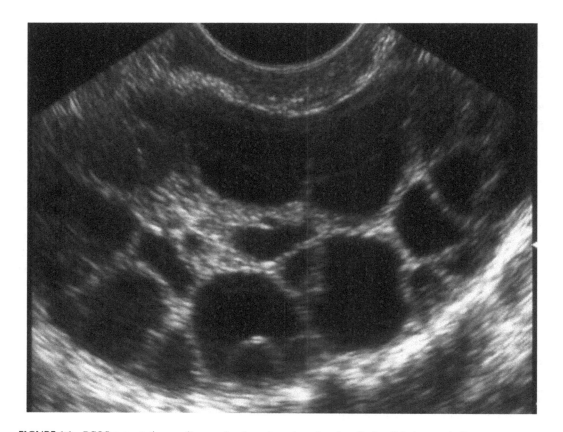

FIGURE 1.1 PCOS presentation on ultrasound: enlarged ovaries, often described as "kissing ovaries".

(From D'Angelo A, Hassan R, Amso NN, Ultrasound features of Ovarian Hyperstimulation Syndrome, in D'Angelo A, Amso NN, eds, *Ultrasound in Assisted Reproduction and Early Pregnancy*, CRC Press, 2020, with permission.)

GnRH from the hypothalamus and the consequent release of luteinizing hormone (LH) and FSH (30). Kisspeptin induces an LH surge that is dependent upon the patient's individual endogenous GnRH/gonadotropin reserves and thus should prevent excessive stimulation of the ovaries. Evidence to date shows kisspeptin to be a safe and effective alternative to hCG trigger for women at risk of OHS, but further large randomized studies are required to conclusively confirm (31, 32).

Coasting refers to the practice of withholding gonadotropins while continuing pituitary suppression in cycles with over-response, allowing the response to settle to "safe levels" prior to triggering administration. Evidence from a large retrospective study indicates that delaying the hCG trigger until estradiol reduces to 3,000 pg/mL is associated with a low risk of OHSS (11). However, on balance there is insufficient evidence available to recommend coasting for the prevention of OHSS (3, 33).

The pathophysiology of ovarian OHSS is largely attributed to an increased vascular permeability of the ovarian and peritoneal capillaries caused by ovarian hypersecretion of VEGF. It has been suggested that treatment with a dopamine receptor agonist such as cabergoline may result in a reduction of VEGF production and a subsequent reduction in OHSS. There is now good evidence available that dopamine agonist administration commencing at the time of hCG trigger for several days reduces the incidence of OHSS (3, 34, 35, 36).

Additional secondary prevention strategies include cycle cancellation (withhold hCG) and cycle segmentation (cryopreservation of embryos). In GnRH agonist co-treated cycles, cancellation of a cycle is a difficult decision for a clinician due to resulting disappointment for the patient, but it may be a necessary step to avoid deleterious consequences for the patient with an extreme ovarian response to stimulation. In segmentation, a bolus of GnRH agonist is administered in an antagonist cycle, oocytes are retrieved, and all embryos are cryopreserved (37, 38). It is important to note that this does not completely eliminate the risk of early-onset OHSS but does avoid the late form of OHSS associated with pregnancy (39).

Treatment of OHSS

The treatment of OHSS is multifaceted and individualized based on disease severity and progression. Once the diagnosis is made, the severity of the condition must be determined. Mild forms of OHSS can be managed on an out-patient basis. For out-patient management to be effective, a plan should be put in place to monitor daily fluid balance, daily weighing, and assessment of increase in umbilical abdominal circumference with serial blood test assessments every 48–72 hours to facilitate an early detection of disease progression. Patients should be provided written information detailing the signs and symptoms of deteriorating OHSS and advised to contact the clinic should they have any concerns. Culdocentesis/paracentesis should be considered to prevent OHSS disease progression on a case-by-case basis.

The criteria for hospitalization due to OHSS are hematocrit >45% and/or any sign of pulmonary or hemodynamic compromise (24). In-patient treatment of OHSS requires fluid management with maintenance of diuresis and administration of albumin if indicated if hypo-albuminemia is present (<28 mg/dL). Administration of anti-coagulant medication is warranted to prevent thromboembolic disease, which is particularly important for patients with a documented history of thrombophilia and thromboembolism. If the condition becomes critical, the patient must be admitted to an intensive care ward. In very critical cases, interruption of an early pregnancy may have to be considered.

Conclusion

The universal adoption of consistently applied criteria by which to define OHSS will ultimately improve medical care. In 2010, Humaidan et al. provided a classification scheme for grading OHSS that incorporates vaginal sonography and laboratory parameters to objectively relate symptoms to severity (10). The authors offered practical, evidence-based guidance to reduce the occurrence of OHSS and cited GnRH antagonist protocols and GnRH agonist trigger as the most important risk reduction strategies and very effective when used in combination (10). Other strategies that show some benefit include the use of cabergoline and cryopreservation of all embryos as opposed to proceeding with embryo transfer. If OHSS prevention strategies are not effective and a patient experiences severe OHSS, fluid resuscitation, supportive care, paracentesis, and prophylactic anti-coagulation are recommended.

Currently, no available method guarantees complete avoidance of OHSS, and there is no universal consensus on the criteria required for applying various preventative strategies. Further research is required in order to predict the risk of OHSS and optimize ART as a safe and effective treatment.

Recommendations

- Women with PCOS, elevated AMH, and high AFC may benefit from ovarian stimulation protocols incorporating GnRH antagonists to reduce the risk of OHSS.
- The use of a GnRH agonist to trigger oocyte maturation prior to oocyte retrieval is recommended to reduce the risk of OHSS if estradiol levels are high or multiple follicular development occurs during stimulation.
- Dopamine agonist administration starting at the time of hCG trigger for several days may be used to reduce the incidence of OHSS.
- Additional strategies which may reduce the risk of developing OHSS include the use of metformin in PCOS patients and elective cryopreservation of embryos.
- Treatment of OHSS includes fluid resuscitation and prophylactic anti-coagulation. When ascites is significant, paracentesis or culdocentesis may be required.

REFERENCES

1. Madill JJ, Mullen NB, Harrison BP. Ovarian hyperstimulation syndrome: A potentially fatal complication of early pregnancy. *J Emerg Med.* 2008;35:283–6.
2. Nastri CO, Ferriani RA, Rocha IA, et al. Ovarian hyper stimulation syndrome: Pathophysiology and prevention. *J Assist Reprod Genet.* 2010;27:121–8.
3. Practice Committee of the American Society for Reproductive Medicine. Prevention and treatment of moderate and severe ovarian hyperstimulation syndrome: A guideline. *Fertility & Sterility.* 2016;106(7);1634–47.
4. Mathur RS, Akande AV, Keay SD, Hunt LP, Jenkins JM. Distinction between early and late ovarian hyperstimulation syndrome. *Fertil Steril.* 2000;73:901–7.
5. Papanikolaou EG, Pozzobon C, Kolibianakis EM, Camus M, Tournaye H, Fatemi HM, Van Steirteghem A, Devroey P. Incidence and prediction of ovarian hyperstimulation syndrome in women undergoing gonadotropin-releasing hormone antagonist in vitro fertilization cycles. *Fertil Steril.* 2006;85:112–20.
6. Navot D, Relou A, Birkenfield A, Rabinowitz R, Brzezinski A, Margalioth EJ. Risk factors and prognostic variables in the ovarian hyperstimulation syndrome. *Am J Obstet Gynecol.* 1988;159:210–15.
7. Brinsden PR, Wada I, Tan SL, Balen A, Jacobs HS. Diagnosis, prevention and management of ovarian hyperstimulation syndrome. *Br J Obstet Gynaecol.* 1995;102;767–72.
8. Enskog A, Henriksson M, Unander M, Nilsson L, Brannstrom M. Prospective study of the clinical and laboratory parameters of patients in whom ovarian hyperstimulation syndrome developed during controlled ovarian hyperstimulation for in vitro fertilization. *Fertil Steril.* 1999;71:808–14.
9. Luke B, Brown MB, Morbeck DE, Hudson SB, Coddington CC, Stern JE. Factors associated with Ovarian Hyperstimulation Syndrome (OHSS) and its effect on Assisted Reproductive Technology (ART) treatment and outcome. *Fertil Steril.* 2009;94:1399–404.
10. Humaidan P, Quartarolo J, Papanikolaou EG. Preventing ovarian hyperstimulation syndrome: Guidance for the clinician. *Fertil Steril.* 2010;94:389–400.
11. Mathur RS, Tan BK. British fertility society policy and practice committee: Prevention of ovarian hyperstimulation syndrome. *Hum Fertil (Camb.).* 2014;17(4):257–68.
12. Delvigne A, Rozenberg S. Epidemiology and prevention of Ovarian Hyperstimulation Syndrome (OHSS): A review. *Hum Reprod Update.* 2002;8:559–77.
13. Navot D, Relou A, Birkenfield A, Rabinowitz R, Brzezinski A, Margalioth EJ. Risk factors and prognostic variables in the ovarian hyperstimulation syndrome. *Am J Obstet Gynecol.* 1988;159:210–15.
14. Asch RH, Li HP, Balmaceda JP, Weckstein LN, Stone SC. Severe ovarian hyperstimulation syndrome in assisted reproductive technology: Definition of high risk groups. *Hum Reprod.* 1991;6:1395–9.
15. Tsampras N, Mathur R. How to avoid ovarian gyperstimulation syndrome. In: Chaper 20 Cheong Y, Tulandi T, Li T-C, editors. *Practical problems in assisted conception.* Cambridge: Cambridge University Press; 2018. pp. 92–6.
16. Goldsman MP, Pedram A, Dominguez CE, Ciuffardi I, Levin E, Asch RH. Increased capillary permeability induced by human follicular fluid: A hypothesis for an ovarian origin of the hyperstimulation syndrome. *Fertil Steril.* 1995;63:268–72.
17. Bergh PA, Navot D. Ovarian hyperstimulation syndrome: A review of pathophysiology. *J Assist Reprod Genet.* 1992;9:429–38.
18. Geva E, Jaffe RB. Role of vascular endothelial growth factor in ovarian physiology and pathology. *Fertil Steril.* 2000;74:429–38.
19. Levin ER, Rosen GF, Cassidenti DL, Yee B, Meldrum D, Wisot A, et al. Role of vascular endothelial cell growth factor in ovarian hyperstimulation syndrome. *J Clin Invest.* 1998;102:1978–85.
20. Neulen J, Yan Z, Raczek S, Weindel K, Keek C, Weich HA, et al. Human chorionic gonadotropin-dependent expression of vascular endothelial growth factor/vascular permeability factor in human granulosa cells: Importance in ovarian hyperstimulation syndrome. *J Clin Endocrinol Metab.* 1995;80:1967–71.
21. Kumbak B, Kahraman S. Efficacy of metformin supplementation during ovarian stimulation of lean PCOS patients undergoing in vitro fertilization. *Acta Obstet Gynecol Scand.* 2009;88:563–8.
22. Swanton A, Lighten A, Granne I, McVeigh E, Lavery S, Trew G, et al. Do women with ovaries of polycystic morphology without any other features of PCOS benefit from short term metformin co-treatment during IVF? A double: Blind, placebo-controlled, randomized trial. *Hum Reprod.* 2011;26:2178–84.
23. Tang T, Glanville J, Orsi N, Barth JH, Balen AH. The use of metformin for women with PCOS undergoing IVF treatment. *Hum Reprod.* 2006;21:1416–25.

24. Palomba S, Falbo A, La Sala GB. Effects of metformin in women with polycystic ovary syndrome treated with gonadotrophins for in vitro fertilization and intracytoplasmic sperm injection cycles: A systematic review and meta-analysis of randomized controlled trials. *BJOG.* 2013;120:267–76.
25. Huang X, Wang P, Tal R, Lv F, Li Y, Zhang X. A systematic review and meta-analysis of metformin among patients with polycystic ovary syndrome undergoing assisted reproductive technology procedures. *Int J Gynaecol Obstet.* 2015;131:111–16.
26. Toftager M, Bogstad J, Bryndorf T, Lossl K, Roskaer J, Holland T, et al. Risk of severe ovarian hyperstimulation syndrome in GnRH antagonist versus GnRH agonist protocol: RCT including 1050 first IVF/ICSI cycles. *Hum Reprod.* 2016.
27. Lainas TG, Sfontouris IA, Zorzovilis IZ, Petsas GK, Lainas GT, Alexopoulou E, et al. Flexible GnRH antagonist protocol versus GnRH agonist long protocol in patients with polycystic ovary syndrome treated for IVF: A prospective Randomised Controlled Trial (RCT). *Hum Reprod.* 2010;25:683–9.
28. Al-Inany HG, Youssef MA, Aboulghar M, Broekmans F, Sterrenburg M, Smit J, et al. Gonadotrophin-releasing hormone antagonists for assisted reproductive technology. *Cochrane Database Syst Rev.* 2011:CD001750.
29. Humaidan P, Nelson SM, Devroey P, Coddington CC, Schwartz LB, Gordon K, Frattarelli JL, Tarlatzis BC, Fatemi HM, Lutjen P, Stegmann BJ. Ovarian hyperstimulation syndrome: Review and new classification criteria for reporting in clinical trials. *Human Reproduction.* 2016;31(9);1997–2004.
30. Irwig MS, Fraley GS, Smith JT, et al. Kisspeptin activation of gonadotropin releasing hormone neurons and regulation of KiSS-1 mRNA in the male rat. *Neuroendocrinology.* 2004;80(4):264–72.
31. Abbara A, Jayasena CN, Christopoulos G, Narayanaswamy S, Izzi-Engbeaya C, Nijher GM, Comninos AN, Peters D, Buckley A, Ratnasabapathy R, et al. Efficacy of kisspeptin-54 to trigger oocyte maturation in women at high risk of Ovarian Hyperstimulation Syndrome (OHSS) during In Vitro Fertilization (IVF) therapy. *J Clin Endocrinol Metab.* 2015;100:3322–31.
32. Abbara A, Islam R, Clarke SA, Jeffers L, Christopoulos G, Comninos AN, Salim R, Lavery SA, Vuong TNL, Humaidan P, Kelsey TW, Trew GH, Dhillo WS. Clinical parameters of ovarian hyperstimulation syndrome following different hormonal triggers of oocyte maturation in IVF treatment. *Clin Endocrinol (Oxf).* 2018 Jun;88(6):920–7.
33. D'Angelo A, Amso NN, Hassan R. Coasting (withholding gonadotrophins) for preventing ovarian hyperstimulation syndrome. *Cochrane Database Syst Rev.* 2017 May 23;5(5):CD002811. doi: 10.1002/14651858.CD002811.pub4.
34. Amir H, Yaniv D, Hasson J, Amit A, Gordon D, Azem F. Cabergoline for reducing ovarian hyperstimulation syndrome in assisted reproductive technology treatment cycles: A prospective randomized controlled trial. *J Reprod Med.* 2015;60:48–54.
35. Carizza C, Abdelmassih V, Abdelmassih S, Ravizzini P, Salgueiro L, Salgueiro PT, et al. Cabergoline reduces the early onset of ovarian hyperstimulation syndrome: A prospective randomized study. *Reprod Biomed Online.* 2008;17:751–5.
36. Leitao VM, Moroni RM, Seko LM, Nastri CO, Martins WP. Cabergoline for the prevention of ovarian hyperstimulation syndrome: Systematic review and meta-analysis of randomized controlled trials. *Fertil Steril.* 2014;101:664–75.
37. Maheshwari A, Bhattacharya S. Elective frozen replacement cycles for all: Ready for prime time? *Hum Reprod.* 2013;28:6–9.
38. Fatemi HM, Popovic-Todorovic B, Humaidan P, Kol S, Banker M, Devroey P, Garcia-Velasco JA. Severe ovarian hyperstimulation syndrome after gonadotropin: Releasing hormone (GnRH) agonist trigger and "freeze-all" approach in GnRH antagonist protocol. *Fertil Steril.* 2014 Apr;101(4):1008–11.
39. D'Angelo A, Amso NN. Embryo Freezing for preventing ovarian hyperstimulation syndrome. *Cochrane Database Syst Rev.* 2007 Jul 18;(3):CD002806. doi: 10.1002/14651858.CD002806.pub2.

2

Evidence of the long term safety of ART and fertility drugs regarding cancer risk

Frida E. Lundberg

With the increasing number of patients undergoing fertility treatments and using fertility drugs, it is essential to understand whether these treatments influence the long term risk of cancer. The most commonly used hormonal medications for ovulation induction in anovulatory women are clomiphene citrate and gonadotropins. Clomiphene citrate inhibits the negative feedback of estrogen on the hypothalamus leading to increased gonadotropin secretion from the pituitary gland, which in turn stimulates the ovaries to induce follicle development and ovulation (1). In assisted reproductive technology (ART) treatments, high and sustained doses of gonadotropins are used to support the growth of multiple follicles during a single cycle, while lower doses of gonadotropins are used for ovulation induction. Both ovulation induction treatments and ART lead to gonadotropin stimulation of the ovaries, causing higher levels of circulating estrogen, which has in turn been suspected to increase the risk of hormone-sensitive cancers.

The current knowledge regarding the possible relationship between ovarian stimulation and cancer risk is based on observational studies, such as case-control and cohort studies, since randomized clinical trials are not feasible in this context. Investigating cancer risk following ovarian stimulation treatments in a non-randomized setting involves several challenges. First of all, the population of women who go through fertility treatments may be at increased risk of cancer due to other factors, such as the underlying infertility, not having children or giving birth at a later age. These characteristics usually co-occur, which may cause selection bias in case-control studies and make it difficult to disentangle the potential effect of treatment in all observational studies. Information on childbirth as well as causes of infertility, both among treated and untreated women, is needed in order to separately estimate potential effects of infertility and treatment. Unfortunately, detailed information on the causes of infertility is not often available, and the results of observational studies may therefore be difficult to interpret. Meta-analyses are used to pool information from several published studies to ideally get more reliable estimates of a studied association. However, meta-analyses will incorporate limitations of the studies included, such as selection bias and unmeasured confounding in observational studies. Meta-analyses are often performed using unadjusted estimates in order to make the results from several studies comparable. In addition, a selective reporting of studies with positive results may lead to bias in meta-analyses (2).

In order to reconstruct the ovarian stimulation history, detailed information on the treatment protocols used, number of treatment cycles, and cumulative doses given to each woman is needed. Studies relying on self-reported treatment information might suffer from recall bias, since cancer patients tend to look for reasons why they developed the disease (3). Infertile women may receive several different types of fertility treatment – for instance, unsuccessful ovulation induction using clomiphene citrate stimulation followed by ART treatment, which could bias the results of studies focusing on one of these treatment types. Few studies to date have been able to quantify the exposure to each type of fertility drug, which is needed to investigate a possible dose-response relationship with cancer risk.

Cancer is also a relatively rare outcome which usually occurs long after the reproductive period, and few studies have follow-up periods long enough to include the age at which cancer is most often diagnosed. In this setting, a small absolute difference in the number of cancer cases can result in a large difference in relative risk.

This chapter will focus on cancers of the breast, ovary and endometrium. These cancer types are known to be associated with hormonal and reproductive factors, and the risk could therefore hypothetically be influenced by hormonal fertility treatments and ART.

Breast cancer

Many established risk factors for breast cancer are related to reproductive health and fertility, such as nulliparity, early menarche, late menopause, higher age at first birth, and not breastfeeding (4, 5). In addition, a transient increase in breast cancer risk has been shown for oral contraceptive use and postmenopausal hormone replacement therapy (6). A unifying hypothesis behind these associations proposes that high cumulative exposure to estrogen increases breast cancer risk regardless of whether estrogen is endogenous or exogenous (7). Aside from the association with nulliparity, infertility has not been shown to be a risk factor for breast cancer (8, 9).

Both clomiphene citrate and gonadotropins have been suspected to influence the risk of breast cancer through increased serum concentrations of endogenous estrogen. Reassuringly, most previous studies have not found a higher risk of breast cancer in women treated with ovulation induction (Table 2.1). Among the cohort studies including women treated with ART (Table 2.2), one study reported a small but significant increase in breast cancer risk among parous women (12), while other studies have found no increased risk. A recently published meta-analysis found no increased risk of breast cancer in women treated with ovarian stimulation, either compared to the general population or to untreated infertile women (13). Overall, these results suggest that ovarian stimulation treatments for infertility are not associated with an increased risk of breast cancer.

Ovarian cancer

Women with early menarche, late menopause, nulliparity or endometriosis have been shown to have a higher risk of ovarian cancer (42, 43). In contrast, the use of oral contraceptives and high age at first as well as last birth are associated with a lower risk of ovarian cancer (44, 45).

Two different theories have been proposed to explain these associations. The *incessant ovulation theory* proposes that the damage and repair of the ovarian epithelium during ovulation leads to an increased ovarian cancer risk, while the *elevated gonadotropins theory* hypothesizes that the higher risk is due to stimulation of the ovarian epithelium by endogenous gonadotropins. Both of these theories suggest that fertility treatments may increase the risk of ovarian cancer, since the treatments increase the levels of circulating gonadotropins and stimulate ovulation (46).

Most cohort studies to date have not found any significant association between ovulation induction treatments and the risk of ovarian cancer (Table 2.3), although many are limited by small numbers of cancer cases. A notable exception is the 2017 study from Norway which found a higher risk of ovarian cancer in women treated with clomiphene citrate, especially among nulliparous women (16). However, the reported associations may be confounded by the cause and severity of the underlying infertility.

Cohort studies which have investigated the associations between ART and ovarian cancer risk are summarized in Table 2.4. A systematic review from 2019, which included 24 cohort and 13 case-control studies, "found no convincing evidence of an increase in the risk of invasive ovarian tumors with fertility drug treatment" (47). However, the authors noted that the certainty of the current evidence was considered very low. Following this review, three large cohort studies have been published which reported higher risks of ovarian cancer following ART treatment (31, 48, 49) and one which did not find a higher risk (50). A Danish study from 2019 also presented risk estimates according to the cause of infertility and found that the higher risk of ovarian cancer after ART was limited to women with endometriosis, while the risk was not increased in women with other causes of infertility (49). Similarly, a UK study found that the higher risk of ovarian cancer among ART-treated women was limited to women with endometriosis and/or low parity, while no increased risk was seen in women treated for male factor or unexplained infertility (31). The Swedish study from 2019 reported a higher risk of ovarian cancer

TABLE 2.1

Cohort Studies on Breast Cancer Risk Following Ovulation Induction

First Author, Year (reference)	Country, Treatment Period	Treatment/ Comparison Group	Cancer Cases	Total Number	Risk (95% CI)	Adjustments
Guleria, 2019 (14)	Denmark, 1995–2011	OI Population	743 19,725	86,231 1,234,070	HR 1.02 (0.95–1.10)	Age, year, parity, age at first birth, gravidity, education, oral contraceptive use
Lundberg, 2017 (15)	Sweden, 2005–2012	CC, Gn Infertile	50 497	26,232 104,836	HR 0.95 (0.71–1.28)	Age, year, parity, age at first birth, education, country of birth, family history, salpingectomy, hysterectomy
Reigstad, 2017 (16)	Norway, 2004–2014	CC Population	140 6,550	38,927 1,314,797	HR 1.12 (0.93–1.35)	Age, year, parity, region of residence
Kessous, 2016 (17)	Israel, 1988–2013	OI Population	16 508	3,214 101,668	Not sign	Time since birth
Brinton, 2014 (18)	US, 5 states, 1965–1988	CC Population Gn Population	284 450 82 450	3,769 ≈5,950 950 ≈5,950	HR 1.05 (0.90–1.22) HR 1.14 (0.89–1.44)	Age, year of first infertility evaluation
Brinton, 2013 (19)	Israel, 1994–2011	CC Infertile	284 133	≈50,930 19,795	HR 0.87 (0.71–1.08)	Age, parity, BMI, smoking, socioeconomic status
Lerner-Geva, 2012 (20)	Israel, 1964–1974	CC, Gn Population	70 83	1,281 1,150	No excess risk	Age, continent of birth
Calderon-Margalit, 2009 (21)	Israel, 1974–1976	OI Population	32 498	567 14,463	HR 1.42 (0.99–2.05)	Age, parity, geographic origin, BMI, socioeconomic status
dos Santos Silva, 2009 (22)	UK, 1963–1999	CC, Gn Infertile	102 72	3,180 3,949	RR 1.27 (0.93–1.75)	Age, year
Orgéas, 2009 (23)	Sweden, 1961–1976	CC, Gn Expected	54 53.5	1,135 –	SIR 1.01 (0.77–1.31)	Age, year, parity, age at first birth
Jensen, 2007 (24)	Denmark, 1963–1998	CC Infertile Gn Infertile	102 229 36 295	405 820 165 1,061	RR 1.08 (0.85–1.39) RR 1.20 (0.82–1.78)	Age, year, parity
Lerner-Geva, 2006 (25)	Israel, 1964–1984	CC, Gn Infertile	73 58	3,076 2,712	RR 1.11 (0.79–1.57)	Age, year, continent of birth
Brinton, 2004 (26)	US, 5 states, 1965–1988	CC Infertile Gn Infertile	108 184 31 261	3,280 5,151 867 7,564	RR 1.02 (0.8–1.3) RR 1.07 (0.7–1.6)	Age, year, study site, family history
Gauthier, 2004 (27)	France, NA	CC, Gn Population	133 2,388	4,834 85,953	RR 0.94 (0.78–1.12)	Age, parity, age at first birth, education, smoking, BMI, family history, benign breast disease, age at menarche, menopausal status
Doyle, 2002 (28)	UK, 1975–1989	OI Infertile	43 11	4,188 1,231	RR 0.95 (0.47–1.92)	Age, year, parity, year of first visit to clinic
Potashnik, 1999 (29)	Israel, 1960–1984	CC, Gn Expected	16 9.6	780 –	SIR 1.65 (0.94–2.68)	Age, year, country of birth
Modan, 1998 (30)	Israel, 1964–1974	CC, Gn Expected	25 22.7	1,309 –	SIR 1.1 (0.7–1.6)	Age, year, country of birth

Abbreviations: *BMI* body mass index, *CC* clomiphene citrate, *CI* confidence interval, *Gn* gonadotropins, *HR* hazard ratio, *NA* not available, *OI* ovulation induction, *OR* odds ratio, *RR* rate ratio, *SIR* standardized incidence ratio, *UK* United Kingdom, *US* United States.

TABLE 2.2

Cohort Studies on Breast Cancer Risk Following ART

First Author, Year (reference)	Country, Treatment Period	Treatment/ Comparison Group	Cancer Cases	Total Number	Risk (95% CI)	Adjustments
Williams, 2018 (31)	UK, 1991–2010	ART Expected	2,578 2,641.2	225,786 –	SIR 0.98 (0.94–1.01)	Age, year
Lundberg, 2017 (15)	Sweden, 1982–2012	ART Infertile	262 853	38,047 87,522	HR 1.01 (0.88–1.17)	Age, year, parity, age at first birth, education, country of birth, family history, salpingectomy, hysterectomy
Reigstad, 2017 (16)	Norway, 2004–2014	ART Population	112 6,578	33,431 1,320,293	HR 1.00 (0.81–1.22)	Age, year, parity, region of residence
Kessous, 2016 (17)	Israel, 1988–2013	ART Population	5 508	1,149 101,668	Not sign	Time since birth
van den Belt-Dusebout, 2016 (32)	The Netherlands, 1989–2013	ART Infertile	619 220	19,158 5,950	HR 1.01 (0.86–1.19)	Age, parity, age at first birth
Luke, 2015 (33)	US, 3 states, 2004–2009	ART Expected	404 487.93	53,859 –	SIR 0.83 (0.75–0.91)	Age, state of residence
Reigstad, 2015 (12)	Norway, 1984–2010	ART Population	138 7,899	16,626 792,208	HR 1.20 (1.01–1.42)	Age, year, parity, age at first birth, region of residence
Brinton, 2013 (19)	Israel, 1994–2011	ART Infertile	140 133	≈22,410 19,795	HR 0.90 (0.71–1.15)	Age, year, study site, gravidity
Stewart, 2012 (34)	Australia, 1983–2002	ART Population	148 236	7,381 13,644	HR 1.10 (0.88–1.36)	Age, age at first birth, multiple birth
Yli-Kuha, 2012 (35)	Finland, 1996–1998	ART Population	55 60	9,175 9,175	OR 0.93 (0.62–1.40)	Age, residence, marital status, socioeconomic status
Källén, 2011 (36)	Sweden, 1982–2006	ART Population	91 13,583	23,192 1,365,179	OR 0.76 (0.62–0.94)	Age and year of delivery, smoking
Pappo, 2008 (37)	Israel, 1986–2003	ART Expected	35 24.8	3,375 –	SIR 1.4 (0.98–1.96)	Age, continent of birth
Kristiansand, 2007 (38)	Sweden, 1981–2001	ART Population	24 3,059	8,716 640,059	RR 0.93 (0.58–1.43)	Age, year, parity, age at first conception, multiple birth
Lerner-Geva, 2003 (39)	Israel, 1984–1992	ART Expected	5 4.88	1,082 –	SIR 1.02 (0.33–2.91)	Age, year, continent of birth
Dor, 2002 (40)	Israel, 1981–1992	ART Expected	11 15.86	5,026 –	SIR 0.69 (0.46–1.66)	Age, year, place of birth
Venn, 1999 (41)	Australia, <1986–1993	ART Expected	87 95.4	20,656 –	SIR 0.91 (0.74–1.13)	Age, year

Abbreviations: *ART* assisted reproductive technology, *CI* confidence interval, *HR* hazard ratio, *OR* odds ratio, *sign.* significant, *SIR* standardized incidence ratio, *UK* United Kingdom, *US* United States.

among parous women treated with ART compared to parous women without infertility (48). When compared to women with infertility who conceived without ART, the risk was smaller but still statistically significant. However, it is likely that the causes and severity of infertility differed between women conceiving with and without the help of ART. The 2020 study from the Netherlands also found a higher risk of ovarian cancer in ART-treated women compared to the general population, but not compared to untreated infertile women (50).

Borderline ovarian tumors (BOTs) are intermediate between benign and invasive ovarian tumors, accounting for around 15% of primary epithelial ovarian tumors (57). These tumors are more common in younger women and have a better prognosis than ovarian cancer. In a 2019 systematic review (47),

TABLE 2.3

Cohort Studies on Ovarian Cancer Risk Following Ovulation Induction

First Author, Year (reference)	Country, Treatment Period	Treatment/ Comparison Group	Cancer Cases	Total Number	Risk (95% CI)	Adjustments
Reigstad, 2017 (16)	Norway, 2004–2014	CC Population	22 609	38,927 1,314,797	HR 1.93 (1.18–3.16)	Age, year, parity, region of residence
Kessous, 2016 (17)	Israel, 1988–2013	OI Population	1 54	3,214 101,668	Not sign.	Time since birth
Brinton, 2013 (19)	Israel, 1994–2011	CC Infertile	20 11	≈50,930 19,795	HR 0.75 (0.36–1.58)	Age, parity, BMI, smoking, socioeconomic status
Trabert, 2013 (51)	US, 5 states, 1965–1988	CC Infertile Gn Infertile	37 48 8 77	3,745 6,080 952 8,873	HR 1.34 (0.86–2.07) HR 1.00 (0.48–2.08)	Year, site, gravidity
Lerner-Geva, 2012 (20)	Israel, 1964–1974	CC, Gn Population	9 9	1,281 1,150	No excess risk	Age, continent of birth
Calderon-Margalit, 2009 (21)	Israel, 1974–1976	OI Population	1 42	567 14,463	HR 0.61 (0.08–4.42)	Age
dos Santos Silva, 2009 (22)	UK, 1963–1999	CC, Gn Infertile	12 8	3,180 3,949	RR 1.42 (0.53–3.99)	Age, year
Jensen, 2009 (52)	Denmark, 1963–1998	Gn Infertile CC Infertile	26 130 58 98	184 1,057 417 824	RR 0.83 (0.50–1.37) RR 1.14 (0.79–1.64)	Age, year, parity
Sanner, 2009 (53)	Sweden, 1961–1975	CC, Gn Expected	9 7.56	1,153 –	SIR 1.19 (0.54–2.25)	Age, indication for fertility treatment
Brinton, 2004 (54)	US, 5 states, 1965–1988	CC Infertile Gn Infertile	15 30 5 40	3,280 5,151 867 7,564	RR 0.82 (0.4–1.5) RR 1.09 (0.4–2.8)	Age, year
Doyle, 2002 (28)	UK, 1975–1989	OI Infertile	4 2	4,188 1,231	RR 0.59 (0.12–3.00)	Age, year, parity, year of first visit to clinic
Potashnik, 1999 (29)	Israel, 1960–1984	CC, Gn Expected	1 0.53	780 –	SIR 1.9 (0.02–10.5)	Age, year, country of birth
Modan, 1998 (30)	Israel, 1964–1974	CC, Gn Expected	6 3.5	1,309 –	SIR 1.7 (0.6–3.8)	Age, year, country of birth

Abbreviations: *BMI* body mass index, *CC* clomiphene citrate, *CI* confidence interval, *Gn* gonadotropins, *HR* hazard ratio, *OI* ovulation induction, *RR* rate ratio, *SIR* standardized incidence ratio, *UK* United Kingdom, *US* United States.

Rizzuto et al. concluded that ovarian stimulation may increase the risk of BOT, although based on low-certainty evidence. Three Nordic cohort studies have reported associations between ovulation induction and risk of BOT separately from ovarian cancer (Table 2.5). One of these studies found a higher risk for BOT based on seven exposed cases (53), while the other two studies reported no increased risk (16, 58).

A few studies have found a higher risk of BOT following ART treatments (Table 2.6), including three which compared to a reference group of untreated infertile women (50, 56, 59). Although these results indicate that women who go through ART may have a slightly higher risk of BOT, the associations could also be due to confounding by the causes of infertility or bias from increased surveillance of ART-treated women. A large UK study reported that the higher risk of BOT was restricted to women with endometriosis or nulliparity, indicating that the association was due to patient characteristics rather than ART treatment itself (31). In the recent study from the Netherlands (50), the authors noted that the higher risk of BOT could be due to unmeasured confounding since no dose-response relationship with number of ART cycles was observed.

TABLE 2.4

Cohort Studies on Ovarian Cancer Risk Following ART

First Author, Year (reference)	Country, Treatment Period	Treatment/ Comparison Group	Cancer Cases	Total Number	Risk (95% CI)	Adjustments
Spaan, 2020 (50)	The Netherlands, 1983–2000	ART Infertile ART Expected	115 37 115 80.6	30,565 9,972 30,565 –	HR 1.02 (0.70–1.50) SIR 1.43 (1.18–1.71)	HR: Age, parity SIR: Age, year
Lundberg, 2019 (48)	Sweden, 1982–2012	ART Infertile ART Population	39 56 39 894	38,025 49,208 38,025 1,252,864	HR 1.79 (1.18–2.71) HR 2.43 (1.73–3.42)	Age, year, parity, age at first birth, education, country of birth, family history, hysterectomy
Vassard, 2019 (49)	Denmark, 1994–2015	ART Population	64 329	58,472 566,858	HR 1.20 (1.10–1.31)	Age, year, parity, education, partnership status
Williams, 2018 (31)	UK, 1991–2010	ART Expected	264 188.1	225,786 –	SIR 1.40 (1.24–1.58)	Age, year
Reigstad, 2017 (16)	Norway, 2004–2014	ART Population	16 615	33,431 1,320,293	HR 1.29 (0.73–2.28)	Age, year, parity, region of residence
Kessous, 2016 (17)	Israel, 1988–2013	ART Population	3 54	1,149 101,668	HR 4.0 (1.2–12.6)	Age, obesity
Luke, 2015 (33)	US, 3 states, 2004–2009	ART Expected	48 40.67	53,859 –	SIR 1.18 (0.87–1.56)	Age, state of residence
Reigstad, 2015 (55)	Norway, 1984–2010	ART Population	16 800	16,525 789,723	HR 1.56 (0.94–2.60)	Age, year, parity, age at first birth, region of residence
Brinton, 2013 (19)	Israel, 1994–2011	ART Infertile	21 11	≈22,410 19,795	HR 1.58 (0.75–3.29)	Age, year, study site, gravidity
Stewart, 2013 (43)	Australia, 1982–2002	ART Infertile	16 22	7,548 14,098	HR 1.36 (0.71–2.62)	Age, socioeconomic status
Yli-Kuha, 2012 (35)	Finland, 1996–1998	ART Population	9 3	9,175 9,175	OR 2.57 (0.69–9.63)	Age, residence, marital status, socioeconomic status
Källén, 2011 (36)	Sweden, 1982–2006	ART Population	26 1,779	23,192 1,365,179	OR 2.09 (1.39–3.12)	Age, year, smoking
Van Leeuwen, 2011 (56)	The Netherlands, 1983–1995	ART Infertile	30 12	19,146 6,006	HR 1.14 (0.54–2.41)	Age, tubal problems
Lerner-Geva, 2003 (39)	Israel, 1984–1992	ART Expected	3 0.60	1,082 –	SIR 5.0 (1.02–14.6)	Age, year, continent of birth
Dor, 2002 (40)	Israel, 1981–1992	ART Expected	1 1.74	5,026 –	SIR 0.57 (0.01–3.20)	Age, year, place of birth
Venn, 1999 (41)	Australia, <1986–1993	ART Expected	7 8.0	20,583 –	SIR 0.88 (0.42–1.84)	Age, year

Abbreviations: *ART* assisted reproductive technology, *CI* confidence interval, *HR* hazard ratio, *OR* odds ratio, *RR* rate ratio, *SIR* standardized incidence ratio, *UK* United Kingdom, *US* United States.

Consequently, there is insufficient evidence to determine whether ovarian stimulation treatments may influence the risk of ovarian cancer or borderline ovarian tumors, or if the reported associations are due to other factors such as the underlying infertility.

Endometrial cancer

The majority of endometrial cancers are estrogen-related and develop under the effect of high levels of estrogen without the opposing action of progesterone (60, 61). Known risk factors include obesity,

TABLE 2.5

Cohort Studies on Borderline Ovarian Tumor Risk Following Ovulation Induction

First Author, Year (reference)	Country, Treatment Period	Treatment/ Comparison Group	BOT Cases	Total Number	Risk (95% CI)	Adjustments
Reigstad, 2017 (16)	Norway, 2004–2014	CC Population	16 623	38,927 1,314,797	HR 0.97 (0.56–1.70)	Age, year, parity, region of residence
Bjørnholt, 2015 (58)	Denmark, 1963–2006	CC Infertile	56 86	440 888	RR 0.96 (0.64–1.44)	Age, year, parity
Sanner, 2009 (53)	Sweden, 1961–1975	CC, Gn Expected	7 1.94	1,153 –	SIR 3.61 (1.45–7.44)	Age

Abbreviations: *CC* clomiphene citrate, *CI* confidence interval, *Gn* gonadotropins, *HR* hazard ratio, *RR* rate ratio, *SIR* standardized incidence ratio.

TABLE 2.6

Cohort Studies on Borderline Ovarian Tumor Risk Following ART

First Author, Year (reference)	Country, Treatment Period	Treatment/ Comparison Group	BOT Cases	Total Number	Risk (95% CI)	Adjustments
Spaan, 2020 (50)	The Netherlands, 1983–2000	ART Infertile ART Expected	79 17 56 25.4	30,565 9,972 30,565 –	HR 1.84 (1.08–3.14) SIR 2.20 (1.66–2.86)	HR: Age, parity, tubal subfertility SIR: Age, year
Lundberg, 2019 (48)	Sweden, 1982–2012	ART Infertile ART Population	27 39 27	38,003 49,183 38,003 1,252,728	HR 1.48 (0.90–2.44) HR 1.91 (1.27–2.86)	Age, year, parity, age at first birth, education, country of birth, family history, hysterectomy
Williams, 2018 (31)	UK, 1991–2010	ART Expected	141 103.7	225,786 –	SIR 1.36 (1.15–1.60)	Age, year
Reigstad, 2017 (16)	Norway, 2004–2014	ART Population	20 619	33,431 1,320,293	HR 1.95 (1.18–3.23)	Age, year, parity, region of residence
Stewart, 2013 (59)	Australia, 1982–2002	ART Infertile	17 14	7,544 14,095	HR 2.46 (1.20–5.04)	Age, year, socioeconomic status
Yli-Kuha, 2012 (35)	Finland, 1996–1998	ART Population	4 4	9,175 9,175	OR 1.68 (0.31–9.27)	Age, residence, marital status, socioeconomic status
Van Leeuwen, 2011 (56)	The Netherlands, 1983–1995	ART Infertile	31 4	19,146 6,006	HR 6.38 (2.05–19.84)	Age, tubal problems

Abbreviations: *ART* assisted reproductive technology, *CC* clomiphene citrate, *CI* confidence interval, *Gn* gonadotropins, *HR* hazard ratio, *OR* odds ratio, *RR* rate ratio, *SIR* standardized incidence ratio, *UK* United Kingdom.

diabetes mellitus, hypertension, and polycystic ovary syndrome (PCOS), as well as nulliparity and late menopause. Using estrogen-only hormone replacement therapy also increases the risk of endometrial cancer. The use of combined oral contraceptives, increased parity and giving birth late in life have been found to have a protective effect (60). Several studies have reported a higher risk of endometrial cancer among infertile women (62–64). This higher risk seems to be restricted to women with ovulatory disturbances or PCOS (63, 64). Some studies have also found a higher risk of endometrial cancer in women with endometriosis (10, 62, 65), although most have not (11, 63, 64, 66, 67).

Ovarian stimulation has also been suggested to influence endometrial cancer risk through increasing serum estrogen levels. A summary of cohort studies on the risk of endometrial cancer following ovulation induction treatment is presented in Table 2.7. A systematic review from 2017 suggested that endometrial

TABLE 2.7

Cohort Studies on Endometrial Cancer Risk Following Ovulation Induction

First Author, Year (reference)	Country, Treatment Period	Treatment/ Comparison Group	Cancer Cases	Total Number	Risk (95% CI)	Adjustments
Reigstad, 2017 (16)	Norway, 2004–2014	CC Population	26 551	38,972 1,314,797	HR 2.91 (1.87–4.53)	Age, year, parity, region of residence
Kessous, 2016 (17)	Israel, 1988–2013	OI Population	4 54	3,214 101,668	Not sign.	Time since birth
Brinton, 2013 (71)	US, 5 states, 1965–1988	CC Population Gn Population	52 66 14 104	3,704 6,010 940 8,774	HR 1.39 (0.96–2.01) HR 1.34 (0.76–2.37)	Year, study site, socioeconomic status
Brinton, 2013 (19)	Israel, 1994–2011	CC Infertile	20 7	≈50,930 19,795	HR 1.01 (0.42–2.42)	Age, parity, BMI, smoking, socioeconomic status
Lerner-Geva, 2012 (20)	Israel, 1964–1974	CC, Gn Infertile	17 13	1,281 1,150	No excess risk	Age, continent of birth
Calderon-Margalit, 2009 (21)	Israel, 1974–1976	OI Population	5 39	567 14,463	HR 3.39 (1.28–8.97)	Age, parity, country of birth, BMI, socioeconomic status
dos Santos Silva, 2009 (22)	UK, 1963–1999	CC, Gn Infertile	18 12	3,180 3,949	RR 1.39 (0.63–3.16)	Age, year
Jensen, 2009 (72)	Denmark, 1965–1998	Gn Infertile CC Infertile	17 66 29 54	184 1,059 417 826	RR 2.21 (1.08–4.50) RR 1.36 (0.83–2.23)	Age, year, parity
Althuis, 2005 (73)	US, 5 states, 1965–1988	CC Infertile	19 20	≈3,000 ≈4,900	RR 1.79 (0.9–3.4)	Age, year, race
Doyle, 2002 (28)	UK, 1975–1989	OI Infertile	3 1	4,188 1,231	RR 0.72 (0.06–8.64)	Age, year, parity, year of first visit to clinic
Potashnik, 1999 (29)	Israel, 1960–1984	CC, Gn Expected	1 0.24	780 –	SIR 2.13 (0.05–23.0)	Age, year, country of birth
Modan, 1998 (30)	Israel, 1964–1974	CC, Gn Expected	13 1.9	1,309 –	SIR 6.8 (3.6–11.5)	Age, year, country of birth

Abbreviations: *BMI* body mass index, *CC* clomiphene citrate, *CI* confidence interval, *Gn* gonadotropins, *HR* hazard ratio, *OI* ovulation induction, *RR* rate ratio, *SIR* standardized incidence ratio, *UK* United Kingdom, *US* United States.

cancer risk may be higher in women treated with clomiphene citrate, especially at very high doses (2000 mg) or more than seven cycles (68). However, the authors noted that the association could be due to the underlying risk factors such as PCOS and that the currently available evidence was of low certainty. A more recent study by Reigstad et. al. (16) also reported a higher risk of endometrial cancer among women treated with clomiphene citrate, especially in nulliparous women and in parous women receiving more than six cycles of treatment. Similar to many previous studies, no information on the cause of infertility or obesity was available, which could bias the results. In addition, this treatment regimen is generally not used today since current guidelines recommend a maximum of six cycles of clomiphene citrate (69, 70).

Most cohort studies to date have not found a significantly higher risk of endometrial cancer following treatment with ART, although the conclusions are often limited by the small number of exposed cancer cases (Table 2.8). In the study from the UK which included 164 endometrial cancer cases among women exposed to ART, no significant increased risk was found compared to the expected rate in the population (31).

Taken together, these results do not suggest any substantial increase in the risk of endometrial cancer following ovarian stimulation treatments. Infertile women treated with high doses and/or multiple cycles

TABLE 2.8

Cohort Studies on Endometrial Cancer Risk Following ART

First Author, Year (reference)	Country, Treatment Period	Treatment/ Comparison Group	Cancer Cases	Total Number	Risk (95% CI)	Adjustments
Williams, 2018 (31)	UK, 1991–2010	ART Expected	164 146.9	225,786 –	SIR 1.12 (0.95–1.30)	Age, year
Reigstad, 2017 (16)	Norway, 2004–2014	ART Population	12 565	33,431 1,320,293	HR 0.76 (0.40–1.45)	Age, year, parity, region of residence
Kessous, 2016 (17)	Israel, 1988–2013	ART Population	3 54	1,149 101,668	HR 4.6 (1.4–15.0)	Age, obesity
Reigstad, 2015 (55)	Norway, 1984–2010	ART Population	5 631	338 21,944	HR 0.69 (0.28–1.68)	Age, year, parity, age at first birth, region of residence
Luke, 2015 (33)	US, 3 states, 2004–2009	ART Expected	49 64.13	53,859 –	SIR 0.76 (0.57–1.01)	Age, state of residence
Brinton, 2013 (19)	Israel, 1994–2011	ART Infertile	15 7	≈22,410 19,795	HR 1.56 (0.63–3.86)	Age, year, study site, gravidity
Yli-Kuha, 2012 (35)	Finland, 1996–1998	ART Population	4 2	9,175 9,175	OR 2.0 (0.37–10.9)	Age, residence, marital status, socioeconomic status
Dor, 2002 (40)	Israel, 1981–1992	ART Expected	2 0.89	5,026 –	SIR 2.25 (0.25–8.11)	Age, year, country of birth
Venn, 1999 (41)	Australia, <1986–1993	ART Expected	5 4.6	20,583 –	SIR 1.09 (0.45–2.61)	Age, year

Abbreviations: *ART* assisted reproductive technology, *CI* confidence interval, *HR* hazard ratio, *OR* odds ratio, *RR* rate ratio, *SIR* standardized incidence ratio, *UK* United Kingdom, *US* United States.

of clomiphene citrate may have a somewhat higher risk of endometrial cancer, although it is not clear whether this association is due to the treatment or the underlying infertility.

Conclusions

- Ovarian stimulation treatments do not seem to be associated with the risk of breast cancer.
- ART treatments do not seem to be associated with the risk of endometrial cancer.
- Infertile women treated with high doses and/or multiple cycles of clomiphene citrate may have a slightly higher risk of endometrial cancer.
- Infertile women treated with ovarian stimulation may have a higher risk of ovarian cancer and borderline ovarian tumors. There is insufficient evidence to conclude whether associations are due to the fertility treatments or other factors such as the underlying infertility.

REFERENCES

1. Macklon NS, Fauser BCJM. Medical approaches to ovarian stimulation for infertility. In: *Yen & Jaffe's reproductive endocrinology*. The Netherlands: Elsevier; 2009. pp. 689–724.
2. Wells GA, Shea B, Higgins JP, Sterne J, Tugwell P, Reeves BC. Checklists of methodological issues for review authors to consider when including non-randomized studies in systematic reviews. *Res Synth Methods*. 2013;4:63–77.
3. Practice Committee of the American Society for Reproductive Medicine. Fertility drugs and cancer: A guideline. *Fertil Steril*. 2016;106(7):1617–26.

4. Warner ET, Colditz GA, Palmer JR, Partridge AH, Rosner BA, Tamimi RM. Reproductive factors and risk of premenopausal breast cancer by age at diagnosis: Are there differences before and after age 40? *Breast Cancer Res Treat.* 2013;142(1):165–75.
5. Collaborative Group on Hormonal Factors in Breast Cancer. Menarche, menopause, and breast cancer risk: Individual participant meta-analysis, including 118 964 women with breast cancer from 117 epidemiological studies. *Lancet Oncol.* 2012;13(11):1141–51.
6. Rojas K, Stuckey A. Breast cancer epidemiology and risk factors. *Clin Obstet Gynecol.* 2016;59(4):651–72.
7. Yager JD, Davidson NE. Estrogen carcinogenesis in breast cancer. *N Engl J Med.* 2006;354:270–82.
8. Cetin I, Cozzi V, Antonazzo P. Infertility as a cancer risk factor: A review. *Placenta.* 2008;29(Suppl B):169–77.
9. Gabriele V, Gapp-Born E, Ohl J, Akladios C, Mathelin C. Infertility and breast cancer: Is there a link? Updated review of the literature and meta-analysis. *Gynécologie Obs Fertil.* 2016;44:113–20.
10. Brøchner Mogensen J, Kjaer SK, Mellemkjaer L, Jensen A. Endometriosis and risks for ovarian, endometrial and breast cancers: A nationwide cohort study. *Gynecol Oncol.* 2016;143(1):87–92.
11. Melin A, Sparén P, Bergqvist A. The risk of cancer and the role of parity among women with endometriosis. *Hum Reprod.* 2007;22(11):3021–6.
12. Reigstad MM, Larsen IK, Myklebust TA, Robsahm TE, Oldereid NB, Omland AK, et al. Risk of breast cancer following fertility treatment: A registry based cohort study of parous women in Norway. *Int J Cancer.* 2015;136(5):1140–8.
13. Barcroft JF, Galazis N, Jones BP, Getreu N, Bracewell-Milnes T, Grewal KJ, et al. Fertility treatment and cancers-the eternal conundrum: A systematic review and meta-analysis. *Hum Reprod.* 2021;36(4):1093–107.
14. Guleria S, Kjaer SK, Albieri V, Frederiksen K, Jensen A. A cohort study of breast cancer risk after 20 years of follow-up of women treated with fertility drugs. *Cancer Epidemiol Biomarkers Prev.* 2019;28:1986–92.
15. Lundberg FE, Iliadou AN, Rodriguez-Wallberg K, Bergh C, Gemzell-Danielsson K, Johansson ALV. Ovarian stimulation and risk of breast cancer in Swedish women. *Fertil Steril.* 2017;108(1):137–44.
16. Reigstad MM, Storeng R, Myklebust TÅ, Oldereid NB, Omland AK, Robsahm TE, et al. Cancer risk in women treated with fertility drugs according to parity status: A registry-based cohort study. *Cancer Epidemiol Biomarkers Prev.* 2017;26(6):953–62.
17. Kessous R, Davidson E, Meirovitz M, Sergienko R, Sheiner E. The risk of female malignancies after fertility treatments: A cohort study with 25-year follow-up. *J Cancer Res Clin Oncol.* 2016;142(1):287–93.
18. Brinton LA, Scoccia B, Moghissi KS, Westhoff CL, Niwa S, Ruggieri D, et al. Long-term relationship of ovulation-stimulating drugs to breast cancer risk. *Cancer Epidemiol Biomarkers Prev.* 2014;23(4):584–93.
19. Brinton LA, Trabert B, Shalev V, Lunenfeld E, Sella T, Chodick G. In vitro fertilization and risk of breast and gynecologic cancers: A retrospective cohort study within the Israeli Maccabi Healthcare Services. *Fertil Steril.* 2013;99(5):1189–96.
20. Lerner-Geva L, Rabinovici J, Olmer L, Blumstein T, Mashiach S, Lunenfeld B. Are infertility treatments a potential risk factor for cancer development? Perspective of 30 years of follow-up. *Gynecol Endocrinol.* 2012;28(10):809–14.
21. Calderon-Margalit R, Friedlander Y, Yanetz R, Kleinhaus K, Perrin MC, Manor O, et al. Cancer risk after exposure to treatments for ovulation induction. *Am J Epidemiol.* 2009;169(3):365–75.
22. dos Santos Silva I, Wark PA, McCormack VA, Mayer D, Overton C, Little V, et al. Ovulation-stimulation drugs and cancer risks: A long-term follow-up of a British cohort. *Br J Cancer.* 2009;100(11):1824–31.
23. Orgéas CC, Sanner K, Hall P, Conner P, Holte J, Nilsson SJ, et al. Breast cancer incidence after hormonal infertility treatment in Sweden: A cohort study. *Am J Obstet Gynecol.* 2009;200(1):72.e1–7.
24. Jensen A, Sharif H, Svare EI, Frederiksen K, Kjaer SK. Risk of breast cancer after exposure to fertility drugs: Results from a large Danish Cohort study. *Cancer Epidemiol Biomarkers Prev.* 2007;16(7):1400–7.
25. Lerner-Geva L, Keinan-Boker L, Blumstein T, Boyko V, Olmar L, Mashiach S, et al. Infertility, ovulation induction treatments and the incidence of breast cancer: A historical prospective cohort of Israeli women. *Breast Cancer Res Treat.* 2006;100:201–12.
26. Brinton LA, Scoccia B, Moghissi KS, Westhoff CL, Althuis MD, Mabie JE, et al. Breast cancer risk associated with ovulation-stimulating drugs. *Hum Reprod.* 2004;19(9):2005–13.

27. Gauthier E, Paoletti X, Clavel-Chapelon F. Breast cancer risk associated with being treated for infertility: Results from the French E3N cohort study. *Hum Reprod*. 2004;19(10):2216–21.
28. Doyle P, Maconochie N, Beral V, Swerdlow AJ, Tan SL. Cancer incidence following treatment for infertility at a clinic in the UK. *Hum Reprod*. 2002;17(8):2209–13.
29. Potashnik G, Lerner-Geva L, Genkin L, Chetrit A, Lunenfeld E, Porath A. Fertility drugs and the risk of breast and ovarian cancers: Results of a long-term follow-up study. *Fertil Steril*. 1999;71(5):853–9.
30. Modan B, Ron E, Lerner-Geva L, Blumstein T, Menczer J, Rabinovici J, et al. Cancer incidence in a cohort of infertile women. *Am J Epidemiol*. 1998;147(11):1038–42.
31. Williams CL, Jones ME, Swerdlow AJ, Botting BJ, Davies MC, Jacobs I, et al. Risks of ovarian, breast, and corpus uteri cancer in women treated with assisted reproductive technology in Great Britain, 1991–2010: Data linkage study including 2.2 million person years of observation. *BMJ*. 2018;362:k2644.
32. van den Belt-Dusebout AW, Spaan M, Lambalk CB, Kortman M, Laven JSE, van Santbrink EJP, et al. Ovarian stimulation for in vitro fertilization and long-term risk of breast cancer. *JAMA*. 2016;316(3):300–12.
33. Luke B, Brown MB, Spector LG, Missmer SA, Leach RE, Williams M, et al. Cancer in women after assisted reproductive technology. *Fertil Steril*. 2015;104(5):1218–26.
34. Stewart LM, Holman CD, Hart R, Bulsara MK, Preen DB, Finn JC. In vitro fertilization and breast cancer: Is there cause for concern? *Fertil Steril*. 2012;98(2):334–40.
35. Yli-Kuha AN, Gissler M, Klemetti R, Luoto R, Hemminki E. Cancer morbidity in a cohort of 9175 Finnish women treated for infertility. *Hum Reprod*. 2012;27(4):1149–55.
36. Källén B, Finnström O, Lindam A, Nilsson E, Nygren KG, Olausson PO. Malignancies among women who gave birth after in vitro fertilization. *Hum Reprod*. 2011;26(1):253–8.
37. Pappo I, Lerner-Geva L, Halevy A, Olmer L, Friedler S, Raziel A, et al. The possible association between IVF and breast cancer incidence. *Ann Surg Oncol*. 2008;15(4):1048–55.
38. Kristiansson P, Bjor O, Wramsby H. Tumour incidence in Swedish women who gave birth following IVF treatment. *Hum Reprod*. 2007;22(2):421–6.
39. Lerner-Geva L, Geva E, Lessing JB, Chetrit A, Modan B, Amit A. The possible association between in vitro fertilization treatments and cancer development. *Int J Gynecol Cancer*. 2003;13(1):23–7.
40. Dor J, Lerner-Geva L, Rabinovici J, Chetrit A, Levran D, Lunenfeld B, et al. Cancer incidence in a cohort of infertile women who underwent in vitro fertilization. *Fertil Steril*. 2002;77(2):324–7.
41. Venn A, Watson L, Bruinsma F, Giles G, Healy D. Risk of cancer after use of fertility drugs with in-vitro fertilisation. *Lancet*. 1999;354(9190):1586–90.
42. Davidson B, Tropé CG. Ovarian cancer: Diagnostic, biological and prognostic aspects. *Women's Heal*. 2014;10(5):519–33.
43. Stewart LM, Holman CD, Aboagye-Sarfo P, Finn JC, Preen DB, Hart R. In vitro fertilization, endometriosis, nulliparity and ovarian cancer risk. *Gynecol Oncol*. 2013;128(2):260–4.
44. Wu AH, Pearce CL, Lee AW, Tseng C, Jotwani A, Patel P, et al. Timing of births and oral contraceptive use influences ovarian cancer risk. *Int J Cancer*. 2017;141(12):2392–9.
45. Whiteman DC, Siskind V, Purdie DM, Green AC. Timing of pregnancy and the risk of epithelial ovarian cancer. *Cancer Epidemiol Biomarkers Prev*. 2003;12(1):42–6.
46. Diergaarde B, Kurta ML. Use of fertility drugs and risk of ovarian cancer. *Curr Opin Obstet Gynecol*. 2014;26(3):125–9.
47. Rizzuto I, Behrens R, Smith L. Risk of ovarian cancer in women treated with ovarian stimulating drugs for infertility. *Cochrane Database Syst Rev*. 2019;6(6):CD008215.
48. Lundberg FE, Johansson ALV, Rodriguez-Wallberg K, Gemzell-Danielsson K, Iliadou AN. Assisted reproductive technology and risk of ovarian cancer and borderline tumors in parous women: A population-based cohort study. *Eur J Epidemiol*. 2019;34(11):1093–101.
49. Vassard D, Schmidt L, Glazer CH, Forman JL, Kamper-Jørgensen M, Pinborg A. Assisted reproductive technology treatment and risk of ovarian cancer-a nationwide population-based cohort study. *Hum Reprod*. 2019;34(1):2290–6.
50. Spaan M, van den Belt-Dusebout AW, Lambalk CB, van Boven HH, Schats R, Kortman M, et al. Long-term risk of ovarian cancer and borderline tumors after assisted reproductive technology. *J Natl Cancer Inst*. 2021;113(6)699–709.
51. Trabert B, Lamb EJ, Scoccia B, Moghissi KS, Westhoff CL, Niwa S, et al. Ovulation-inducing drugs and ovarian cancer risk: Results from an extended follow-up of a large US infertility cohort. *Fertil Steril*. 2013;100(6):1660–6.

52. Jensen A, Sharif H, Frederiksen K, Kjaer SK. Use of fertility drugs and risk of ovarian cancer: Danish population based cohort study. *Br Med J.* 2009;338:b249.
53. Sanner K, Conner P, Bergfeldt K, Dickman P, Sundfeldt K, Bergh T, et al. Ovarian epithelial neoplasia after hormonal infertility treatment: Long-term follow-up of a historical cohort in Sweden. *Fertil Steril.* 2009;91(4):1152–8.
54. Brinton LA, Lamb EJ, Moghissi KS, Scoccia B, Althuis MD, Mabie JE, et al. Ovarian cancer risk after the use of ovulation-stimulating drugs. *Obstet Gynecol.* 2004;103(6):1194–203.
55. Reigstad MM, Larsen IK, Myklebust TA, Robsahm TE, Oldereid NB, Omland AK, et al. Cancer risk among parous women following assisted reproductive technology. *Hum Reprod.* 2015;30(8):1952–63.
56. van Leeuwen FE, Klip H, Mooij TM, van de Swaluw AM, Lambalk CB, Kortman M, et al. Risk of borderline and invasive ovarian tumours after ovarian stimulation for in vitro fertilization in a large Dutch cohort. *Hum Reprod.* 2011;26(12):3456–65.
57. Sun Y, Xu J, Jia X. The diagnosis, treatment, prognosis and molecular pathology of borderline ovarian tumors: Current status and perspectives. *Cancer Manag Res.* 2020;12:3651–9.
58. Bjørnholt SM, Kjaer SK, Nielsen TS, Jensen A. Risk for borderline ovarian tumours after exposure to fertility drugs: Results of a population-based cohort study. *Hum Reprod.* 2015;30(1):222–31.
59. Stewart LM, Holman CD, Finn JC, Preen DB, Hart R. In vitro fertilization is associated with an increased risk of borderline ovarian tumours. *Gynecol Oncol.* 2013;129(2):372–6.
60. Ignatov A, Ortmann O. Endocrine risk factors of endometrial cancer: Polycystic ovary syndrome, oral contraceptives, infertility, tamoxifen. *Cancers (Basel).* 2020;12(7):1766.
61. Ali AT. Reproductive factors and the risk of endometrial cancer. *Int J Gynecol Cancer.* 2014;24(3):384–93.
62. Yang HP, Cook LS, Weiderpass E, Adami H-O, Anderson KE, Cai H, et al. Infertility and incident endometrial cancer risk: A pooled analysis from the epidemiology of endometrial cancer consortium (E2C2). *Br J Cancer.* 2015;112(5):925–33.
63. Lundberg FE, Iliadou AN, Rodriguez-Wallberg K, Gemzell-Danielsson K, Johansson ALV. The risk of breast and gynecological cancer in women with a diagnosis of infertility: A nationwide population-based study. *Eur J Epidemiol.* 2019;34(5):499–507.
64. Murugappan G, Li S, Lathi RB, Baker VL, Eisenberg ML. Risk of cancer in infertile women: Analysis of US claims data. *Hum Reprod.* 2019;34(5):894–902.
65. Yu HC, Lin CY, Chang WC, Shen BJ, Chang WP, Chuang CM. Increased association between endometriosis and endometrial cancer: A nationwide population-based retrospective cohort study. *Int J Gynecol Cancer.* 2015;25(3):447–52.
66. Poole EM, Lin WT, Kvaskoff M, De Vivo I, Terry KL, Missmer SA. Endometriosis and risk of ovarian and endometrial cancers in a large prospective cohort of U.S. nurses. *Cancer Causes Control.* 2017;28:437–45.
67. Rowlands IJ, Nagle CM, Spurdle AB, Webb PM. Gynecological conditions and the risk of endometrial cancer. *Gynecol Oncol.* 2011;123:537–41.
68. Skalkidou A, Sergentanis TN, Gialamas SP, Georgakis MK, Psaltopoulou T, Trivella M, et al. Risk of endometrial cancer in women treated with ovary-stimulating drugs for subfertility. *Cochrane Database Syst Rev.* 2017;3:CD010931.
69. National Collaborating Centre for Women's and Children's Health (UK). *Fertility: Assessment and treatment for people with fertility problems.* London: Royal College of Obstetricians and Gynaecologists; 2013.
70. Gottlieb C, Fridström M. *Ofrivillig barnlöshet.* Stockholm: Svensk förening för obstetrik och gynekologi; 2010.
71. Brinton LA, Westhoff CL, Scoccia B, Lamb EJ, Trabert B, Niwa S, et al. Fertility drugs and endometrial cancer risk: Results from an extended follow-up of a large infertility cohort. *Hum Reprod.* 2013;28(10):2813–21.
72. Jensen A, Sharif H, Kjaer SK. Use of fertility drugs and risk of uterine cancer: Results from a large Danish population-based cohort study. *Am J Epidemiol.* 2009;170(11):1408–14.
73. Althuis MD, Moghissi KS, Westhoff CL, Scoccia B, Lamb EJ, Lubin JH, et al. Uterine cancer after use of clomiphene citrate to induce ovulation. *Am J Epidemiol.* 2005;161:607–15.

3

Maternal and obstetric outcomes after IVF indicated by a male factor

Begoña Prieto and Maria Diaz-Nuñez

ICSI

Perinatal outcomes

Safety in assisted reproductive technology (ART) techniques has an increasing importance, as up to 6% of newborns in Europe are conceived by ART (1). Intracytoplasmic sperm injection (ICSI) was developed to solve severe male factor cases, but its use has been extended to other indications such as advanced maternal age, fertilization of cryopreserved oocytes (2), in vitro maturation (IVM) oocytes, low number of oocytes (3), and preimplantation genetic testing (PGT) cycles. In a great majority ICSI is performed but also conventional in vitro fertilization (IVF) as well. The latest data confirm an increasing global use of ICSI in two out of three ART cycles (1, 4).

Although a great majority of children born are healthy, ART-derived pregnancies are associated with worse obstetric and perinatal outcomes when compared with spontaneously conceived pregnancies. This is related to the increase in multiple pregnancies due to multiple embryo transfer (5, 6). In order to reduce perinatal risks in ART pregnancies, embryo transfer policy has changed during last decade towards single embryo transfer (SET) (7). SET dramatically decreases short and long term risks in children, while live birth rates remain similar as double embryo transfer (DET) (8, 9).

When adverse outcomes are analyzed in singletons, it is complicated to separate the contribution of ART technique from infertility per se (10). In order to evaluate the effect of ART techniques on children's health, may be using natural conception as a control is not the best approach. Bernsten suggests subfertile parents (with a time to pregnancy of more than a year), which have poorer perinatal outcomes (11), or children born after intrauterine insemination (IUI) (when mild ovarian stimulation is needed) are a better control group. However, the influence of different ART methods can be studied in siblings, as long as several parental factors keep stable (12, 13). Some studies have shown that IVF singletons have an increased risk of adverse outcome compared to their non-IVF siblings (5). When comparing ICSI and standard IVF, most studies have found similar risks of preterm birth, very preterm birth, low birth weight and very low birth weight and perinatal or neonatal mortality in singletons. However, a lower risk of preterm birth was found with ICSI singletons (adjusted odds ratio 0.80, 95% CI: 0.69–0.93) (5).

Maternal and obstetric outcomes

Regarding maternal outcome, IVF is associated with an increased risk of severe maternal morbidity compared with deliveries from fertile couples (vaginal: AOR 2.27; cesarean: AOR 1.67) and subfertile couples (vaginal: AOR 1.97; cesarean: AOR 1.75). Among twins, cesarean IVF deliveries have significantly greater severe maternal morbidity compared to cesarean fertile deliveries (AOR, 1.48) (14). Various studies showed that ART pregnancies had an increased risk of postpartum hemorrhage (15, 16) and had a higher probability of cesarean section, retained placenta and failure of labor induction (17). However, a recently published study finds no differences in the incidence of first-trimester complications such as early miscarriage, ectopic pregnancy, vanishing twins, and bleeding between male factor IVF cycles and unexplained infertility cycles. The study authors could not find significant differences in the second and third trimester in preeclampsia, placenta previa, gestational diabetes mellitus and preterm labor between study groups (18).

Embryo vitrification is an excellent tool in the IVF laboratory, and the number of frozen embryo transfers (FETs) has increased, as well as pregnancy rates (1). Many studies showed no difference in the risk of stillbirth and perinatal mortality and suggested better perinatal outcomes in FET compared to fresh embryo transfer (ET), such as reduced risks of preterm birth or low birth weight (5, 19, 20). However, a higher risk of being large for gestational age and having a birth weight more than 4000 g (macrosomia) and a risk of hypertensive disorders in pregnancy were related to FET (21).

Children follow-up

Regarding long term health in IVF-conceived children, various studies described an increase in developmental delay (22), differences in IQ tests (23) and in mental retardation risk (24) or neurologic deficits and special needs (5). These differences are not statistically significant when data are corrected only to singletons. A higher risk of autism spectrum disease and attention deficit hyperactivity disorder has also been described, but this association seems to be lost as well when data are corrected to singletons (25–27).

There is some controversy about the association between imprinting disorders and ART – some studies show a higher incidence of imprinting disorders such as Silver-Russell syndrome and Beckwith-Wiedemann syndrome in ART children when compared to spontaneously conceived children (28–30), while others defend no association (31). Further studies will be needed to shed light on this issue.

Concerning cardiovascular and metabolic risks in ART singletons, several studies have described an increased body fat, blood pressure, and fasting glucose compared to singletons born from fertile or subfertile parents (32–36) and an increase in cardiovascular birth defects (37), suboptimal cardiac diastolic function under stress conditions and higher aortic and carotid intima-media thickness (38, 39).

There are also some data indicating worse semen quality in young adults born from ICSI, who were 3 times more likely to suffer oligozoospermia, but no clear association was found with their father's semen parameters (40).

PESA/TESE

Perinatal outcomes

Substantial data on children born from Percutaneous Epididymal Sperm Aspiration (PESA) and Testicular Sperm Aspiration/Testicular Sperm Extraction (TESA/TESE) are missing in the literature, with most studies of a retrospective nature.

Two papers described the increased chromosomal aberrations in testicular spermatozoa from patients with nonobstructive azoospermia (NOA) (41, 42). There could thus be an increased risk of congenital anomaly in children born after ICSI with testicular spermatozoa when compared to the rate of <4% of congenital abnormalities present in the general population of the same racial group (43).

In a study of 466 children born after ICSI with epididymal and testicular sperm TESE/PESA/TESA (TPT) compared with control (8.967 children born after ICSI with ejaculated sperm, 17.592 IVF and 63.854 natural conception [NC]), the sex ratio (male/female) was significantly lower for children born TPT (0.89) compared with conventional IVF (1.11; $P = 0.017$) (44). The total rate of congenital malformations in the TPT group was 7.7% and did not differ significantly from any of the control groups. However, singleton TPT showed an increased rate of cardiac malformations (3.6%) compared with singleton after IVF (1.4%; $P = 0.04$) and NC (1.1%; $P = 0.02$). The rate of hypospadias in the TPT group did not differ significantly compared with the control groups. This study also describes an increase in the rate of neoplasms in bones or joint cartilages, including osteosarcomas, in twins born after ICSI with TESA/TESE sperm (1.14%) compared with ICSI with ejaculated sperm (0.13%; $P = 0.03$) and NC (0.21%; $P = 0.04$). However, this increase was not significant when compared with conventional IVF (0.21%) (44).

Although some studies found higher rates of aneuploid (69.7%) and mosaic (31.2%) embryos in the NOA (45), others did not find any statistical differences in abnormal karyotypes and major malformation rates in offspring between the ICSI with ejaculated sperm group and the ICSI with TESA/TESE group (46, 47). In total, there were 55/1973 (2.8%) abnormal karyotypes in children derived from ICSI with ejaculated sperm, 0/31 (0%) with epididymal sperm and 5/91 (2.6%) with TESA/TESE. Major malformations were found in 543/12.377 (4.4%) in children from ICSI with ejaculated sperm, 17/533 (3.2%) with epididymal sperm and 31/670 (4.6%) with TESA/TESE (47). The studies on chromosome aberrations were too small to be conclusive (48).

Children follow-up

In a prospective study that evaluates at the age of 5 years the behavioral, cognitive and motor performance and physical development, only four children (3.8%) had developmental problems/delays (49). Two of them were diagnosed with a form of autism, which is a relatively high prevalence compared to the prevalence in the general population (1%–2%) (50). The authors conclude that long term effects on development and health in children born after these procedures seem to reassure us on the safety of these techniques (49).

Obstetric outcomes

The risk of spontaneous abortion showed a nonsignificant tendency to be higher for testicular sperm than for epididymal sperm (48).

The mean gestational age in the TPT singletons (279 + 12 days) was significantly higher compared with IVF (276 + 18 days; $P = 0.02$) with little clinical relevance. Cesarean sections were performed after IVF (27.3% for singletons) and ICSI (25.1% for singletons) with ejaculated sperm compared with the TPT group (16.4% for singletons) (44).

Similar neonatal outcomes (stillbirths, perinatal and neonatal mortality) for children conceived by ICSI with epididymal sperm were found to that of children conceived by ICSI with ejaculated sperm (44, 46, 51–53).

In a study the ICSI outcomes were compared among obstructive azoospermia, donor sperm and NOA – there was no difference in neonatal outcomes once a live birth was achieved (54, 55).

Donor sperm

Obstetric and perinatal outcomes

Regarding birth defects or chromosomal abnormalities, no differences have been observed from the general population. The available information on the psychosocial development of these children up to the age of 8–10 years appears to be reassuring (56).

In the study comparing perinatal outcomes between cycles using donor and nondonor sperm, there was no significant difference in preterm birth per singleton live birth (11.5% vs. 11.8%; adjusted relative risk, 0.98, 95% confidence interval, 0.90–1.06); however, low birth weight delivery was slightly lower in donor sperm cycles (8.8% vs. 9.4%; adjusted relative risk, 0.91, 95% confidence interval [CI], 0.83–0.99) (57). In another study, the same results were obtained, and no differences were found in the high birth weight delivery following donor sperm versus partner sperm IVF/ICSI (58). There was also no difference in the miscarriage rates (59).

The risk of gestational hypertensive disorders is higher among women who conceived using donor sperm compared to those who used their partner's sperm (60). In the meta-analysis, where 2.342 pregnancies conceived with donor sperm versus 8.556 with a partner's sperm were analyzed, the women who had conceived with donor sperm had an increased risk of developing preeclampsia (blood pressure levels ≥140/90 mm Hg measured on at least two occasions at least 4–6 hours apart, and proteinuria coexisted) compared with those who had used their partner's sperm (odds ratio [OR] 1.63, 95% CI 1.36–1.95). No difference was observed in the risk of gestational hypertension (OR 0.94, 95% CI 0.43–2.03, blood pressure levels ≥140/90 mm Hg measured on at least two occasions at least 4–6 hours apart) (61). See Table 3.1.

Characteristics of the Meta-Analyses Revised

First Author	Year		Obstetric and Maternal Outcomes	Perinatal Outcomes	Control Group	Risk Assessment
Pinborg	2013	IVF vs. ICSI	**Preterm birth*** *ICSI*: AOR 0.80, 95% CI:0.69–0.93			AOR
Luke	2017	ICSI vs. fertile couples	**Maternal morbidity*** *ICSI*: vaginal: AOR 2.27; cesarean: AOR 1.67 *Subfertile couples*: vaginal: AOR 1.97; cesarean: AOR 1.75 Twins: Cesarean: AOR, 1.48		Natural pregnancies	AOR
Fedder	2013	TESE/PESA/TESA vs. control	**Gestational age*** TPT (279 + 12 days) IVF (276 + 18; $P = 0.02$) **Cesarean sections*** TPT (16.4%) IVF (27.3%) ICSI (25.1%)	Sex ratio: TPT: 0.89; IVF: 1.11 ($P = 0.017$) Cardiac malformations: TPT: 3.5%; IVF: 1.4% ($P = 0.04$); NC: 1.1% ($P = 0.02$)	ICSI, IVF and natural conception	
Fedder	2007	PESA/TESA vs. control		Neoplasms in bones or joint cartilages: TESA/TESE (1.14%), ICSI (0.13; $P = 0.03$), NC (0.21%; $P = 0.04$) IVF (0.21%; NS)	ICSI with ejaculated sperm, IVF and NC	
Woldringh	2010	TESA/TESE, epididymal sperm and ICSI		Abnormal karyotypes: ICSI: 2.8% Epididymal sperm: 0% TESA/TESE: 2.6% Major malformations: ICSI: 4.4% Epididymal sperm: 3.2% TESA/TESE: 4.6%		
Meijerink Gerkowicz	2016 2018	TESE Donor vs. partner sperm	**Preterm birth*** Donor sperm (11.5%) Partner sperm (11.8%) AOR: 0.98, 95% CI: 0.90–1.06 **Low birth weight*** Donor sperm (8.8%) Partner sperm (9.4%) (AOR 0.91, 95% CI: 0.83–0.99)	Developmental problems/delays: 3.8%		AOR
González-Comadran	2014	Donor vs. partner sperm	**Preeclampsia** OR 1.63, 95% CI: 1.36–1.95 **Gestational hypertension** OR 0.94, 95% CI 0.43–2.03			OR

* Singletons.

Abbreviations: *AOR* adjusted odds ratio, *CI* confidence interval, *ICSI* intracytoplasmic sperm injection, *IVF* in vitro fertilization, *NS* not significant, *OR* odds ratio.

Conclusions

- In conclusion, despite many studies showing the evident relation between worse obstetric outcome in ART-derived pregnancies compared to spontaneous conception, the latest studies suggest that this outcome may not be related to male factor.
- Children conceived by ART techniques show a slight increased risk of adverse outcome, especially preterm birth and low birth weight.
- Regarding long term child health, existing data suggest that metabolic and cardiovascular risk profiles could be altered.
- In PESA/TESE, there are no differences in neonatal outcomes, and the total rate of congenital malformations do not differ significantly compared to other types of ART conception and natural conception.
- Studies on chromosomal aberrations in PESA/TESE are too small to be conclusive, and behavioral, cognitive and motor development appear to be reassuring.
- Concerning donor sperm, there are no differences in birth defects, chromosomal abnormalities, psychosocial development and perinatal outcomes. However, low-birth-weight delivery was lower in donor sperm cycles and there was a higher risk of developing preeclampsia.

REFERENCES

1. Calhaz-Jorge C, De Geyter C, Kupka MS, de Mouzon J, Erb K, Mocanu E, Motrenko T, Scaravelli G, Wyns C, Goossens V. Assisted reproductive technology in Europe, 2013: Results generated from European registers by ESHRE: European IVF monitoring Consortium (EIM): European Society of Human Reproduction and Embryology (ESHRE). *Hum Reprod.* 2017 Oct 1;32(10):1957–73.
2. Porcu E, Fabbri R, Seracchioli R, Ciotti PM, Magrini O, Flamigni C. Birth of a healthy female after intracytoplasmic sperm injection of cryopreserved human oocytes. *Fertil Steril.* 1997 Oct;68(4):724–6.
3. Pereira N, Palermo GD. Intracytoplasmic sperm injection: History, indications, technique, and safety. In: Palermo GD, Sills ES, editors. *Intracytoplasmic sperm injection: Indications, techniques, and applications.* 1st ed. Cham, Switzerland: Springer Nature; 2018. pp. 9–22.
4. Dyer S, Chambers GM, de Mouzon J, Nygren KG, Zegers-Hochschild F, Mansour R, Ishihara O, Banker M, Adamson GD. International committee for monitoring assisted reproductive technologies world report: Assisted reproductive technology 2008, 2009 and 2010. *Hum Reprod.* 2016 Jul;31(7):1588–609.
5. Pinborg A, Wennerholm UB, Romundstad LB, et al. Why do singletons conceived after assisted reproduction technology have adverse perinatal outcome? Systematic review and meta-analysis. *Hum Reprod Update.* 2013;19:87–104.
6. Adams D, Clark R, Davies M, De Lacey S. A meta-analysis of neonatal health outcomes from oocyte donation. *J Dev Orig Health Dis.* 2016;7:257–72.
7. Henningsen AA, Gissler M, Skjaerven R, Bergh C, Tiitinen A, Romundstad LB, Wennerholm UB, Lidegaard O, Nyboe Andersen A, Forman JL, Pinborg A. Trends in perinatal health after assisted reproduction: A Nordic study from the CoNARTaS group. *Hum Reprod.* 2015 Mar;30(3):710–16.
8. Thurin A, Hausken J, Hillensjo T, Jablonowska B, Pinborg A, Strandell A, Bergh C. Elective single-embryo transfer versus double-embryo transfer in in vitro fertilization. *N Engl J Med.* 2004;351:2392–402.
9. Thurin-Kjellberg A, Olivius C, Bergh C. Cumulative live-birth rates in a trial of single-embryo or double-embryo transfer. *N Engl J Med.* 2009;361:1812–13.
10. Berntsen S, Söderström-Anttila V, Wennerholm UB, Laivuori H, Loft A, Oldereid NB, Romundstad LB, Bergh C, Pinborg A. The health of children conceived by ART: "The chicken or the egg?" *Hum Reprod Update.* 2019 Mar 1;25(2):137–58.
11. Zhu JL, Basso O, Obel C, et al. Infertility, infertility treatment, and congenital malformations: Danish national birth cohort. *BMJ.* 2006;333:679.
12. Romundstad LB, Romundstad PR, Sunde A, von Düring V, Skjaerven R, Gunnell D, Vatten LJ. Effects of technology or maternal factors on perinatal outcome after assisted fertilisation: A population-based cohort study. *Lancet.* 2008 Aug 30;372(9640):737–43.

13. Henningsen AK, Pinborg A, Lidegaard Ø, Vestergaard C, Forman JL, Andersen AN. Perinatal outcome of singleton siblings born after assisted reproductive technology and spontaneous conception: Danish national sibling-cohort study. *Fertil Steril.* 2011 Mar 1;95(3):959–63.
14. Luke B. Pregnancy and birth outcomes in couples with infertility with and without assisted reproductive technology: With an emphasis on US population-based studies. *Am J Obstet Gynecol.* 2017 Sep;217(3):270–81.
15. Fauser BCJM, Devroey P, Diedrich K, Balaban B, Bonduelle M, Delemarre-van de Waal HA, et al. Health outcomes of children born after IVF/ICSI: A review of current expert opinion and literature. *Reprod Biomed.* 2014 Feb;28(2):162–82. Online.
16. Le Ray C, Pelage L, Seco A, Bouvier-Colle MH, Chantry AA, Deneux-Tharaux C, Epimoms Study Group. Risk of severe maternal morbidity associated with in vitro fertilisation: A population-based study. *BJOG.* 2019 Jul;126(8):1033–41.
17. Vannuccini S, Clifton VL, Fraser IS, Taylor HS, Critchley H, Giudice LC, et al. Infertility and reproductive disorders: Impact of hormonal and inflammatory mechanisms on pregnancy outcome. *Hum Reprod Update.* 2016 Feb;22(1):104–15.
18. Amouyal M, Boucekine M, Paulmyer-Lacroix O, Agostini A, Bretelle F, Courbiere B. No specific adverse pregnancy outcome in singleton pregnancies after Assisted Reproductive Technology (ART) for unexplained infertility. *J Gynecol Obstet Hum Reprod.* 2020 Jan;49(1):101623.
19. Maheshwari A, Pandey S, Shetty A, Hamilton M, Bhattacharya S. Obstetric and perinatal outcomes in singleton pregnancies resulting from the transfer of frozen thawed versus fresh embryos generated through in vitro fertilization treatment: A systematic review and meta-analysis. *Fertil Steril.* 2012 Aug;98(2):368–77.e1–9.
20. Zhao J, Xu B, Zhang Q, Li YP. Which one has a better obstetric and perinatal outcome in singleton pregnancy, IVF/ICSI or FET?: A systematic review and meta-analysis. *Reprod Biol Endocrinol.* 2016 Aug 30;14(1):51.
21. Maheshwari A, Pandey S, Amalraj Raja E, Shetty A, Hamilton M, Bhattacharya S. Is frozen embryo transfer better for mothers and babies? Can cumulative meta-analysis provide a definitive answer? *Hum Reprod Update.* 2018 Jan 1;24(1):35–58.
22. Strömberg B, Dahlquist G, Ericson A, Finnström O, Köster M, Stjernqvist K. Neurological sequelae in children born after in-vitro fertilisation: A population-based study. *Lancet.* 2002 Feb 9;359(9305):461–5.
23. Knoester M, Helmerhorst FM, Vandenbroucke JP, van der Westerlaken LA, Walther FJ, Veen S. Cognitive development of singletons born after intracytoplasmic sperm injection compared with in vitro fertilization and natural conception: Leiden artificial reproductive techniques follow-up project. *Fertil Steril.* 2008 Aug;90(2):289–96.
24. Sandin S, Nygren KG, Iliadou A, Hultman CM, Reichenberg A. Autism and mental retardation among offspring born after in vitro fertilization. *JAMA.* 2013 Jul 3;310(1):75–84.
25. Kallen AJ, Finnstrom OO, Lindam AP, Nilsson EM, Nygren KG, Otterblad Olausson PM. Is there an increased risk for drug treated attention deficit/hyperactivity disorder in children born after in vitro fertilization? *Eur J Paediatr Neurol.* 2011;15:247–53.
26. Kissin DM, Zhang Y, Boulet SL, Fountain C, Bearman P, Schieve L, Yeargin-Allsopp M, Jamieson DJ. Association of Assisted Reproductive Technology (ART) treatment and parental infertility diagnosis with autism in ART-conceived children. *Hum Reprod.* 2015;30:454–65.
27. Liu L, Gao J, He X, Cai Y, Wang L, Fan X. Association between assisted reproductive technology and the risk of autism spectrum disorders in the offspring: A meta-analysis. *Sci Rep.* 2017;7:46207.
28. Lazaraviciute G, Kauser M, Bhattacharya S, Haggarty P, Bhattacharya S. A systematic review and meta-analysis of DNA methylation levels and imprinting disorders in children conceived by IVF/ICSI compared with children conceived spontaneously. *Hum Reprod Update.* 2014 Nov–Dec;20(6):840–52.
29. Tenorio J, Romanelli V, Martin-Trujillo A, Fernandez GM, Segovia M, Perandones C, Perez Jurado LA, Esteller M, Fraga M, Arias P, et al. Clinical and molecular analyses of Beckwith-Wiedemann syndrome: Comparison between spontaneous conception and assisted reproduction techniques. *Am J Med Genet A.* 2016;170:2740–9.
30. Vermeiden JP, Bernardus RE. Are imprinting disorders more prevalent after human in vitro fertilization or intracytoplasmic sperm injection? *Fertil Steril.* 2013;99:642–51.
31. Lidegaard O, Pinborg A, Andersen AN. Imprinting diseases and IVF: Danish National IVF cohort study. *Hum Reprod.* 2005;20:950–4.

32. Hart R, Norman RJ. The longer-term health outcomes for children born as a result of IVF treatment: Part I – General health outcomes. *Hum Reprod Update.* 2013 May–June;19(3):232–43.
33. Ceelen M, et al. Body composition in children and adolescents born after in vitro fertilization or spontaneous conception. *J Clin Endocrinol Metab.* 2007;92:3417–23.
34. Ceelen M, van Weissenbruch MM, Roos JC, et al. Cardiometabolic differences in children born after in vitro fertilization: Follow-up study. *J Clin Endocrinol Metab.* 2008;93:1682–8.
35. Belva F, Painter R, Bonduelle M, et al. Are ICSI adolescents at risk for increased adiposity? *Hum Reprod.* 2012;27:257–64.
36. La Bastide-Van Gemert S, Seggers J, Haadsma ML, et al. Is ovarian hyperstimulation associated with higher blood pressure in 4-year-old IVF offspring? Part II: An explorative causal inference approach. *Hum Reprod.* 2014;29:510–7.
37. Henningsen AA, Berg C, Skjaerven R, Tiitinen A, Wennerholm UB, Romundstad LB, Gissler M, Opdahl S, Nyboe Andersen A, Lidegaard O, et al. Trends over time in congenital malformations in live-born children conceived after assisted reproductive technology. *Acta Obstet Gynecol Scand.* 2018;97:816–23.
38. Scherrer U, Rimoldi SF, Rexhaj E, Stuber T, Duplain H, Garcin S, de Marchi SF, Nicod P, Germond M, Allemann Y, et al. Systemic and pulmonary vascular dysfunction in children conceived by assisted reproductive technologies. *Circulation.* 2012;125:1890–6.
39. Valenzuela-Alcaraz B, Crispi F, Bijnens B, Cruz-Lemini M, Creus M, Sitges M, Bartrons J, Civico S, Balasch J, Gratacos E. Assisted reproductive technologies are associated with cardiovascular remodeling in utero that persists postnatally. *Circulation.* 2013;128:1442–50.
40. Belva F, Bonduelle M, Roelants M, Michielsen D, Van Steirteghem A, Verheyen G, Tournaye H. Semen quality of young adult ICSI offspring: The first results. *Hum Reprod.* 2016 Dec;31(12):2811–20.
41. Bernardini L, Gianaroli L, Fortini D, et al. Frequency of hyperhypohaploidy and diploidy in ejaculate, epididymal and testicular germcells of infertile patients. *Hum Reprod.* 2000;15:2165–72.
42. Martin RH, Greene C, Rademaker A, et al. Chromosome analysis of spermatozoa extracted from testes of men with non-obstructive azoospermia. *Hum Reprod.* 2000;15:1121–4.
43. Holmes LB. Current concepts in genetics: Congenital malformations. *N Engl J Med.* 1976;295:204–7.
44. Fedder J, Loft A, Parner ET, Rasmussen S, Pinborg A. Neonatal outcome and congenital malformations in children born after ICSI with testicular or epididymal sperm: A controlled national cohort study. *Hum Reprod.* 2013 Jan;28(1):230–40.
45. Rubio C, Rodrigo L, Perez-Cano I, Mercader A, Meteu E, Buendia P, Remohi J, Simon C, Pellicer A. FISH screening of aneuploidies in preimplantation embryos to improve IVF outcome. *Reprod Biomed Online.* 2005;11:497–506.
46. Belva F, De Schrijver F, Tournaye H, Liebaers I, Devroey P, Haentjens P, Bonduelle M. Neonatal outcome of 724 children born after ICSI using non-ejaculated sperm. *Hum Reprod.* 2011;26:1752–8.
47. Woldringh GH, Besselink DE, Tillema AH, Hendriks JC, Kremer JA. Karyotyping, congenital anormalies and follow-up of children afer intracytoplasmic sperm injection with non-ejaculated sperm: A systematic review. *Hum Reprod Update.* 2010 Jan–Feb;16(1):12–19.
48. Holte TO, Hofmann B, Lie RT, Norderhaug IN, Romundstad P, Saeterdal I, Orstavik KH, Tanbo T. *Male infertility: Intracytoplasmic Sperm Injection (ICSI) using surgically retrieved sperm from the testis or the epididymis.* Oslo, Norway: Knowledge Centre for the Health Services at The Norwegian Institute of Public Health (NIPH); 2007 Jan. Report from Norwegian Knowledge Centre for the Health Services (NOKC) No. 07-2007.
49. Meijerink AM, Ramos L, Janssen AJ, Maas-van Schaaijk NM, Meissner A, Repping S, Mochtar MH, Braat DD, Fleischer K. Behavioral, cognitive, and motor performance and physical development of five-year-old children who were born after intracytoplasmic sperm injection with the use of testicular sperm. *Fertil Steril.* 2016 Dec;106(7):1673–82.e5.
50. Christensen DL, Baio J, Van Naarden Braun K, Bilder D, Charles J, Constantino JN, et al. Prevalence and characteristics of autism spectrum disorder among children aged 8 years: Autism and developmental disabilities monitoring network, 11 sites, United States, 2012. *MMWR Surveill Summ.* 2016;65:1–23.
51. Woldringh GH, Horvers M, Janssen AJWM, Reuser JJCM, de Groot SAF, Steiner K, D'Hauwers KW, Wetzels AMM, Kremer JAM. Follow-up of children born after ICSI with epididymal spermatozoa. *Hum Reprod.* 2011;26:1759–67.
52. Oldereid NB, Hanevik HI, Bakkevig I, Romundstad LB, Magnus O, Hazekamp J, Hentemann M, Eikeland SN, Skrede S, Reitan IR, et al. Pregnancy outcome according to male diagnosis after ICSI with non-ejaculated sperm compared with ejaculated sperm controls. *Reprod Biomed Online.* 2014;29:417–23.

53. Guo YH, Dong RN, Su YC, Li J, Zhang YJ, Sun YP. Follow-up of children born after intracytoplasmic sperm injection with epididymal and testicular spermatozoa. *Chin Med J (Engl)*. 2013;126(11):2129–33.
54. Yu Y, Xi Q, Pan Y, Jiang Y, Zhang H, Li L, Liu R. Pregnancy and neonatal outcomes in azoospermic men after intracytoplasmic sperm injection using testicular sperm and donor sperm. *Med Sci Monit*. 2018 Oct 1;24:6968–74.
55. Tsai Y-R, Huang F-J, Lin P-Y, Kung F-T, Lin Y-J, Lan K-C. Clinical outcomes and development of children born to couples with obstructive and nonobstructive azoospermia undergoing testicular sperm extraction-intracytoplasmic sperm injection: A comparative study. *Taiwan J Obstet Gynecol*. 2015 Apr;54(2):155–9.
56. Lansac J, Royere D. Follow-up studies of children born after frozen sperm donation. *Hum Reprod Update*. 2001 Jan–Feb;7(1):33–7.
57. Gerkowicz SA, Crawford SB, Hipp HS, Boulet SL, Kissin DM, Kawwass JF. Assisted reproductive technology with donor sperm: National trends and perinatal outcomes. *Am J Obstet Gynecol*. 2018 Apr;218(4):421.e1–e10.
58. Kamath MS, Antonisamy B, Hepsy Y, Selliah HY, La Marca A, Sesh Kamal Sunkara SK. Perinatal outcomes following IVF with use of donor versus partner sperm. *Reprod Biomed Online*. 2018 June;36(6):705–10.
59. Yu B, Fritz R, Xie X, Negassa A, Jindal S, Vega M, Buyuk E. The impact of using donor sperm in assisted reproductive technology cycles on perinatal outcomes. *Fertil Steril*. 2018 Dec;110(7):1285–9.
60. Kyrou D, Kolibianakis EM, Devroey P, Fatemi HM. Is the use of donor sperm associated with a higher incidence of preeclampsia in women who achieve pregnancy after intrauterine insemination? *Fertil Steril*. 2010 Mar 1;93(4):1124–7.
61. González-Comadran M, Urresta Avila J, Saavedra Tascón A, Jimenéz R, Solà I, Brassesco M, Carreras R, Checa MÁ. The impact of donor insemination on the risk of preeclampsia: A systematic review and meta-analysis. *Eur J Obstet Gynecol Reprod Biol*. 2014 Nov;182:160–6.

4

The long term outcomes of children conceived through ART

Kenny A. Rodriguez-Wallberg and Panagiotis Tsiartas

Introduction

The number of couples seeking infertility treatments using assisted reproductive techniques (ART) has continuously increased over the years (1, 2). Numerous publications on early life data of children conceived through ART are available, and despite the fact that the existent surveillance data are reassuring, it is shown that both infertility and ART pregnancies are associated with increased risks of poor perinatal outcomes in the short term (3–7). The literature regarding the long term outcomes of children born after ART, on the other hand, is still limited, despite the large cohorts of children and adolescents born after ART worldwide. In this chapter the current literature regarding long term outcomes after ART treatments and, more specifically, after in vitro fertilization/intracytoplasmic sperm injection (IVF/ICSI) is summarized. The data reported on the following aspects are discussed: neurodevelopmental outcomes, cardiovascular, respiratory, gastrointestinal, endocrine, skin and sensory organ disorders, growth and metabolism, health of ICSI-conceived children, and overall mortality.

Neurodevelopmental outcomes (Table 4.1)

Psychomotor development and behavior

Two recent reviews have reported that children conceived through ART vs. natural conception (NC) presented with similar outcomes regarding psychomotor development, behavior, social functioning and language development (8, 9).

Cognitive development

A systematic review (10) focusing on cognitive development has reported conflicting results, mainly due to methodological limitations, including selection bias and/or failure to address confounding by family background. Moreover, a meta-analysis based on these studies could not be performed due to heterogeneity in the assessment of cognitive outcomes. However, three high-quality studies from Sweden, the Netherlands and England considered in the review suggest that children born after IVF may have some negative influence on cognitive development, such as increased risk of developmental delay and needing of habilitation services, lower intelligence test results or mental retardation (11–13). Although when restricting the analysis to singletons, excluding by this way twin pregnancies associated with higher risk of preterm birth and its complications, the statistical significance disappeared (10). A few more follow-up and retrospective studies from Denmark and Sweden have reported reassuring results with no statistically significant differences between ART and NC children in terms of neurological deficits, special needs, cognitive function, mental retardation, and school or academic performance (14–17).

TABLE 4.1

Summary of the Published Studies on Neurodevelopmental Outcomes in Children Conceived after ART

	Study Size	Study Type and Country	Conclusion of the Study
		Psychomotor Development and Behavior	
Berntsen et al., 2019	3 systematic reviews included.	Review	IVF/ICSI vs. NC: no difference
Bergh et al., 2020	3 systematic reviews included.	Review	IVF/ICSI vs. NC: no difference
		Cognitive Development	
Rumbold et al., 2017	35 studies included.	Systematic review	IVF/ICSI vs. NC: no difference in singletons
Strömberg et al., 2002	IVF: n = 5680 NC: n = 11,360	Retrospective cohort – Sweden	IVF vs. NC: need of habilitation services (OR 1.7, 95% CI 1.3–2.2) Singletons IVF vs. NC: need of habilitation services (OR 1.4, 95% CI 1–2.1)
Knoester et al., 2008	IVF: n = 83 ICSI: n = 86 NC: n = 85	Follow-up – Netherlands	Children between 5 and 8 years of age: ICSI singletons vs. NC: lower IQ scores (adjusted mean difference IQ 3.6 95% CI −0.8 to 8
Sandin et al., 2013	IVF: n = 19 445 ICSI: n = 11,514 NC: n = 2,510,166	Follow-up – England using Swedish registry data	Children born between 1982 and 2007 and followed up until 2009 (10-year follow-up): IVF/ICSI singletons vs. NC: no difference ICSI singletons vs. NC: higher risk for mental retardation (frozen embryos: RR 2.36 95% 1.04–5.36 and fresh embryos: RR 1.6 95% CI 1–2.57)
Spangmose et al., 2017	ART: n = 4766 NC: n = 12,724	Follow-up – Denmark	Adolescents born between 1995 and 1998 aged 15–16 years: Singletons ART vs. NC: lower academic performance (adjusted mean difference −0.15 CI −0.29-(−0.02))
Spangmose et al., 2019	Fresh ET: n = 6072 Frozen ET: n = 423	Retrospective cohort – Denmark	Children born from 1995 to 2001: Fresh vs. frozen ET: no difference
Norrman et al., 2018	ART: n = 8323 NC: n = 1,499,667	Retrospective cohort – Sweden	Children born between 1985 and 2001: ART vs. NC: no difference
Norrman et al., 2020	IVF: n = 11,713 ICSI: n = 6953 NC: n = 2,022,995	Retrospective cohort – Sweden	Children born between 1985 and 2015: ICSI vs. IVF: no difference

(Continued)

TABLE 4.1 (Continued)
Summary of the Published Studies on Neurodevelopmental Outcomes in Children Conceived after ART

	Study Size	Study Type and Country	Conclusion of the Study
ASD and ADHD			
Källén et al., 2011	IVF: n = 28,158 NC: n = 2,417,886	Retrospective cohort – Sweden	**Children born between 1982 and 2005:** **Singletons IVF vs. NC:** no difference
Hvidtjørn et al., 2011	IVF: n = 14,991 NC: n = 555,810	Follow-up – Denmark	**Children born between 1995 and 2003 and followed up to the age of 4–13 years:** **IVF vs. NC:** no difference
Sandin et al., 2013	IVF: n = 19,445 ICSI: n = 11,514 NC: n = 2,510,166	Follow-up – England using Swedish registry data	**Children born between 1982 and 2007 with 10-year follow-up:** **General ART vs. NC:** no difference
Fountain et al., 2015	ART: n = 48,865 NC: n = 5,877,386	Retrospective cohort – USA	**Children born between 1997 and 2011:** **Singletons ART vs. NC:** no difference
Liu et al., 2017	11 studies included	Meta-analysis	**ART vs. NC:** higher percentage of ASD (RR 1.35 95% CI 1.09–1.68)
Kissin et al., 2015	IVF: n = 13,753 ICSI: n = 21,728	Follow-up – USA	Children born between 1997 and 2006 with 5-year follow-up: ICSI vs. IVF: higher autism risk after ICSI (adjusted HRR 1.65 95% CI 1.08–2.52)
Cerebral Palsy (CP)			
Strömberg et al., 2002	IVF: n = 5680 NC: n = 11,360	Retrospective cohort – Sweden	**IVF vs. NC:** most common diagnosis (OR 3.7 95% CI 2–6.6) **Singletons IVF vs. NC:** most common diagnosis (OR 2.8 95% CI 1.3–5.8)
Källén et al., 2010	IVF: n = 31,614 NC: n = 2,623,514	Retrospective cohort – Sweden	**Children born between 1982 and 2007:** **Singletons IVF vs. NC:** no difference
Hvidtjørn et al., 2010	ART: n = 33,139 NC: n = 555,827	Follow-up – Denmark	**Children born between 1995 and 2003 and followed up between 1995 and 2009:** **Singletons IVF vs. NC:** no difference
Pinborg et al., 2010	IVF: n = 11,286 NC: n = 4800	Follow-up – Denmark	**Children born between 1995 and 2006 and followed up between 1995 and 2007:** **IVF/ICSI vs. NC:** higher CP rates between total fresh and non-ART groups
Goldsmith et al., 2018	IVF/ICSI: n = 1927 NC: n = 203,352	Retrospective cohort – Australia	**Children born between 1994 and 2002:** **ART vs. NC:** higher prevalence (adjusted OR 2.7 95% CI 1–6.9)
Epilepsy			
Kettner et al., 2017	IVF/ICSI: n = 8490 NC: n = 541,641	Retrospective cohort – Denmark	**Children born between 1995 and 2003 and followed up until 2013:** **IVF/ICSI vs. NC:** higher risk of idiopathic generalized epilepsy (HR 1.43 95% CI 0.99–2.05)

Autism spectrum disorder (ASD) and attention deficit hyperactivity disorder (ADHD)

A weak association has been found with ADHD in children born after IVF; however, the significant difference disappeared after adjustment for infertility length and when only singletons were analyzed (18). Additionally, a few studies reporting no increased risk for ASD in singletons born after ART have appeared (13, 19, 20). However, a meta-analysis from Liu et al. that included 11 studies (3 cohorts and 8 case-control studies) have shown that ART is associated with a higher risk for ASD in the offspring (21). Similarly, one population-based retrospective study that included 42,383 children born after IVF/ICSI reported a higher risk for ASD in singleton children conceived through ICSI vs. those conceived using standard IVF. Although the exact mechanism of the association between ICSI and neurobehavioral disorders, including ASD, is yet to be determined, it has been suggested that epigenetic modifications resulting from either the procedure itself or characteristics of the patients using the procedure may play a role in this higher ASD risk. However, according to this study, the risk of ASD was lower when parents had unexplained infertility (among singletons) or tubal factor infertility (among multiples). The inverse association of unexplained and tubal factor infertility with ASD diagnosis might be related to the younger age of patients going through ART (22).

Cerebral palsy (CP)

An increased risk of CP has been reported in a retrospective cohort study among children born after IVF that included 5680 children (11). Likewise, there was an increased risk for CP among children after IVF, but this disappeared when adjusted for multiple pregnancies and gestational age at delivery (23, 24). A Danish study showed an increased risk of CP in singletons born after fresh embryo transfer compared with NC-conceived children (25). A recent registry study with a limited number of children born after ART showed an increased prevalence of CP among extremely preterm singletons (26).

Epilepsy

A Danish nationwide birth cohort study found no overall increased risk of childhood epilepsy among children born after IVF/ICSI, but the risk of idiopathic generalized epilepsy was slightly increased (27).

In summary, conflicting results exist for most neurodevelopmental outcomes concerning a possible association with ART. However, many of the identified risk associations disappeared after adjustment for multiple births. A need of larger studies is imminent for ASD, CP, and epilepsy in order to clarify the risk association with ART.

Cardiovascular disorders (Table 4.2)

The long term cardiovascular risks in ART children have not been extensively studied. The published studies so far are based on small cohorts, and the risk of selection bias among both ART and NC children is high. A meta-analysis published in 2015 including 19 studies (9 prospective and 10 retrospective studies) showed that the levels of systolic and diastolic blood pressure were higher in the offspring after IVF/ICSI than after NC (28). A population-based study from Israel showed that the hospitalizations up to the age of 18 years involving cardiovascular disease were not different between IVF-conceived children and NC. Furthermore, no difference in the cumulative incidence of cardiovascular diseases was found between these groups (29). A small cross-sectional study where 17 children aged 10–14 years born after IVF were assessed found results supporting abnormal vascular health (30). In summary, limited data suggest a potential increase in blood pressure, as well as suboptimal cardiovascular function among ART-conceived children. The exact mechanism by which IVF may affect vascular health of offspring is not yet elucidated, and it is possibly multifactorial. The supraphysiological levels of steroid hormones after IVF and epigenetic changes after ART during embryonic development have been associated with vascular dysfunction and could possibly partially explain the higher risk of cardiovascular diseases after IVF (31, 32).

Respiratory disorders (Table 4.2)

A limited number of studies assessing the risk of developing respiratory diseases in ART children have been reported. Reassuring results regarding the prevalence of asthma and allergic rhinitis were seen in a study where 158 children born after IVF were compared with children born after NC and showed no difference in the prevalence of these conditions (33). However, a registry study that included 31 918 children born after IVF showed an increased risk for asthma that was higher for preterm than term

TABLE 4.2

Summary of the Published Studies on Cardiovascular and Respiratory Outcomes in Children Conceived after ART

	Study Size	Study Type and Country	Conclusion of the Study
Cardiovascular Disorders			
Guo et al., 2017	19 studies included IVF/ICSI: n = 2112 NC: n = 4096	Review and meta-analysis	**IVF/ICSI vs. NC**: higher blood pressure levels (weighted mean differences 1.88 mmHg 95% CI 0.27–3.49)
Shiloh et al., 2019	IVF: n = 2603 NC: n = 237,863	Retrospective cohort – Israel	**Children born between 1991 and 2014 and followed up to the age of 18 years:** **IVF vs. NC**: no difference in hospitalization rates for cardiovascular causes
Zhang et al., 2019	IVF: n = 17 NC: n = 42	Cross-sectional pilot – USA	**Children born between 2004 and 2008 aged 10–14 years:** **IVF vs. NC**: thicker common carotid artery intima-media thickness, higher elastic modulus, higher $\beta_{stiffness}$, higher peak velocity
Respiratory Disorders			
Cetinkaya et al., 2009	IVF: n = 158 NC: n = 102	Prospective – Turkey	**Children's mean age at follow-up: 4.6 ± 2.1 years:** **IVF vs. NC**: no difference
Kallen at el., 2013	IVF: n = 31,918 NC: n = 2,596,810	Retrospective cohort – Sweden	**Children born between 1982 and 2007 and followed up between 2005 and 2009:** **IVF vs. NC**: increased risk of asthma (aOR 1.28 95% CI 1.23–1.34). Adjustment for infertility duration eliminated the effect
Carson et al., 2013	ART: n = 104 NC: n = 6575	Prospective – UK	**Children born between 2000 and 2002 and followed up to the age of 5 and 7 years:** **ART vs. NC**: increased risk for asthma (aOR 2.65 95% CI 1.48–4.76) and wheezing (aOR 1.97 95% CI 1.1–3.5) at 5 years and 7 years, respectively (aOR 1.84 95% CI 1.03–3.28; aOR 1.5 95% CI 0.77–2.92)
Forton et al., 2019	IVF/ICSI: n = 15 NC: n = 30	Prospective case control – Belgium	**Adolescents and young adults aged 11–24 years old born between 2015 and 2018:** **IVF/ICSI vs. NC**: lower pulmonary vascular distensibility coefficient α and a blunted exercise-induced increase in pulmonary capillary volume

singletons. After adjustment for infertility duration, the effect was eliminated, suggesting that the main risk factor was parental subfertility (34). Another prospective study including 104 children born after ART and based on a follow-up survey at 5 and 7 years of age showed that children born after ART may experience asthma more often and use antiasthmatic drugs at 5 years of age compared with them born after NC. The same association, although diminished, was also present at 7 years of age (35). A prospective case-control study that included 15 apparently healthy adolescents conceived by IVF/ICSI showed slight alterations in pulmonary vascular distensibility assessed by two different methods, suggesting decreased pulmonary vascular reserve, with no associated impact on right ventricular function or aerobic exercise capacity (36). In summary, the studies in this area are still limited, although the existing data suggest that the main risk factor for developing asthma after ART is parental subfertility.

Gastrointestinal disorders (Table 4.3)

The literature on long term gastrointestinal complications in ART offspring is limited. A population-based cohort study from Israel that included 2,603 children born after IVF, showed that hospitalization rates because of overall gastrointestinal morbidity were significantly higher in children conceived after IVF compared with children born after NC (37).

TABLE 4.3

Summary of the Published Studies on Gastrointestinal and Endocrine Outcomes and Metabolism in Children Conceived after ART

	Study Size	Study Type and Country	Conclusion of the Study
Gastrointestinal Disorders			
Schachor et al., 2020	IVF: n = 2,603 NC: n = 237,863	Retrospective cohort – Israel	**Children born between 1991 and 2014 followed up to the age of 18 years:** **IVF vs. NC:** higher hospitalization rates involving gastrointestinal morbidity. IVF was noted as an independent risk factor for pediatric gastrointestinal morbidity (aHR 1.27 95% CI 1.08–1.5)
Endocrine Disorders and Metabolism			
Steiner et al., 2020	IVF: n = 2,603 NC: n = 237,863	Retrospective cohort – Israel	**Children born between 1991 and 2014 and followed up to the age of 18 years:** **IVF vs. NC:** no difference in hospitalization rates for endocrine disorders
Sakka et al., 2009	IVF: n = 106 NC: n = 68	Cross sectional – Greece	**Children's mean age at follow-up: 8.8 ± 2.9 years:** **Conventional IVF vs. NC:** mild TSH resistance with elevation of serum TSH (subclinical hypothyroidism)
Ceelen et al., 2008	IVF: n = 225 NC: n = 225	Follow-up – Netherlands	**Children born between 1986 and 1995 and followed up to the age of 8–18 years:** **IVF vs. NC:** higher fasting glucose levels
Guo et al., 2017	19 studies included.	Systematic review and meta-analysis	**IVF/ICSI vs. NC:** higher fasting insulin levels
Kettner et al., 2016	IVF: n = 8490 NC: n = 541,641	Retrospective cohort – Denmark	**Children born between 1995–2003 and followed up until 2013:** **IVF vs. NC:** no difference in type 1 diabetes
Norrman et al., 2020	IVF: n = 47,938 NC: n = 3,090,602	Retrospective cohort – Sweden	**Children born between 1985 and 2015:** **IVF vs. NC:** higher risk of type 1 diabetes in children born after frozen embryo transfer

Endocrine disorders and metabolism (Table 4.3)

Despite the fact that infertility can be often caused by endocrine etiologies, the current literature on endocrine disorders and metabolic risks in ART-conceived children is limited. The majority of the published studies have a cohort design with potential selection bias among the included ART and NC children. Furthermore, metabolic diseases are not common among young adults and children, and data about children conceived with ART are not commonly included in these registries. Hospitalization rates up to the age of 18 years involving endocrine disorders were not significantly different between IVF and NC children in a retrospective study from Israel (38). Nevertheless, significant higher levels of thyroid-stimulating hormone (TSH) and fasting glucose levels have been seen among IVF-conceived children in a cross-sectional study from Greece at 8 years of age and in a follow-up study from Netherlands at 8–18 years of age (39, 40). Contrarily, comparable body mass index (BMI), low-density lipoprotein, cholesterol, and fasting glucose levels have been seen in one meta-analysis between IVF/ICSI and NC children (28). The evidence regarding the risk of developing type 1 diabetes in ART children is limited. No increased risk of type 1 diabetes has been seen in two studies; however, children conceived after frozen/thawed cycles had a higher risk compared with children born after NC (41, 42). In summary, limited data suggest potentially deteriorated metabolic profiles in ART children. The evidence for developing type 1 diabetes in IVF-conceived children is in general reassuring, although there might be an increased risk for children born after frozen/thawed cycles.

Skin disorders (Table 4.4)

Only one study from Israel evaluated the risk of long term eruptive dermatological morbidity among children born after ART. This retrospective cohort study showed higher rates of cutaneous eruption–related hospitalizations of ART children as compared with NC children. This increased incidence although most prominent between 2 and 5 years, remained constant up to the age of 18 years (43).

Vision and hearing disorders (Table 4.4)

There are few studies on vision and hearing in children born after ART. These studies showed no significant difference in the development of hearing and vision between children born after ICSI and NC (44, 45). However, one study from Israel reported significantly higher hospitalization rates involving ophthalmic morbidity among children born after ART compared to them born after NC up to the age of 18 years (46). In summary, the results on vision and hearing disturbances in children conceived after ART are so far reassuring even though these data are based on small and limited studies.

Growth (Table 4.4)

Children born after IVF are more likely to have an increased risk of adverse pregnancy outcomes in terms of preterm delivery and low birth weight compared to children born after NC (47). Although this altered growth pattern is mainly seen after multiple pregnancies through the transfer of more than one embryo, even singletons conceived after ART have a higher risk of being born with a lower birth weight and of being small for gestational age (48). The exact reasons for this impaired growth are largely unknown; however, early childhood catch-up is common and has been associated with a risk of obesity, cardiovascular disease, and diabetes later in life (49–53). The majority of available studies investigating the long term growth have not found significant differences between ART and NC children, and this has been confirmed by a recent systematic review and meta-analysis from Denmark that included 3,972 children born after IVF/ICSI and 11,012 born after NC. This study showed a significantly lower weight of children born after IVF/ICSI up to preschool age; however, the long term height was comparable

The long term outcomes of children

TABLE 4.4

Summary of the Published Studies on Skin, Vision, and Hearing Outcomes and Growth in Children Conceived after ART

		Skin Disorders	
	Study Size	**Study Type and Country**	**Conclusion of the Study**
Krieger et al., 2018	ART: n = 4,324 NC: n = 237,863	Retrospective cohort – Israel	**Children born between 1991 and 2014:** **ART vs. NC**: increased risk of long term eruptive dermatological morbidity
		Vision and Hearing	
Wikstrand et al., 2006	ICSI: n = 137 NC: n = 159	Case control matched – Sweden	**Children born between 1994 and 1996 and followed up to the age of 5 years:** **ICSI vs. NC**: no difference in visual function and/or ocular morphology
Ludwig et al., 2010	ICSI: n = 276 NC: n = 273	Prospective – Germany	**Children followed up to the age of 4–6 years:** **ICSI vs. NC**: no difference in the development of hearing and vision
Tsumi et al., 2020	ART: n = 4364 NC: n = 239,318	Retrospective cohort – Israel	**Children born between 1991 and 2014 and followed up to the age of 18 years:** **ART vs. NC**: higher hospitalization rate and ophthalmic morbidity involving ophthalmic causes
		Growth	
Jackson et al., 2004	15 studies included.	Meta-analysis	**IVF vs. NC**: higher risk for low and very low birth weight
Pinborg et al., 2013	65 studies included.	Systematic review and meta-analysis	**ART vs. NC**: higher risk for low and very low birth weight
Bay et al., 2019	20 studies included. IVF/ICSI: n = 3,972 NC: n = 11,012	Systematic review and meta-analysis	**IVF/ICSI vs. NC**: Significantly lower weight up to preschool age but no difference in long term height
Magnus et al., 2021	ART: n = 1,721 NC: n = 79 740	Prospective – Norway	**Children born between 1992 and 2001 and followed up to the age of 17 years:** **ART vs. NC**: no difference at the age of 17

to that of NC children. Long term height was unrelated to mode of conception (54). In line with these findings were the results of a cohort study from Norway that included 79,740 children born after NC and 1,721 ART children and showed no significant difference in growth by age 17 (55). In summary, the results on growth of children conceived after ART are so far reassuring and suggest that there is no difference compared with NC children.

Long term health of ICSI-conceived children (Table 4.5)

The use of ICSI escalated globally the last years for all causes of infertility, although there is evidence that shows no benefit compared with conventional IVF. The long term effects on ICSI-conceived children are still not clear. Studies on neurodevelopment showed that ICSI-conceived children have the same outcomes as children conceived after IVF and NC (56, 57). A modest increase in the risk of mental retardation and autism has been reported in ICSI-conceived children; however, these findings are conflicting and have not been replicated by larger studies (58, 59). No differences were found in growth, cancer risk, vision, and hearing of ICSI-conceived children compared with children conceived after NC (44, 45, 56, 58). Increased numbers of surgical interventions, illnesses during childhood, and hospitalizations have

TABLE 4.5

Summary of the Published Studies on Long Term Outcomes of ICSI-Conceived Children and Overall Mortality in Children Conceived after ART

ICSI-Conceived Children

	Study Size	Study Type and Country	Conclusion of the Study
Catford et al., 2017	34 studies included	Systematic review	ICSI vs. IVF: no difference in neurodevelopmental outcomes, growth, and physical health
Catford et al., 2018	48 studies included	Systematic review	ICSI vs. NC: no difference in neurodevelopment, growth, vision, hearing, and higher risk for impaired general health, particularly metabolic and reproductive health
Rumbold et al., 2019		Review	ICSI: modest increase in risk of mental retardation and autism and accelerated postnatal growth and risk of adiposity. Impaired spermatogenesis has been also described. Need for larger studies
Ackerman et al., 2014	ART: n = 122 IVF/ICSI: n = 30 NC: n = 1,872	Case control – USA	Children between 4 and 18 years of age: ART vs. NC: no difference in autism-associated gene-disrupting events
Wikstrand et al., 2006	ICSI: n = 137 NC: n = 159	Case control – Sweden	Children born between 1994 and 1996 and followed up to the age of 5 years: ICSI vs. NC: no difference in visual function and/or ocular morphology
Ludwig et al., 2010	ICSI: n = 276 NC: n = 273	Prospective – Germany	Children followed up to the age of 4–6 years: ICSI vs. NC: no difference in the development of hearing and vision
Bonduelle et al., 2004	ICSI: n = 300 NC: n = 300	Prospective – Belgium	Children followed up at 5 years of age: ICSI vs. NC: no difference in growth and chronic illnesses. More ICSI children underwent surgical interventions and required physiotherapy and dietary therapy
Bonduelle et al., 2005	ICSI: n = 540 IVF: n = 437 NC: n = 538	Case control – Multicenter European	Children followed up to the age of 5 years: ICSI/IVF vs. NC: higher need of health care resources
Ludwig et al., 2009	ICSI: n = 276 NC: n = 273	Prospective – Germany	Children born between 1998 and 2000 and followed up to the age of 4-6 years: ICSI vs. NC: increased urogenital surgeries in ICSI boys. No difference in general health
Belva and Bonduelle et al., 2018	ICSI: n = 126 NC: n = 133	Case control – Belgium	Young adults at age of 18 years born between 1992 and 1996: ICSI vs. NC: no difference in the markers of metabolic syndrome
Belva and De Schepper et al., 2018	ICSI: n = 127 NC: n = 138	Retrospective – Belgium	Young adults at age of 18 years born between 1992 and 1996: ICSI vs. NC: higher peripheral fat deposition in men conceived by ICSI
Belva et al., 2016	ICSI: n = 54 NC: n = 57	Retrospective – Belgium	Young adults between 18 and 22 years born between 1992 and 1996: ICSI vs. NC: lower semen quantity and quality in young adults born after ICSI
Belva et al., 2017	ICSI: n = 54 NC: n = 57	Retrospective – Belgium	Young adults between 18 and 22 years born between 1992–1996: ICSI vs. NC: lower inhibin B and higher FSH levels in ICSI-conceived men

Overall Mortality

Henningsen et al., 2014	ART: n = 62 485 NC: n = 362 798	Case control – data from Nordic countries	Children born between 1982 and 2007: ART vs. NC: increased risk of stillbirth in singletons before 28 gestational weeks
Rodriguez-Wallberg et al., 2020	ART: n = 43,506 NC: n = 2,803,602	Prospective – Sweden	Children born between 1983 and 2012 and followed up to the age of 19 years: ART vs. NC: increased risk of infant mortality after transfer of frozen embryos

been described among ICSI-conceived children (60–62). Two studies presented higher peripheral fat deposition among ICSI-conceived young men, but the cardiometabolic parameters were comparable to those after NC (63, 64). Recently, impaired spermatogenesis and altered reproductive hormone levels were found among men aged between 18 and 22 years conceived by ICSI compared to age-matched controls (58, 65, 66). In summary, the current inconsistent and sparse literature on the long term health of ICSI-conceived children underscores the need for lifelong follow-up studies for these children and for large studies comparing the outcomes between groups of ICSI-conceived children after male and non-male infertility causes. Male factor infertility accounts for about half the cases of couple infertility, and in around 50% of cases its etiology remains unknown. However, microdeletions of the Y chromosome are the most frequent genetic causes of male factor infertility and can be transmitted to the male offspring after ART, affecting their fertility (67).

Overall mortality (Table 4.5)

The majority of deaths in ART children occur early in life during the neonatal period because of causes related to preterm birth and malformations (68). A Swedish large nationwide prospective population-based study that included 43,506 singletons born after ART compared them with NC singletons and found an increased risk of infant mortality in ART-conceived children (defined as death of the child at any point from birth up to 1 year of age) compared with children born after NC. Most causes of death in ART singletons were associated with prematurity and its complications. Mortality was higher in the group of children conceived using frozen/thawed embryos. This study cohort has been followed up to teenage years (median 15.9 years). The data are reassuring, as beyond the infant period, no increased risk for higher mortality was found (69).

Conclusions

- Children born after ART, when restricted to singletons, have a similar outcome for many conditions as their NC peers.
- For some outcomes, particularly cardiovascular diseases and diabetes, studies show some higher risk for ART singletons or subgroups of ART singletons.
- The continuous surveillance of children born after ART is obligatory, since the cohorts of children and adolescents born after ART worldwide are large.

REFERENCES

1. Adamson GD, de Mouzon J, Chambers GM, Zegers-Hochschild F, Mansour R, Ishihara O, et al. International committee for monitoring assisted reproductive technology: World report on assisted reproductive technology, 2011. *Fertil Steril.* 2018;110(6):1067–80.
2. European IVFMCftESoHR, Embryology, Calhaz-Jorge C, de Geyter C, Kupka MS, de Mouzon J, et al. Assisted reproductive technology in Europe, 2012: Results generated from European registers by ESHRE. *Human Reproduction (Oxford, England).* 2016;31(8):1638–52.
3. Draper ES, Kurinczuk JJ, Abrams KR, Clarke M. Assessment of separate contributions to perinatal mortality of infertility history and treatment: A case-control analysis. *Lancet.* 1999;353(9166):1746–9.
4. Basso O, Baird DD. Infertility and preterm delivery, birthweight, and caesarean section: A study within the Danish National Birth Cohort. *Human Reproduction (Oxford, England).* 2003;18(11):2478–84.
5. Helmerhorst FM, Perquin DA, Donker D, Keirse MJ. Perinatal outcome of singletons and twins after assisted conception: A systematic review of controlled studies. *BMJ.* 2004;328(7434):261.
6. Kallen B, Finnstrom O, Nygren KG, Otterblad Olausson P. In vitro fertilization in Sweden: Maternal characteristics. *Acta obstetricia et gynecologica Scandinavica.* 2005;84(12):1185–91.

7. Davies MJ, Moore VM, Willson KJ, Van Essen P, Priest K, Scott H, et al. Reproductive technologies and the risk of birth defects. *N Engl J Med*. 2012;366(19):1803–13.
8. Berntsen S, Soderstrom-Anttila V, Wennerholm UB, Laivuori H, Loft A, Oldereid NB, et al. The health of children conceived by ART: "The chicken or the egg?" *Hum Reprod Update*. 2019;25(2):137–58.
9. Bergh C, Wennerholm UB. Long-term health of children conceived after assisted reproductive technology. *Ups J Med Sci*. 2020;125(2):152–7.
10. Rumbold AR, Moore VM, Whitrow MJ, Oswald TK, Moran LJ, Fernandez RC, et al. The impact of specific fertility treatments on cognitive development in childhood and adolescence: A systematic review. *Human Reproduction (Oxford, England)*. 2017;32(7):1489–507.
11. Strömberg B, Dahlquist G, Ericson A, Finnström O, Köster M, Stjernqvist K. Neurological sequelae in children born after in-vitro fertilisation: A population-based study. *Lancet*. 2002;359(9305):461–5.
12. Knoester M, Helmerhorst FM, Vandenbroucke JP, van der Westerlaken LA, Walther FJ, Veen S. Cognitive development of singletons born after intracytoplasmic sperm injection compared with in vitro fertilization and natural conception. *Fertil Steril*. 2008;90(2):289–96.
13. Sandin S, Nygren KG, Iliadou A, Hultman CM, Reichenberg A. Autism and mental retardation among offspring born after in vitro fertilization. *JAMA*. 2013;310(1):75–84.
14. Spangmose AL, Malchau SS, Schmidt L, Vassard D, Rasmussen S, Loft A, et al. Academic performance in adolescents born after ART-a nationwide registry-based cohort study. *Human Reproduction (Oxford, England)*. 2017;32(2):447–56.
15. Spangmose AL, Malchau SS, Henningsen AA, Forman JL, Rasmussen S, Loft A, et al. Academic performance in adolescents aged 15–16 years born after frozen embryo transfer compared with fresh embryo transfer: A nationwide registry-based cohort study. *BJOG*. 2019;126(2):261–9.
16. Norrman E, Petzold M, Bergh C, Wennerholm UB. School performance in singletons born after assisted reproductive technology. *Human Reproduction (Oxford, England)*. 2018;33(10):1948–59.
17. Norrman E, Petzold M, Bergh C, Wennerholm UB. School performance in children born after ICSI. *Human Reproduction (Oxford, England)*. 2020;35(2):340–54.
18. Källén AJ, Finnström OO, Lindam AP, Nilsson EM, Nygren KG, Otterblad Olausson PM. Is there an increased risk for drug treated attention deficit/hyperactivity disorder in children born after in vitro fertilization? *Eur J Paediatr Neurol*. 2011;15(3):247–53.
19. Hvidtjorn D, Grove J, Schendel D, Schieve LA, Svaerke C, Ernst E, et al. Risk of autism spectrum disorders in children born after assisted conception: A population-based follow-up study. *J Epidemiol Community Health*. 2011;65(6):497–502.
20. Fountain C, Zhang Y, Kissin DM, Schieve LA, Jamieson DJ, Rice C, et al. Association between assisted reproductive technology conception and autism in California, 1997–2007. *Am J Public Health*. 2015;105(5):963–71.
21. Liu L, Gao J, He X, Cai Y, Wang L, Fan X. Association between assisted reproductive technology and the risk of autism spectrum disorders in the offspring: A meta-analysis. *Scientific Reports*. 2017;7:46207.
22. Kissin DM, Zhang Y, Boulet SL, Fountain C, Bearman P, Schieve L, et al. Association of Assisted Reproductive Technology (ART) treatment and parental infertility diagnosis with autism in ART-conceived children. *Human Reproduction (Oxford, England)*. 2015;30(2):454–65.
23. Hvidtjorn D, Grove J, Schendel D, Svaerke C, Schieve LA, Uldall P, et al. Multiplicity and early gestational age contribute to an increased risk of cerebral palsy from assisted conception: A population-based cohort study. *Human Reproduction (Oxford, England)*. 2010;25(8):2115–23.
24. Källén AJ, Finnström OO, Lindam AP, Nilsson EM, Nygren KG, Olausson PM. Cerebral palsy in children born after in vitro fertilization: Is the risk decreasing? *Eur J Paediatr Neurol*. 2010;14(6):526–30.
25. Pinborg A, Loft A, Aaris Henningsen AK, Rasmussen S, Andersen AN. Infant outcome of 957 singletons born after frozen embryo replacement: The Danish National Cohort study 1995–2006. *Fertil Steril*. 2010;94(4):1320–7.
26. Goldsmith S, McIntyre S, Badawi N, Hansen M. Cerebral palsy after assisted reproductive technology: A cohort study. *Dev Med Child Neurol*. 2018;60(1):73–80.
27. Kettner LO, Kesmodel US, Ramlau-Hansen CH, Bay B, Ritz B, Matthiesen NB, et al. Fertility treatment and childhood epilepsy: A nationwide cohort study. *Epidemiology*. 2017;28(3):412–18.

28. Guo XY, Liu XM, Jin L, Wang TT, Ullah K, Sheng JZ, et al. Cardiovascular and metabolic profiles of offspring conceived by assisted reproductive technologies: A systematic review and meta-analysis. *Fertil Steril*. 2017;107(3):622–31 e5.
29. Shiloh SR, Sheiner E, Wainstock T, Walfisch A, Segal I, Landau D, et al. Long-term cardiovascular morbidity in children born following fertility treatment. *J Pediatr*. 2019;204:84–8 e2.
30. Zhang WY, Selamet Tierney ES, Chen AC, Ling AY, Fleischmann RR, Baker VL. Vascular health of children conceived via in vitro fertilization. *J Pediatr*. 2019;214:47–53.
31. Xu GF, Zhang JY, Pan HT, Tian S, Liu ME, Yu TT, et al. Cardiovascular dysfunction in offspring of ovarian-hyperstimulated women and effects of estradiol and progesterone: A retrospective cohort study and proteomics analysis. *J Clin Endocrinol Metab*. 2014;99(12):E2494–503.
32. Rexhaj E, Paoloni-Giacobino A, Rimoldi SF, Fuster DG, Anderegg M, Somm E, et al. Mice generated by in vitro fertilization exhibit vascular dysfunction and shortened life span. *J Clin Invest*. 2013;123(12):5052–60.
33. Cetinkaya F, Gelen SA, Kervancioglu E, Oral E. Prevalence of asthma and other allergic diseases in children born after in vitro fertilisation. *Allergol Immunopathol (Madr)*. 2009;37(1):11–13.
34. Kallen B, Finnstrom O, Nygren KG, Otterblad Olausson P. Asthma in Swedish children conceived by in vitro fertilisation. *Arch Dis Child*. 2013;98(2):92–6.
35. Carson C, Sacker A, Kelly Y, Redshaw M, Kurinczuk JJ, Quigley MA. Asthma in children born after infertility treatment: Findings from the UK Millennium Cohort Study. *Human Reproduction (Oxford, England)*. 2013;28(2):471–9.
36. Forton K, Motoji Y, Pezzuto B, Caravita S, Delbaere A, Naeije R, et al. Decreased pulmonary vascular distensibility in adolescents conceived by in vitro fertilization. *Human Reproduction (Oxford, England)*. 2019;34(9):1799–808.
37. Shachor N, Wainstock T, Sheiner E, Harlev A. Fertility treatments and gastrointestinal morbidity of the offspring. *Early Hum Dev*. 2020;144:105021.
38. Steiner N, Wainstock T, Sheiner E, Walfisch A, Segal I, Haim A, et al. Long-term endocrine disorders in children born from pregnancies conceived following fertility treatments. *Early Hum Dev*. 2020;148:105132.
39. Sakka SD, Malamitsi-Puchner A, Loutradis D, Chrousos GP, Kanaka-Gantenbein C. Euthyroid hyperthyrotropinemia in children born after in vitro fertilization. *Journal of Clinical Endocrinology and Metabolism*. 2009;94(4):1338–41.
40. Ceelen M, van Weissenbruch MM, Vermeiden JP, van Leeuwen FE, Delemarre-van de Waal HA. Cardiometabolic differences in children born after in vitro fertilization: Follow-up study. *Journal of Clinical Endocrinology and Metabolism*. 2008;93(5):1682–8.
41. Kettner LO, Matthiesen NB, Ramlau-Hansen CH, Kesmodel US, Bay B, Henriksen TB. Fertility treatment and childhood type 1 diabetes mellitus: A nationwide cohort study of 565,116 live births. *Fertil Steril*. 2016;106(7):1751–6.
42. Norrman E, Petzold M, Clausen TD, Henningsen AK, Opdahl S, Pinborg A, et al. Type 1 diabetes in children born after assisted reproductive technology: A register-based national cohort study. *Human Reproduction (Oxford, England)*. 2020;35(1):221–31.
43. Krieger Y, Wainstock T, Sheiner E, Harlev A, Landau D, Horev A, et al. Long-term pediatric skin eruption-related hospitalizations in offspring conceived via fertility treatment. *Int J Dermatol*. 2018;57(3):317–23.
44. Wikstrand MH, Stromland K, Flodin S, Bergh C, Wennerholm UB, Hellstrom A. Ophthalmological findings in children born after intracytoplasmic sperm injection. *Acta Ophthalmol Scand*. 2006;84(2):177–81.
45. Ludwig AK, Hansen A, Katalinic A, Sutcliffe AG, Diedrich K, Ludwig M, et al. Assessment of vision and hearing in children conceived spontaneously and by ICSI: A prospective controlled, single-blinded follow-up study. *Reprod Biomed Online*. 2010;20(3):391–7.
46. Tsumi E, Lavy Y, Sheiner E, Barrett C, Harlev A, Hagbi Bal M, et al. Assisted reproductive technology and long-term ophthalmic morbidity of the offspring. *J Dev Orig Health Dis*. 2020:1–5.
47. Jackson RA, Gibson KA, Wu YW, Croughan MS. Perinatal outcomes in singletons following in vitro fertilization: A meta-analysis. *Obstet Gynecol*. 2004;103(3):551–63.

48. Pinborg A, Wennerholm UB, Romundstad LB, Loft A, Aittomaki K, Soderstrom-Anttila V, et al. Why do singletons conceived after assisted reproduction technology have adverse perinatal outcome? Systematic review and meta-analysis. *Hum Reprod Update.* 2013;19(2):87–104.
49. Barker DJ, Gluckman PD, Godfrey KM, Harding JE, Owens JA, Robinson JS. Fetal nutrition and cardiovascular disease in adult life. *Lancet.* 1993;341(8850):938–41.
50. Barker DJ, Fall CH. Fetal and infant origins of cardiovascular disease. *Arch Dis Child.* 1993;68(6):797–9.
51. Barker DJ, Hales CN, Fall CH, Osmond C, Phipps K, Clark PM. Type 2 (non-insulin-dependent) diabetes mellitus, hypertension and hyperlipidaemia (syndrome X): Relation to reduced fetal growth. *Diabetologia.* 1993;36(1):62–7.
52. Eriksson JG, Forsen T, Tuomilehto J, Winter PD, Osmond C, Barker DJ. Catch-up growth in childhood and death from coronary heart disease: Longitudinal study. *BMJ.* 1999;318(7181):427–31.
53. Ceelen M, van Weissenbruch MM, Prein J, Smit JJ, Vermeiden JP, Spreeuwenberg M, et al. Growth during infancy and early childhood in relation to blood pressure and body fat measures at age 8–18 years of IVF children and spontaneously conceived controls born to subfertile parents. *Human Reproduction (Oxford, England).* 2009;24(11):2788–95.
54. Bay B, Lyngso J, Hohwu L, Kesmodel US. Childhood growth of singletons conceived following in vitro fertilisation or intracytoplasmic sperm injection: A systematic review and meta-analysis. *BJOG.* 2019;126(2):158–66.
55. Magnus MC, Wilcox AJ, Fadum EA, Gjessing HK, Opdahl S, Juliusson PB, et al. Growth in children conceived by ART. *Human Reproduction (Oxford, England).* 2021;36(4):1074–1082.
56. Catford SR, McLachlan RI, O'Bryan MK, Halliday JL. Long-term follow-up of intra-cytoplasmic sperm injection-conceived offspring compared with in vitro fertilization-conceived offspring: A systematic review of health outcomes beyond the neonatal period. *Andrology.* 2017;5(4):610–21.
57. Catford SR, McLachlan RI, O'Bryan MK, Halliday JL. Long-term follow-up of ICSI-conceived offspring compared with spontaneously conceived offspring: A systematic review of health outcomes beyond the neonatal period. *Andrology.* 2018;6(5):635–53.
58. Rumbold AR, Sevoyan A, Oswald TK, Fernandez RC, Davies MJ, Moore VM. Impact of male factor infertility on offspring health and development. *Fertil Steril.* 2019;111(6):1047–53.
59. Ackerman S, Wenegrat J, Rettew D, Althoff R, Bernier R. No increase in autism-associated genetic events in children conceived by assisted reproduction. *Fertil Steril.* 2014;102(2):388–93.
60. Bonduelle M, Bergh C, Niklasson A, Palermo GD, Wennerholm UB, Collaborative Study Group of Brussels G, et al. Medical follow-up study of 5-year-old ICSI children. *Reprod Biomed Online.* 2004;9(1):91–101.
61. Bonduelle M, Wennerholm UB, Loft A, Tarlatzis BC, Peters C, Henriet S, et al. A multi-centre cohort study of the physical health of 5-year-old children conceived after intracytoplasmic sperm injection, in vitro fertilization and natural conception. *Human Reproduction (Oxford, England).* 2005;20(2):413–19.
62. Ludwig AK, Katalinic A, Thyen U, Sutcliffe AG, Diedrich K, Ludwig M. Physical health at 5.5 years of age of term-born singletons after intracytoplasmic sperm injection: Results of a prospective, controlled, single-blinded study. *Fertil Steril.* 2009;91(1):115–24.
63. Belva F, Bonduelle M, Provyn S, Painter RC, Tournaye H, Roelants M, et al. Metabolic syndrome and its components in young adults conceived by ICSI. *Int J Endocrinol.* 2018;2018:8170518.
64. Belva F, De Schepper J, Roelants M, Tournaye H, Bonduelle M, Provyn S. Body fat content, fat distribution and adipocytokine production and their correlation with fertility markers in young adult men and women conceived by Intracytoplasmic Sperm Injection (ICSI). *Clin Endocrinol (Oxf).* 2018;88(6):985–92.
65. Belva F, Bonduelle M, Roelants M, Michielsen D, Van Steirteghem A, Verheyen G, et al. Semen quality of young adult ICSI offspring: The first results. *Human Reproduction (Oxford, England).* 2016;31(12):2811–20.
66. Belva F, Roelants M, De Schepper J, Van Steirteghem A, Tournaye H, Bonduelle M. Reproductive hormones of ICSI-conceived young adult men: The first results. *Human Reproduction (Oxford, England).* 2017;32(2):439–46.
67. Krausz C, Degl'Innocenti S. Y chromosome and male infertility: Update, 2006. *Front Biosci.* 2006;11:3049–61.

68. Henningsen AA, Wennerholm UB, Gissler M, Romundstad LB, Nygren KG, Tiitinen A, et al. Risk of stillbirth and infant deaths after assisted reproductive technology: A Nordic study from the CoNARTaS group. *Human Reproduction (Oxford, England)*. 2014;29(5):1090–6.
69. Rodriguez-Wallberg KA, Lundberg FE, Ekberg S, Johansson ALV, Ludvigsson JF, Almqvist C, et al. Mortality from infancy to adolescence in singleton children conceived from assisted reproductive techniques versus naturally conceived singletons in Sweden. *Fertil Steril*. 2020;113(3):524–32.

5

Maternal and obstetric outcomes after transfer of cryopreserved embryos

Anne Lærke Spangmose, Anna-Karina Aaris Henningsen, and Anja Pinborg

Abbreviations

aOR	Adjusted odds ratio
ART	Assisted reproductive technology
BMI	Body mass index
BW	Birth weight
CoNARTaS	Committee of Nordic ART and Safety
eFET	Elective frozen/thawed embryo transfer
FET	Frozen/thawed embryo transfer
FSH	Follicle-stimulating hormone
GDM	Gestational diabetes mellitus
GnRH	Gonadotropin-releasing hormone
hCG	Human chorionic gonadotropin
HDP	Hypertensive disorders in pregnancy
ICSI	Intracytoplasmic sperm injection
IUI	Intrauterine insemination
IVF	In vitro fertilization
LBW	Low birth weight
LGA	Large for gestational age
LH	Luteinizing hormone
mNC-FET	Modified natural cycle FET
NC-FET	Natural cycle FET
OHSS	Ovarian hyperstimulation syndrome
OR	Odds ratio
PCOS	Polycystic ovary syndrome
PGT	Preimplantation genetic testing
PPH	Postpartum hemorrhage
PPROM	Preterm prelabor rupture of membranes
PTB	Preterm birth
RCT	Randomized controlled trial
RR	Relative risk
SC	Spontaneous conception
SD	Standard deviation
SGA	Small for gestational age
tNC-FET	True natural cycle FET
VEGF	Vascular endothelial growth factor
VLBW	Very low birth weight
VPTB	Very preterm birth

Introduction

In 1983, Trounson and Mohr reported the first pregnancy after frozen/thawed embryo transfer (FET) worldwide, initially using the slow-freeze technique (1). Since then the rate of FET cycles has steadily increased, as FET enables freezing of surplus embryos, reduces the need for repeated oocyte retrievals, and allows time for results from preimplantation genetic testing to return (2). Furthermore, FET almost eliminates the risk of late-onset ovarian hyperstimulation syndrome (OHSS) when used in a "GnRH agonist trigger + elective FET" strategy. Finally, and maybe most importantly, FET promotes the use of single embryo transfer, as live birth rates are shown to be comparable for double fresh embryo transfer and elective single embryo transfer with an FET in a subsequent cycle (3–5). Thus FET is a key tool to reduce multiple births after assisted reproductive technology (ART) treatment and the associated maternal and obstetric complications.

At the beginning of the decade, vitrification of human embryos has tremendously increased post-thaw embryo survival rates and pregnancy rates following FET (6–14). The proportion of frozen embryo replacements (FERs) in Europe relative to all transfer cycles has increased from 12% in 1997 to 27% in 2016 (Figure 5.1).

Frozen embryo transfer (FET)

Obstetric and perinatal outcomes following FET

Adjusted risk estimates on obstetric outcomes in pregnancies after FET vs. fresh embryo transfer from systematic reviews, including meta-analyses, are shown in Table 5.1.

A recent meta-analysis found that in pregnancies after FET, the relative risk (RR) of hypertensive disorder of pregnancy (HDP) was higher (RR 1.29 [95% CI 1.07–1.56]) compared to those after fresh

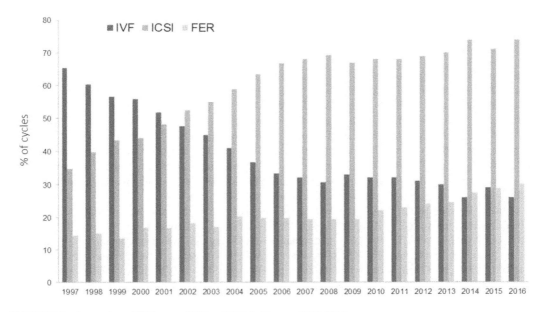

FIGURE 5.1 Proportion of IVF versus ICSI and FER in Europe, 1997–2016.

[From Wyns et al. 2020 (15).]

TABLE 5.1

Systematic Review and Meta-Analyses Presenting Pooled Risk Estimates of Maternal and Obstetric Outcomes in Pregnancies after FET versus Fresh Embryo Transfer

	Maheshwari (2012)	Pinborg (2013)	Zhao (2016)*	Maheshwari (2018)	Roque (2019)
Comparison group	FET vs. Fresh	FET vs. Fresh	FET vs. Fresh	FET vs. Fresh	eFET* vs. Fresh
Risk estimate	RR (95% CI)	aOR (95% CI)	OR (95% CI)	RR (95% CI)	RR (95% CI)
Pregnancy-induced hypertension	–	–	–	1.29 (1.07–1.56)	1.03 (0.48–2.18)
Preeclampsia	–	–	–	–	1.79 (1.03–3.09)
Preterm birth	0.84 (0.78–0.90)	0.85 (0.76–0.94)	1.14 (1.02–1.28) Inverse: 0.88 (0.78–0.98)	0.90 (0.84–0.97)	1.13 (0.93–1.36)
Low birth weight	0.69 (0.62–0.76)	–	1.48 (1.37, 1.60) Inverse: 0.68 (0.63–0.73)	0.72 (0.67–0.77)	(No difference in mean birth weight)
Small for gestational age	0.45 (0.30–0.66)	–	–	0.61 (0.56–0.67)	–
Large for gestational age	–	–	–	1.54 (1.48–1.61)	–
High birth weight	–	–	–	1.85 (1.46–2.33)	–
Perinatal deaths	0.68 (0.48–0.96)	–	1.11 (0.85–1.46) Inverse: 0.90 (0.68–1.18)	0.92 (0.78–1.08)	–
Congenital anomalies	1.05 (0.81–1.35)	–	–	1.01 (0.87–1.16)	0.88 (0.46–1.69)

* Including randomized controlled trials.

Abbreviations: *FET* frozen embryo transfer, *RR* risk ratio, *aOR* adjusted odds ratio, *CI* confidence intervals.

embryos (16). The increased risk of preeclampsia was confirmed in a systematic review based on pregnancies from elective freezing (eFET) versus fresh embryo transfer (RR 1.79 [95% CI 1.03–3.09]) (17). Based on Nordic data from the Committee of Nordic ART and Safety (CoNARTaS) in mothers having siblings, one from FET and one from fresh embryo transfer, the risk of HDP was higher after FET cycles compared with fresh cycles within the same mother (OR 2.63 [95% CI 1.73–3.99]) (18).

Initial systematic reviews and meta-analyses showed reassuring obstetric outcomes in pregnancies and children conceived following FET in comparison with fresh embryo transfers and even a reduced risk of preterm birth (PTB), low birth weight (LBW), and small for gestational age (SGA), while the risks of stillbirth and perinatal deaths were similar as after fresh ART cycles (19–22).

An updated systematic review and meta-analysis including 26 studies and nearly 300,000 births confirmed that the relative risk of PTB (RR 0.90 [95% CI 0.84–0.97]), LBW (RR 0.72 [95% CI 0.67–0.77]), and SGA (RR 0.61 [95% CI 0.56–0.67]) in pregnancies following FET was lower than in pregnancies following fresh embryo transfer (16). The same study showed no difference in risk of congenital anomalies (RR 1.01 [95% CI 0.87–1.16]) or perinatal mortality (RR 0.92 [95% CI 0.78–1.08]) in singleton pregnancies from FET when compared with those after fresh embryo transfer (16).

Multiples studies have documented that FET children have a higher mean birth weight than children born after transfer of fresh embryos and children born after spontaneous conception (16, 19, 23–25). In 2010 Pelkonen et al. were the first to report that FET was associated with an increased risk of being born large for gestational age (LGA). Recently a meta-analysis demonstrated that the risk of LGA is increased

1.5-fold and 1.3-fold compared to children born after fresh cycles and spontaneous conception (26, 27) and a 1.7-fold and 1.4-fold increased risk of high birth weight, respectively (26).

The findings of an altered growth profile in children born after FET have furthermore been illustrated in studies using sibling designs, where singleton siblings conceived after different conception methods have been compared. The strength of these studies is that the mother, and thereby the maternal factors, are kept steady. This helps differentiate the effect of the conception method on child outcomes. All sibling studies confirm that cryopreservation of embryos results in a higher mean birth weight and an increased risk of being born LGA and macrosomic (28–31).

Maternal and obstetric outcomes following eFET

Risk estimates on maternal and obstetric outcomes in pregnancies after eFET vs. fresh embryo transfer from randomized controlled trials (RCTs) are shown in Table 5.2.

The shift towards an eFET strategy has been highly debated recently. The pros claim an impairment of the endometrium in the fresh cycle with ovarian hyper-response and multiple corpora lutea and high levels of sex steroids due to the gonadotrophin stimulation in the fresh embryo transfer cycle, whereas the cons focus on the negative implications of postponement of embryo transfer, prolonged wait time to pregnancy, and the increased risk of preeclampsia and high birth weight in the offspring from FET pregnancies (32).

Recently, a systematic review has shown that an eFET strategy may be beneficial, with higher live birth rates in women with a hyper-response to gonadotrophin stimulation, while in women with a normo-ovarian response, a fresh embryo transfer strategy with strict cancellation criteria when at risk of OHSS seems to result in a similar live birth rate but shorter time to live birth and similar risk of OHSS (17).

Five recent large RCTs on eFET vs. fresh embryo transfer with pregnancy and live birth rates as their primary outcomes included maternal and obstetric results as secondary outcomes (Table 5.2) (33–37). The first RCT published in 2016 found a higher mean birth weight and a higher risk of preeclampsia in the eFET group in Chinese women with polycystic ovary syndrome (PCOS) (33). A further two RCTs only included normo-ovulatory women with no PCOS, one Chinese and one Vietnamese (34, 35). The Chinese study found similar maternal and obstetric outcomes (34), while the Vietnamese study confirmed the higher mean birth weight as was observed in the first Chinese study including women with PCOS, and furthermore found fewer neonates born SGA in the eFET group compared with the fresh embryo transfer group (33, 35). A third recent Chinese study on women with a regular menstrual cycle based on single blastocyst transfer confirmed the threefold increased risk of preeclampsia and a significantly higher birth weight in eFET vs. fresh embryo transfer, as was observed also by the first Chinese study on women with PCOS (33, 36). A recent systematic review and meta-analysis looked at maternal risks in women with a regular menstrual cycle excluding women with PCOS and comparing only pregnancies after eFET vs. fresh embryo transfer (38). In their meta-analyses, the risk estimates on PTB were RR 1.06 (95% CI 0.85–1.33), pregnancy-induced hypertension RR 0.90 (95% CI 0.48–1.67), and preeclampsia RR 1.68 (95% CI 1.03–2.75) (38).

Summary

Systematic reviews with more than 25,000 FET pregnancies confirm that singleton babies conceived after FET are at lower risk of PTB, SGA, and LBW while more likely to be LGA and born with high birth weight. Women pregnant after FET have an increased risk of HDP and preeclampsia. Other maternal and obstetric outcomes such as antepartum hemorrhage, perinatal mortality, and congenital anomalies are not increased in pregnancies from FET.

Slow-freeze and vitrification

To enhance elective single embryo transfer, thereby reducing the number of multiple births after ART, an efficient cryopreservation program in ART clinics is of the utmost importance. This can facilitate a single embryo transfer strategy, with freezing of surplus embryos and preventing OHSS, when eFET is applied in

TABLE 5.2
Randomized Controlled Trials Presenting Risk Estimates of Maternal and Obstetric Outcomes in Pregnancies after eFET vs. Fresh Embryo Transfer

	Chen (2016)	Shi (2018)	Vuong (2018)	Wei (2019)	Stormlund (2020)	Meta-Analyses Jin (2020)
Number of included women	1,508	2,157	782	1,650	460	Including results from Shi, Vuong, and Wei
Included women	With PCOS	Normo-ovulatory	Normo-ovulatory	Normo-ovulatory	Normo-ovulatory	Normo-ovulatory
FET cycle	Programmed FET	74.2% NC-FET 25.8% programmed FET	Programmed FET	62.5% NC-FET 36.4% programmed FET 1.2% other*	mNC-FET	NC-FET and programmed FET
Risk estimate	Rate ratio (95% CI)	Rate ratio (95% CI)	Relative risk (95% CI)	Relative risk (95% CI)	Numbers, percentages, or mean and SD, and p-value	Relative risk
Pregnancy-induced hypertension	1.97 (0.68–5.71)	0.75 (0.24–2.36)**	0.60 (0.15–2.51)**	1.17 (0.48–2.84)**	eFET: 2/57 (3.5%) Fresh: 2/55 (3.6%) P = 1.00	0.90 (0.48–1.67)
Preeclampsia	3.12 (1.26–7.73)	1.35 (0.76–2.39)**	1.99 (0.18–21.91)**	3.07 (1.03–9.11)**	eFET: 4/57 (7.0%) Fresh: 4/55 (7.3%) P = 1.00	1.68 (1.03–2.75)
Postpartum hemorrhage	—	—	—	6.20 (0.78–49.37)	eFET: 3/57 (5.3%) Fresh: 3/55 (5.5%) P = 1.00	—
Cesarean sections	—	—	No significant difference	—	eFET: 12/57 (21.1%) Fresh: 20/55 (36.4%) P = 0.07	—
Preterm birth	1.17 (0.87–1.57)	1.17 (0.88–1.55)**	0.83 (0.46–1.51)**	0.97 (0.58–1.60)**	eFET: 0/56 (0.0%) Fresh: 6/54 (11.1%) P = 0.01	1.06 (0.85–1.33)
Mean birth weight	Significantly higher in eFET	No significant difference	Significantly higher in eFET singletons	Significantly higher in eFET singletons	eFET: 3,586 g (SD 610) Fresh: 3,117 g (SD 641) P < 0.001	—

	Chen (2016)	Shi (2018)	Vuong (2018)	Wei (2019)	Stormlund (2020)	Meta-Analyses Jin (2020)
Low birth weight	–	–	–	–	eFET: 3/56 (5.4%) Fresh: 8/53 (15.1%) P = 0.12	–
Small for gestational age	–	–	0.21 (0.06–0.74)	0.69 (0.43–1.11)	eFET: 4/56 (7.1%) Fresh: 9/52 (17.3%) P = 0.14	–
Large for gestational age	–	–	2.33 (0.61–8.96)	1.60 (1.13–2.26)	eFET: 4/56 (7.1%) Fresh: 0/52 (0.0%) P = 0.12	–
Neonatal or perinatal deaths	No significant difference	0.50 (0.09–2.74)[a]	–	–	eFET: 1/57 (1.8%)[b] Fresh: 1/55 (1.8%)[b] P = 1.00	–
Congenital anomalies	1.24 (0.68–2.28)	0.62 (0.34–1.15)	–	0.83 (0.37–1.87)	–	–

* Minimal ovarian stimulation cycles.
** Estimates and 95% CI from meta-analyses by Jin et al. 2020.
[a] Neonatal death.
[b] Perinatal death.

Abbreviations: *eFET* elective frozen embryo transfer, *PCOS* polycystic ovarian syndrome, *CI* confidence intervals, *P* p-value.

women at risk of this severe complication. Two cryopreservation methods are routinely used: slow-freezing and vitrification. Slow-freezing allows for freezing to occur at a sufficiently slow rate to permit adequate cellular dehydration while minimizing intracellular ice formation. Vitrification allows the solidification of the cell(s) and the extracellular milieu into a glass-like state without the formation of ice. Due to the high efficacy, today vitrification has become the most widespread method for cryopreservation of human embryos.

Maternal and obstetric outcomes

Several studies have compared maternal and obstetric outcomes after vitrification and slow-freeze of embryos, with diverging findings. In 2013, a large Chinese cohort study showed children born after day 3 vitrified embryos had a higher mean birth weight than children born after transfer of day 3 slow-freeze embryos (39). A few years later, a Finnish group found similar mean birth weights in children born after day 2–3 vitrification versus slow-freeze embryos but lower miscarriage rates and higher post-thaw embryo survival rates in the vitrification group. Hence they concluded that vitrification is superior to slow-freeze (40). A large population-based cohort with data from Australia and New Zealand compared vitrified blastocysts (n = 20,887) to slow-freeze blastocysts (n = 12,852) and found higher clinical pregnancy rates and delivery rates for vitrified blastocysts but similar perinatal outcomes for the two groups (41). A recent large Nordic cohort study compared 3,650 children born after vitrified blastocyst with 8,123 children born after slow-freeze day 2–3 embryos and found children born after vitrified blastocysts to have a higher risk of PTB (<37 weeks) (42). All other main maternal and obstetric outcomes did not differ between the two groups (42). A prospective randomized trial from 2014 found implantation rates to be similar between the two cryo-techniques, but embryos thawed after vitrification had higher post-thawing survival rates (43). The same year Debroek et al. published their results from an RCT showing higher live birth rates per embryo thawed in the vitrification group versus the slow-freeze group (RR 3.23 [95% CI 1.59–4.81]) and higher implantation rate (RR 2.76 [95% CI 1.59–4.81]) for vitrified embryos (14). However, when a recent systematic review and meta-analysis from 2017 compared the outcomes from vitrified versus slow-freeze embryos, they found only a trend towards better clinical pregnancy rates and live birth rates after vitrification but no strong statistical significance for vitrification to be superior to slow-freezing of embryos. Still, they found a significant improvement in the post-thaw embryo survival after vitrification compared with slow-freezing (RR 1.59 [95% CI 1.30–1.93]) (13).

Summary

With the current evidence available, vitrification must overall be considered the best choice of cryopreservation for human embryos compared with slow-freezing. Nevertheless, continual focus and data collection on outcomes after both cryopreservation methods seem reasonable, as only very few studies have compared maternal and obstetric outcomes in pregnancies after slow-freezing and vitrification.

Programmed and natural cycle

In an FET cycle, the endometrium can be primed according to different protocols depending on whether the woman has a regular cycle. For regular cycling women, FET can be performed in a natural cycle (NC-FET) either in a true natural cycle (tNC-FET) or a modified natural cycle (mNC-FET), whereas programmed FET cycle, also called artificial FET or substituted FET, is used for logistic reasons or for women not presenting with a regular cycle. Further FET can be performed in a stimulated cycle with ovulation induction by either aromatase inhibitors, clomiphene, or gonadotrophin stimulation.

The NC-FET is performed in a physiological endocrine environment with one corpus luteum present. In tNC-FET, the transfer of the frozen/thawed embryo is timed by the peak in luteinizing hormone (LH) and/or by monitoring the size of the growing follicle by frequent ultrasound scans without exogenous ovulation induction. In mNC-FET, human chorionic gonadotropin (hCG) administration is used for ovulation induction.

Programmed FET cycles include priming of the endometrium with estradiol in the follicular phase and adding progesterone in the luteal phase. Hence suppression of the hypothalamic-pituitary axis occurs and no corpus luteum is created, contrary to a NC-FET.

Recent studies have suggested that the endometrium preparation protocol in FET cycles influences the maternal adaptation to pregnancy and thus maternal and obstetric outcomes (44–57). The underlying mechanisms are not yet fully understood; however, the presence or absence of a corpus luteum is thought to play an important role. This hypothesis was initially suggested by Conrad and Baker in 2013 and later supported by several studies (44–50). In NC-FET or mNC-FET luteal-phase progesterone may rescue the endometrium in patients with insufficient corpus luteum function; however, there is still no consensus on whether pregnancies in natural or modified natural cycle FET may benefit from luteal-phase progesterone supplementation to avoid higher miscarriage rates (58–60).

In a naturally conceived pregnancy, the corpus luteum is the primary source of the hormone secretion such as estrogen, progesterone, relaxin, and vascular endothelial growth factor (VEGF) in the early pregnancy, and it has been hypothesized that altered levels of these hormones in a pregnancy, where no corpus luteum is developed, may lead to an altered risk profile in both maternal and obstetric outcome compared with pregnancies after a NC-FET (44–57). Estrogen and progesterone are crucial for the development of a normal placenta; hence altered levels of these sex-steroid hormones, as seen in a programmed FET cycle, may lead to placenta-related complications (47, 48). Relaxin and VEGF, both vasoactive hormones, play an important role in the vascular function and circulatory adaptions in pregnancy (45, 47–50). In human pregnancies, relaxin levels are undetectable in the absence of a corpus luteum, and as relaxin is a potent vasodilator, deficient levels of circulation relaxin are one plausible biological explanation for a part of the effect of an absent corpus luteum (46–48).

In a prospective cohort study including a limited number of patients, women with no corpus luteum lacked the physiological drop in mean arterial pressure in the first trimester compared with women with one corpus luteum present (48). Furthermore, women with no corpus luteum had impaired peripheral endothelial function, increased arterial stiffness, and reduced angiogenic and nonangiogenic circulating endothelial progenitor cells, suggesting an impact on endothelial homeostasis and repair capacity (48). Compromised maternal cardiovascular function during pregnancy in women conceiving in the absence of a corpus luteum has been confirmed in other studies; however, all had limited sample sizes (45, 49, 50).

Maternal outcomes

Eight cohort studies on the risk of maternal outcomes in pregnancies after different FET protocols have been published (Tables 5.3 and 5.4) (50–57).

Obstetric outcomes

Obstetric outcomes in pregnancies after different FET protocols are presented in Tables 5.3 and 5.4) (51, 54–57),

The risk of postterm birth (gestational weeks >41 or >42) was significantly increased after programmed FET cycles in three large studies compared with NC-FET (54, 55), tNC-FET (51), or stimulated cycles (51), with aOR ranging from 1.59 to 5.68 (51, 54, 55). The association between FET protocol and postterm birth was not confirmed in other studies (56, 57). A large Japanese study including over 75,000 women undergoing programmed FET cycles found the risk of PTB to be significantly increased after programmed FET cycles with an aOR 1.12 (95% CI 1.05–1.40) (54).

In two studies, the risk of high birth weight (>4,500 g) was significantly increased in children born after a programmed FET cycle when compared with tNC-FET (aOR 1.62 [95% CI 1.16–2.09]) (51), stimulated cycles (aOR 1.40 [95% CI 1.03–1.90]) (51), or NC-FET (aOR 1.95 [95% CI 1.09–3.48]) (56).

Summary

Eight cohort studies have compared maternal and obstetric outcomes after programmed FET cycles and NC-FET. All studies investigating the risk of HDP and cesarean section found the risk to be increased

TABLE 5.3

Characteristics of Studies Comparing Maternal and Obstetric Outcomes in Pregnancies Resulting from 0 versus 1 Corpus Luteum

	Birth Cohort	Country	0 Corpus Luteum	Singleton Deliveries 1 Corpus Luteum	Design
Saito (2017)	2013	Japan	Hormone replacement cycle n = 10,235 *Cycles including: not described*	NC-FET n = 6,287 *Cycles including: clomiphene citrate, human menopausal gonadotropin, or FSH*	Retrospective cohort
Ginström Ernstad (2019)	2005–2015	Sweden	Programmed FET n = 1,446 *Cycles including: estrogen and progesterone with or without suppression with a GnRH agonist/antagonist*	tNC-FET n = 6,297 *Cycles including: no exogenous hormones* Stimulated cycles n = 1,983 *Cycles including: mNC-FET (hCG-trigger), ovulation induction (clomiphene citrate or letrozole with/without hCG), gonadotropin stimulation (FSH or human menopausal gonadotropin with/without GnRH-agonist/antagonist), luteal support (progesterone with/without hCG)*	Retrospective cohort
Jing (2019)	2013–2016	Sweden	Programmed FET n = 787[a] *Cycles including: estrogen and progesterone*	NC-FET n = 2,802[a] *Cycles including: no exogenous hormones in the follicular phase, luteal phase with vaginal progesterone*	Retrospective cohort
Saito (2019)	2013–2016	Japan	Hormone replacement cycle n = 75,474 *Cycles including: estrogen and progesterone*	NC-FET n = 29,760 *Cycles including: hCG-trigger or luteal support*	Retrospective cohort
von Versen-Höynck (2019)	2011–2017	USA	Programmed FET n = 94 *Cycles including: estrogen and progesterone*	mNC-FET n = 127 *Cycles including: hCG trigger and luteal phase with vaginal progesterone* SC with known subfertility, IUI, mNC-FET n = 290 *IUI cycles including: clomiphene, letrozole, or gonadotropins*	Prospective cohort
Asserhøj (2020)	2006–2014	Denmark	Programmed FET n = 357 *Cycles including: progesterone and/or estrogen with or without suppression with a GnRH agonist/antagonist*	NC-FET n = 779 *Cycles including: no exogenous hormones or hCG trigger*	Retrospective cohort
Makhijani (2020)	2013–2018	USA	Programmed FET n = 391 *Cycles including: estrogen and progesterone with suppression with a GnRH agonist*	NC-FET n = 384 *Cycles including: no exogenous hormones in the follicular phase, luteal phase with vaginal progesterone*	Retrospective cohort
Wang (2020)	2013–2018	China	Programmed FET n = 4,162 *Cycles including: estrogen and progesterone*	NC-FET n = 10,211 *Cycles including: with or without hCG trigger; luteal phase with vaginal progesterone*	Retrospective cohort

[a] Both singleton and multiple deliveries, adjusting for plurality.

TABLE 5.4

Cohort Studies Presenting Risk Estimates of Maternal Outcomes in Pregnancies Resulting from 0 versus 1 Corpus Luteum

	Saito (2017)	Ginström Ernstad (2019)	Jing (2019)	Saito (2019)	von Versen-Höynck (2019)	Asserhøj (2020)	Makhijani (2020)	Wang (2020)
Reference group	Hormone replacement cycle*	Programmed FET	Programmed FET	Hormone replacement cycle	Programmed FET	Programmed FET	Programmed FET	Programmed FET
Comparison group	NC-FET	a: tNC-FET b: Stimulated cycles	NC-FET	NC-FET	a: mNC-FET b: SC with known subfertility, IUI, or mNC-FET	NC-FET	NC-FET	NC-FET
Risk estimate	aOR (95% CI)[a]	aOR (95% CI)[b]	aOR (95% CI)[c]	aOR (95% CI)[d]	aOR (95% CI)[e]	aOR (95% CI)[f]	aOR (95% CI)[g]	aOR (95% CI)[h]
Hypertensive disorders in pregnancy	—	a: 1.78 (1.43–2.21) b: 1.61 (1.22–2.10)	1.86 (1.38–2.50)	1.43 (1.14–1.80)	—	1.87 (1.17–3.00)	2.39 (1.37–4.17)	—
Preeclampsia	—	—	—	—	a: 3.55 (1.20–11.94) b: 2.73 (1.14–6.49)	2.40 (1.43–4.02)	—	2.55 (2.06–3.16)
Severe preeclampsia	—	—	—	—	a: 15.05 (2.59–286.27) b: 6.45 (1.94–25.09)	—	—	—
Placenta previa	—	a: 0.71 (0.36–1.37) b: 1.00 (0.46–2.16)	—	1.00 (0.64–1.56)	—	1.10 (0.46–2.62)	1.50 (0.57–3.89)	Not increased***
Placenta abruption	—	a: 0.93 (0.37–2.35) b: 0.56 (0.16–1.99)	—	1.58 (0.43–5.88)	—	1.19 (0.45–3.16)	1.11 (0.12–10.15)	Not increased***
Placenta accreta	—	—	—	6.91 (2.87–16.66)	—	—	2.98 (0.25–34.95)	—
Postpartum hemorrhage	—	a: 2.63 (2.20–3.13) b: 2.87 (2.29–3.60)	—	—	—	2.24 (1.68–2.99)**	2.02 (0.49–8.30)	2.94 (1.44–5.99)
Cesarean sections	1.64 (1.52–1.76)	a: 1.39 (1.21–1.60) b: 1.27 (1.08–1.50)	1.67 (1.37–2.04)	1.69 (1.55–1.84)	—	1.52 (1.15–2.01)	1.44 (1.04–2.01)	Not increased***

(*Continued*)

TABLE 5.4 (Continued)

Cohort Studies Presenting Risk Estimates of Maternal Outcomes in Pregnancies Resulting from 0 versus 1 Corpus Luteum

	Saito (2017)	Ginström Ernstad (2019)	Jing (2019)	Saito (2019)	von Versen-Höynck (2019)	Asserhøj (2020)	Makhijani (2020)	Wang (2020)
Preterm prelabor rupture of membranes	–	–	–	1.87 (0.82–4.28)	–	1.19 (0.81–1.74)	2.39 (1.37–4.17)	
Gestational diabetes mellitus	–	–	–	0.52 (0.40–0.68)	–	–	1.69 (0.95–2.99)	Not increased[***]

[*] Cycles not described.
[**] Not adjusted for culture duration.
[***] Data not shown.

Logistic regression analyses adjusted for:
[a] Maternal age, culture duration, child's sex, number of embryos transferred, use of assisted hatching, and cause of infertility.
[b] Maternal age, BMI, parity, smoking, child's sex, year of birth of child, chronic hypertension, maternal educational level, years of involuntary childlessness, cause of infertility, IVF/ICSI, freezing method, culture duration, and number of gestational sacs.
[c] BMI, endometrial thickness on translate day, basal FSH level, culture duration, the day of development of frozen embryos, plurality, and HDP (when appropriate).
[d] Maternal age, culture duration, number of embryos transferred, use of assisted hatching, and cause of infertility.
[e] Maternal age, BMI, parity, history of hypertension, PCOS, and diabetes mellitus (pregestational and gestational).
[f] Maternal age, parity, child's sex, year of birth of child, IVF/ICSI, culture duration, and single embryo transfer.
[g] Maternal age, BMI, parity, smoking, diabetes mellitus, chronic hypertension, cause of infertility, number of embryos transferred, and PGT.
[h] Maternal age; BMI; cause of infertility: primary infertility; IVF/ICSI; number of embryos transferred; endometrial thickness; number of antral follicle count; blood pressure; baseline FSH, LH, and total testosterone; fasting glucose level.

Abbreviations: *FET* frozen embryo transfer, *NC-FET* natural cycle-FET, *tNC-FET* true natural cycle-FET, *mNC-FET* modified natural cycle-FET, *SC* spontaneous conception, *IUI* intrauterine insemination, *aOR* adjusted odds ratio, *CI* confidence interval, *BMI* body mass index, *IVF* in vitro fertilization, *ICSI* intracytoplasmic sperm injection, *FSH* follicle-stimulating hormone, *HDP* hypertensive disorders in pregnancy, *PCOS* polycystic ovary syndrome, *PGT* preimplantation genetic testing, *LH* luteinizing hormone.

after programmed FET cycles. Current evidence also indicates an increased risk of preeclampsia, postpartum hemorrhage (PPH), high birth weight, and postterm birth after programmed FET. Other maternal and obstetric outcomes such as placenta previa, placenta abruption, LBW, SGA, LGA, or low Apgar score are seemingly not affected in pregnancies after programmed FET cycles.

Epigenetic changes and FET

Epigenetics involves various processes altering gene activity without changing the primary nucleotide sequence of the DNA molecule. A common process for controlling gene activity is DNA methylation, causing activation or repression of gene expression (61). The human genome undergoes several phases of epigenetic programming during gametogenesis and early embryo development coinciding with ART, which makes a potential association difficult to entangle. Genomic imprinting is essential for the normal development of the embryo, and disrupted imprinting can result in imprinting disorders influencing fetal growth. The potential induction of epigenetic alterations during early embryonic development as the embryo is frozen and thawed has been discussed. Still, a lot of uncertainty remains. It has been shown that children born after FET have higher levels of insulin-like growth factor I and II (IGH-1 and 2), as well as lower levels of insulin-like growth factor binding protein 3 (IGFBP-3) (62). Obviously, the effect of both subfertility and ART on epigenetic instability is complex. Several studies have found overall methylation error rates to be significantly higher in children conceived after ART (63–67). Still, the potential health implications of epigenetic changes associated with ART should not be overinterpreted, as there is still no evidence of any functional consequence or altered health outcomes in adulthood (68). However, it seems well documented that ART children have an increased risk of imprinting disorders (67, 69–71), but in a recent Nordic study on the risk of imprinting disorders in ART children, none of the children identified with imprinting disorders in the ART group were conceived after transfer of cryopreserved embryos (72).

Discussion

Singleton babies conceived after FET are at lower risk of PTB, SGA, and LBW, but at increased risk of being born with a high birth weight or LGA compared with singletons conceived after fresh embryo transfer. However, women pregnant after FET have an increased risk of HDP. Other maternal and obstetric outcomes such as antepartum hemorrhage, perinatal mortality, and congenital anomalies are not affected in pregnancies from FET.

Causal hypotheses

A possible explanation for the increased risk of HDP and preeclampsia in FET pregnancies relates to the endometrial priming with estradiol and progesterone in programmed FET cycles where no corpus luteum is present. There seems to be strong evidence of an increased risk of HDP in programmed FET cycles compared with NC-FET, and current evidence also indicates a higher risk of preeclampsia after programmed FET cycles. Nonetheless, secondary outcomes from RCTs on eFET versus fresh cycles are not convincing regarding the impact of the type of FET protocol on the increased risk of HDP or preeclampsia in FET compared with fresh pregnancies (33–37). Further, the risk of selection bias must be considered when interpreting the results from the cohort studies on outcomes after programmed FET cycles, as the type of FET protocol is highly dependent on the cause of infertility, as all patients with anovulatory infertility are treated in programmed FET (such as patients with PCOS). On the other hand, programmed FET is by far the most used protocol in many clinical settings, as this protocol provides the opportunity to plan exactly the date of warming and transfer of the frozen embryo.

Also, the higher risk of LGA and higher birth weight in FET babies are hypothesized to be explained by the proportion of FET pregnancies with absence of a corpus luteum. However, as two out of three RCTs reported a significantly higher birth weight in children following eFET in natural cycles compared with children from fresh cycles, the "missing corpus luteum" theory is not the sole explanation for the high birth weight in FET pregnancies (34, 36, 37). Another explanation for the higher birth weight in FET children may be a selection process with higher-quality embryos surviving the freezing and thawing procedure; however, mean birth weight in FET also exceeds natural conception, hence it is less likely that the higher mean BW is caused by a positive selection. A third hypothesis is that a potential asynchrony between the endometrium and the embryo might be present in FET cycles with an influence on fetal growth and development leading to the increased birth weight. Further, it has been speculated that in most FET cycles, the embryo is transferred in a more natural uterine environment compared with fresh cycles, where the levels of sex steroids due to gonadotrophin stimulation is very high. If the IVF embryo per se is prone to overgrowth, this may be blurred in fresh cycles due to the impairment of the endometrium, while in the frozen cycles the endometrium is more receptive. Supportive of this theory is the "large cattle syndrome" that was observed in animal studies in the early days of IVF (73). Finally, an explanation could be that the cryopreservation techniques per se cause epigenetic modifications in the embryo at the early embryonic stages, hence affecting the growth potential of the fetus. However, studies on epigenetic changes in FET children are sparse. Further, evidence on the potential health implications of epigenetic modifications in FET children should not be overinterpreted, as no studies have shown any functional consequence or altered health outcomes in adulthood.

Implications

HDP and preeclampsia imply a direct risk to the health of the mother and unborn child. Preeclampsia is the main cause of maternal death and is also related to fetal growth restriction and preterm birth, either spontaneously or caused by iatrogenic delivery (74). High birth weight increases the risk of shoulder dystocia, perineal lacerations, postpartum hemorrhage, cesarean sections, and neonatal hypoglycemia (26). The implications of the increased risk of LGA and high birth weight in children born after FET may affect childhood health and risk of obesity in both childhood and adult life.

Long term implications of LGA or high birth weight has been investigated in several studies (75, 76). A meta-analysis based on six prospective cohort studies found no significant difference in the risk of coronary heart disease in children with high birth weight (>4,000 g) compared to children with normal birth weight (2,500–4,000 g) (OR 0.89 [95% CI 0.79–1.01]) (75). Further, a meta-analysis by Zhang and co-workers including 31 studies on the association between high birth weight or LGA and blood pressure or hypertension showed that systolic and diastolic blood pressure were positively associated with high birth weight in younger children (6–12 years of age), while in older adults (41–60 years of age) the reverse association was found. The same pattern was seen for the relative risk of hypertension. The authors describe the phenomenon as a "catch-down" effect in the elevation of blood pressure that is observed in subjects with high birth weight as they grow older. Hence, older individuals with high birth weight are less likely to develop hypertension than those with normal birth weight (76).

Conclusions

- Embryo cryopreservation is a key tool in ART, as it promotes the use of single embryo transfer, thus reducing multiple births and the associated maternal and obstetric complications.
- The "GnRH agonist trigger + e-FET" strategy almost eliminates the risk of late-onset OHSS.
- Though it seems that FET pregnancies increase the risk of HDP, preeclampsia, LGA, and high birth weight, it is important to keep in mind that the risk of PTB, SGA, and LBW is decreased in FET pregnancies.
- HDP and preeclampsia in FET pregnancies might be partly prevented by the use of NC-FET.
- In anovulatory women, an alternative to programmed FET cycles is to create a corpus luteum by stimulation with low-dose gonadotrophins or aromatase inhibitors, aiming for mono-ovulation, which might be a better strategy regarding safety aspects of the mother and child (77).

- In pregnancies where no ovulation can be induced, like in oocyte donation FET, in women with premature ovarian insufficiency, or when programmed FET is used for planning of blastocyst warming and transfer, low-dose aspirin from early pregnancy may be considered for patients at high risk of preeclampsia, i.e., women with advanced maternal age (78).

TABLE 5.5

Cohort Studies Presenting Risk Estimates of Obstetric Outcomes in Pregnancies Resulting from 0 versus 1 Corpus Luteum

	Saito (2017)	Ginström Ernstad (2019)	Saito (2019)	Asserhøj (2020)	Wang (2020)
Reference group	Hormone replacement cycle*	Programmed FET	Hormone replacement cycle	Programmed FET	Programmed FET
Comparison group	NC-FET	a: tNC-FET b: Stimulated cycles	NC-FET	NC-FET	NC-FET
Risk estimate	aOR (95% CI)[a]	aOR (95% CI)[b]	aOR (95% CI)[c]	aOR (95% CI)[d]	aOR (95% CI)[e]
Low birth weight	–	a: 0.88 (0.62–1.26) b: 0.83 (0.55–1.27)	–	–	Not increased***
Very low birth weight	–	a: 1.01 (0.46–2.20) b: 0.92 (0.36–2.35)	–	–	Not increased***
High birth weight	–	a: 1.62 (1.26–2.09) b: 1.40 (1.03–1.90)	–	1.95 (1.09–3.48)**	Not increased***
Preterm birth	–	a: 1.09 (0.85–1.40) b: 1.15 (0.84–1.57)	1.12 (1.05–1.40)	0.91 (0.56–1.49)	Not increased***
Very preterm birth	–	a: 1.23 (0.67–2.24) b: 1.54 (0.70–3.42)	–	1.94 (0.82–4.57)	
Postterm birth	5.68 (3.30–9.80)	a: 1.59 (1.27–2.01) b: 1.98 (1.47–2.68)	3.28 (1.73–6.19)	1.27 (0.60–2.66)**	Not increased***
Small for gestational age	1.14 (0.99–1.32)	a: 0.91 (0.62–1.35) b: 0.89 (0.56–1.43)	–	1.47 (0.71–3.04)	Not increased***
Large for gestational age	–	a: 1.27 (0.99–1.61) b: 1.10 (0.82–1.47)	–	1.19 (0.70–2.03)	Not increased***
Low Apgar score 5 min	–	a: 1.09 (0.78–1.51) b: 1.46 (0.94–2.24)	–	–	

* Cycles not described.
** Not adjusted for culture duration.
*** Data not shown.

Logistic regression analyses adjusted for:
[a] Maternal age, culture duration, child's sex, number of embryos transferred, use of assisted hatching, and cause of infertility.
[b] Maternal age, BMI, parity, smoking, child's sex, year of birth of child, chronic hypertension, maternal educational level, years of involuntary childlessness, cause of infertility, IVF/ICSI, freezing method, culture duration, and number of gestational sacs.
[c] Maternal age, culture duration, number of embryos transferred, use of assisted hatching, and cause of infertility.
[d] Maternal age, parity, child's sex, year of birth of child, IVF/ICSI, culture duration, and single embryo transfer.
[e] Maternal age; BMI; cause of infertility; primary infertility; IVF/ICSI; number of embryos transferred; endometrial thickness; number of antral follicle count; blood pressure; baseline FSH, LH, and total testosterone; fasting glucose level.

Abbreviations: *FET* frozen embryo transfer, *NC-FET* natural cycle-FET, *tNC-FET* true natural cycle-FET, *aOR* adjusted odds ratio, *CI* confidence interval, *BMI* body mass index, *IVF* in vitro fertilization, *ICSI* intracytoplasmic sperm injection, *FSH* follicle-stimulating hormone, *LH* luteinizing hormone.

REFERENCES

1. Trounson A, Mohr L. Human pregnancy following cryopreservation, thawing and transfer of an eight-cell embryo. *Nature*. 1983;305(5936):707–9. doi: 10.1038/305707a0 [published Online First: 1983/10/20].
2. Ferraretti AP, Nygren K, Andersen AN, et al. Trends over 15 years in ART in Europe: An analysis of 6 million cycles. *Hum Reprod Open*. 2017;2017(2):hox012. doi: 10.1093/hropen/hox012 [published Online First: 2017/08/29].
3. Thurin A, Hausken J, Hillensjo T, et al. Elective single-embryo transfer versus double-embryo transfer in in vitro fertilization. *N Engl J Med*. 2004;351(23):2392–402. doi: 10.1056/NEJMoa041032 [published Online First: 2004/12/03].
4. Lopez-Regalado ML, Clavero A, Gonzalvo MC, et al. Randomised clinical trial comparing elective single-embryo transfer followed by single-embryo cryotransfer versus double embryo transfer. *Eur J Obstet Gynecol Reprod Biol*. 2014;178:192–8. doi: 10.1016/j.ejogrb.2014.04.009 [published Online First: 2014/05/07].
5. Kamath MS, Mascarenhas M, Kirubakaran R, et al. Number of embryos for transfer following in vitro fertilisation or intra-cytoplasmic sperm injection. *Cochrane Database Syst Rev*. 2020;8:CD003416. doi: 10.1002/14651858.CD003416.pub5 [published Online First: 2020/08/23].
6. Mukaida T, Nakamura S, Tomiyama T, et al. Successful birth after transfer of vitrified human blastocysts with use of a cryoloop containerless technique. *Fertil Steril*. 2001;76(3):618–20. doi: 10.1016/s0015-0282(01)01968-9 [published Online First: 2001/09/05].
7. Yokota Y, Sato S, Yokota M, et al. Birth of a healthy baby following vitrification of human blastocysts. *Fertil Steril*. 2001;75(5):1027–9. doi: 10.1016/s0015-0282(01)01685-5 [published Online First: 2001/05/04].
8. Saito H, Ishida GM, Kaneko T, et al. Application of vitrification to human embryo freezing. *Gynecol Obstet Invest*. 2000;49(3):145–9. doi: 10.1159/000010236 [published Online First: 2000/03/24].
9. Kuleshova LL, Lopata A. Vitrification can be more favorable than slow cooling. *Fertil Steril*. 2002;78(3):449–54. doi: 10.1016/s0015-0282(02)03305-8 [published Online First: 2002/09/07].
10. AbdelHafez FF, Desai N, Abou-Setta AM, et al. Slow freezing, vitrification and ultra-rapid freezing of human embryos: A systematic review and meta-analysis. *Reprod Biomed Online*. 2010;20(2):209–22. doi: 10.1016/j.rbmo.2009.11.013 [published Online First: 2010/02/02].
11. Balaban B, Urman B, Ata B, et al. A randomized controlled study of human Day 3 embryo cryopreservation by slow freezing or vitrification: Vitrification is associated with higher survival, metabolism and blastocyst formation. *Hum Reprod*. 2008;23(9):1976–82. doi: 10.1093/humrep/den222 [published Online First: 2008/06/12].
12. Rezazadeh Valojerdi M, Eftekhari-Yazdi P, Karimian L, et al. Vitrification versus slow freezing gives excellent survival, post warming embryo morphology and pregnancy outcomes for human cleaved embryos. *J Assist Reprod Genet*. 2009;26(6):347–54. doi: 10.1007/s10815-009-9318-6 [published Online First: 2009/06/11].
13. Rienzi L, Gracia C, Maggiulli R, et al. Oocyte, embryo and blastocyst cryopreservation in ART: Systematic review and meta-analysis comparing slow-freezing versus vitrification to produce evidence for the development of global guidance. *Hum Reprod Update*. 2017;23(2):139–55. doi: 10.1093/humupd/dmw038 [published Online First: 2016/11/10].
14. Debrock S, Peeraer K, Fernandez Gallardo E, et al. Vitrification of cleavage stage day 3 embryos results in higher live birth rates than conventional slow freezing: A RCT. *Hum Reprod*. 2015;30(8):1820–30. doi: 10.1093/humrep/dev134 [published Online First: 2015/06/20].
15. Wyns C, Bergh C, Calhaz-Jorge C, et al. ART in Europe, 2016: Results generated from European registries by ESHRE. *Hum Reprod Open*. 2020;2020(3):hoaa032. doi: 10.1093/hropen/hoaa032 [published Online First: 2020/08/08].
16. Maheshwari A, Pandey S, Amalraj Raja E, et al. Is frozen embryo transfer better for mothers and babies? Can cumulative meta-analysis provide a definitive answer? *Hum Reprod Update*. 2018;24(1):35–58. doi: 10.1093/humupd/dmx031.
17. Roque M, Haahr T, Geber S, et al. Fresh versus elective frozen embryo transfer in IVF/ICSI cycles: A systematic review and meta-analysis of reproductive outcomes. *Hum Reprod Update*. 2019;25(1):2–14. doi: 10.1093/humupd/dmy033 [published Online First: 2018/11/06].

18. Opdahl S, Henningsen AA, Tiitinen A, et al. Risk of hypertensive disorders in pregnancies following assisted reproductive technology: A cohort study from the CoNARTaS group. *Hum Reprod.* 2015;30(7):1724–31. doi: 10.1093/humrep/dev090 [published Online First: 2015/05/01].
19. Wennerholm UB, Soderstrom-Anttila V, Bergh C, et al. Children born after cryopreservation of embryos or oocytes: A systematic review of outcome data. *Hum Reprod.* 2009;24(9):2158–72. doi: 10.1093/humrep/dep125 [published Online First: 2009/05/22].
20. Maheshwari A, Pandey S, Shetty A, et al. Obstetric and perinatal outcomes in singleton pregnancies resulting from the transfer of frozen thawed versus fresh embryos generated through in vitro fertilization treatment: A systematic review and meta-analysis. *Fertil Steril.* 2012;98(2):368–77.e1–9. doi: 10.1016/j.fertnstert.2012.05.019 [published Online First: 2012/06/16].
21. Pinborg A, Wennerholm U, Romundstad L, et al. Why do singletons conceived after assisted reproduction technology have adverse perinatal outcome? Systematic review and meta-analysis. *Hum Reprod Update.* 2013;19:87–104.
22. Zhao J, Xu B, Zhang Q, et al. Which one has a better obstetric and perinatal outcome in singleton pregnancy, IVF/ICSI or FET?: A systematic review and meta-analysis. *Reprod Biol Endocrinol.* 2016;14(1):51. doi: 10.1186/s12958-016-0188-3 [published Online First: 2016/09/01].
23. Wennerholm UB, Henningsen AK, Romundstad LB, et al. Perinatal outcomes of children born after frozen-thawed embryo transfer: A Nordic cohort study from the CoNARTaS group. *Hum Reprod.* 2013;28(9):2545–53. doi: 10.1093/humrep/det272.
24. Spijkers S, Lens JW, Schats R, et al. Fresh and frozen-thawed embryo transfer compared to natural conception: Differences in perinatal outcome. *Gynecol Obstet Invest.* 2017;82(6):538–46. doi: 10.1159/000468935 [published Online First: 2017/05/16].
25. Terho. Birth weight and large-for-gestational-age in singletons born after frozen compared to fresh embryo transfer by gestational week: A Nordic register study from the CoNARTaS group. 2020.
26. Berntsen S, Pinborg A. Large for gestational age and macrosomia in singletons born after Frozen/Thawed Embryo Transfer (FET) in Assisted Reproductive Technology (ART). *Birth Defects Res.* 2018;110(8):630–43. doi: 10.1002/bdr2.1219 [published Online First: 2018/05/02].
27. Pelkonen S, Koivunen R, Gissler M, et al. Perinatal outcome of children born after frozen and fresh embryo transfer: The Finnish cohort study 1995–2006. *Hum Reprod.* 2010;25(4):914–23. doi: 10.1093/humrep/dep477 [published Online First: 2010/02/04].
28. Henningsen AK, Pinborg A, Lidegaard O, et al. Perinatal outcome of singleton siblings born after assisted reproductive technology and spontaneous conception: Danish national sibling-cohort study. *Fertil Steril.* 2011;95(3):959–63. doi: 10.1016/j.fertnstert.2010.07.1075 [published Online First: 2010/09/04].
29. Pinborg A, Henningsen A, Loft A, et al. Large baby syndrome in singletons born after Frozen Embryo Transfer (FET): Is it due to maternal factors or the cryotechnique? *Hum Reprod.* 2014;29(3):618–27. doi: 10.1093/humrep/det440.
30. Luke B, Brown MB, Wantman E, et al. Increased risk of large-for-gestational age birthweight in singleton siblings conceived with in vitro fertilization in frozen versus fresh cycles. *J Assist Reprod Genet.* 2017;34(2):191–200. doi: 10.1007/s10815-016-0850-x [published Online First: 2016/12/03].
31. Westvik-Johari. Perinatal health after fresh and frozen embryo transfer in assisted reproduction: Separating parental and treatment contributions. 2020.
32. Blockeel C, Campbell A, Coticchio G, et al. Should we still perform fresh embryo transfers in ART? *Hum Reprod.* 2019;34(12):2319–29. doi: 10.1093/humrep/dez233 [published Online First: 2019/12/06].
33. Chen ZJ, Shi Y, Sun Y, et al. Fresh versus frozen embryos for infertility in the polycystic ovary syndrome. *N Engl J Med.* 2016;375(6):523–33. doi: 10.1056/NEJMoa1513873 [published Online First: 2016/08/11].
34. Shi Y, Sun Y, Hao C, et al. Transfer of fresh versus frozen embryos in ovulatory eomen. *N Engl J Med.* 2018;378(2):126–36. doi: 10.1056/NEJMoa1705334 [published Online First: 2018/01/11].
35. Vuong LN, Dang VQ, Ho TM, et al. IVF transfer of fresh or frozen embryos in women without polycystic ovaries. *N Engl J Med.* 2018;378(2):137–47. doi: 10.1056/NEJMoa1703768 [published Online First: 2018/01/11].

36. Wei D, Liu JY, Sun Y, et al. Frozen versus fresh single blastocyst transfer in ovulatory women: A multicentre, randomised controlled trial. *Lancet.* 2019;393(10178):1310–18. doi: 10.1016/s0140-6736(18)32843-5 [published Online First: 2019/03/05].
37. Stormlund S, Sopa N, Zedeler A, et al. Freeze-all versus fresh blastocyst transfer strategy during in vitro fertilisation in women with regular menstrual cycles: Multicentre randomised controlled trial. *BMJ.* 2020;370:m2519. doi: 10.1136/bmj.m2519 [published Online First: 2020/08/08].
38. Jin X, Liu G, Jiao Z, et al. Pregnancy outcome difference between fresh and frozen embryos in women without polycystic ovary syndrome: A systematic review and meta-analysis. *Reprod Sci.* 2020. doi: 10.1007/s43032-020-00323-2 [published Online First: 2020/10/03].
39. Liu SY, Teng B, Fu J, et al. Obstetric and neonatal outcomes after transfer of vitrified early cleavage embryos. *Hum Reprod.* 2013;28(8):2093–100. doi: 10.1093/humrep/det104 [published Online First: 2013/04/10].
40. Kaartinen N, Kananen K, Huhtala H, et al. The freezing method of cleavage stage embryos has no impact on the weight of the newborns. *J Assist Reprod Genet.* 2016;33(3):393–99. doi: 10.1007/s10815-015-0642-8 [published Online First: 2016/01/11].
41. Li Z, Wang YA, Ledger W, et al. Clinical outcomes following cryopreservation of blastocysts by vitrification or slow freezing: A population-based cohort study. *Hum Reprod.* 2014;29(12):2794–801. doi: 10.1093/humrep/deu246 [published Online First: 2014/10/16].
42. Ginstrom Ernstad E, Spangmose AL, Opdahl S, et al. Perinatal and maternal outcome after vitrification of blastocysts: A Nordic study in singletons from the CoNARTaS group. *Hum Reprod.* 2019;34(11):2282–89. doi: 10.1093/humrep/dez212 [published Online First: 2019/11/07].
43. Fasano G, Fontenelle N, Vannin AS, et al. A randomized controlled trial comparing two vitrification methods versus slow-freezing for cryopreservation of human cleavage stage embryos. *J Assist Reprod Genet.* 2014;31(2):241–7. doi: 10.1007/s10815-013-0145-4 [published Online First: 2013/12/10].
44. Conrad KP, Baker VL. Corpus luteal contribution to maternal pregnancy physiology and outcomes in assisted reproductive technologies. *Am J Physiol Regul Integr Comp Physiol.* 2013;304(2):R69–72. doi: 10.1152/ajpregu.00239.2012 [published Online First: 2012/10/27].
45. Conrad KP, Petersen JW, Chi YY, et al. Maternal cardiovascular dysregulation during early pregnancy after in vitro fertilization cycles in the absence of a corpus luteum. *Hypertension.* 2019;74(3):705–15. doi: 10.1161/HYPERTENSIONAHA.119.13015 [published Online First: 2019/07/30].
46. Conrad KP, Graham GM, Chi YY, et al. Potential influence of the corpus luteum on circulating reproductive and volume regulatory hormones, angiogenic and immunoregulatory factors in pregnant women. *Am J Physiol Endocrinol Metab.* 2019;317(4):E677–85. doi: 10.1152/ajpendo.00225.2019 [published Online First: 2019/08/14].
47. von Versen-Höynck F, Strauch NK, Liu J, et al. Effect of mode of conception on maternal serum relaxin, creatinine, and sodium concentrations in an infertile population. *Reprod Sci.* 2019;26(3):412–19. doi: 10.1177/1933719118776792 [published Online First: 2018/06/05].
48. von Versen-Höynck F, Narasimhan P, Selamet Tierney ES, et al. Absent or excessive corpus luteum number is associated with altered maternal vascular health in early pregnancy. *Hypertension.* 2019;73(3):680–90. doi: 10.1161/hypertensionaha.118.12046 [published Online First: 2019/01/15].
49. von Versen-Höynck F, Häckl S, Selamet Tierney ES, et al. Maternal vascular health in pregnancy and postpartum after assisted reproduction. *Hypertension.* 2020;75(2):549–60. doi: 10.1161/hypertensionaha.119.13779 [published Online First: 2019/12/17].
50. von Versen-Höynck F, Schaub AM, Chi YY, et al. Increased preeclampsia risk and reduced aortic compliance with in vitro fertilization cycles in the absence of a corpus luteum. *Hypertension.* 2019;73(3):640–9. doi: 10.1161/hypertensionaha.118.12043 [published Online First: 2019/01/15].
51. Ginstrom Ernstad E, Wennerholm UB, Khatibi A, et al. Neonatal and maternal outcome after frozen embryo transfer: Increased risks in programmed cycles. *Am J Obstet Gynecol.* 2019;221(2):126 e1–e18. doi: 10.1016/j.ajog.2019.03.010 [published Online First: 2019/03/27].
52. Jing S, Li XF, Zhang S, et al. Increased pregnancy complications following frozen-thawed embryo transfer during an artificial cycle. *J Assist Reprod Genet.* 2019;36(5):925–33. doi: 10.1007/s10815-019-01420-1 [published Online First: 2019/03/30].
53. Makhijani R, Bartels C, Godiwala P, et al. Maternal and perinatal outcomes in programmed versus natural vitrified-warmed blastocyst transfer cycles. *Reprod Biomed Online.* 2020;41(2):300–8. doi: 10.1016/j.rbmo.2020.03.009 [published Online First: 2020/06/09].

54. Saito K, Kuwahara A, Ishikawa T, et al. Endometrial preparation methods for frozen-thawed embryo transfer are associated with altered risks of hypertensive disorders of pregnancy, placenta accreta, and gestational diabetes mellitus. *Hum Reprod*. 2019;34(8):1567–75. doi: 10.1093/humrep/dez079 [published Online First: 2019/07/13].
55. Saito K, Miyado K, Yamatoya K, et al. Increased incidence of post-term delivery and Cesarean section after frozen-thawed embryo transfer during a hormone replacement cycle. *J Assist Reprod Genet*. 2017;34(4):465–70. doi: 10.1007/s10815-017-0869-7 [published Online First: 2017/01/22].
56. Asserhøj LL, Spangmose AL, Henningsen AA, et al. Adverse obstetric and perinatal outcomes in 1,136 singleton pregnancies conceived after programmed Frozen Embryo Transfer (FET) compared with natural cycle FET. *Fertil Steril*. 2020.
57. Wang Z, Liu H, Song H, et al. Increased risk of pre-eclampsia after frozen-thawed embryo transfer in programming cycles. *Front Med (Lausanne)*. 2020;7:104. doi: 10.3389/fmed.2020.00104 [published Online First: 2020/04/24].
58. Ghobara T, Gelbaya TA, Ayeleke RO. Cycle regimens for frozen-thawed embryo transfer. *Cochrane Database Syst Rev*. 2017;7(7):Cd003414. doi: 10.1002/14651858.CD003414.pub3 [published Online First: 2017/07/05].
59. Groenewoud ER, Cantineau AE, Kollen BJ, et al. What is the optimal means of preparing the endometrium in frozen-thawed embryo transfer cycles? A systematic review and meta-analysis. *Hum Reprod Update*. 2013;19(5):458–70. doi: 10.1093/humupd/dmt030 [published Online First: 2013/07/04].
60. Horowitz E, Mizrachi Y, Finkelstein M, et al. A randomized controlled trial of vaginal progesterone for luteal phase support in modified natural cycle: Frozen embryo transfer. *Gynecol Endocrinol*. 2020:1–6. doi: 10.1080/09513590.2020.1854717 [published Online First: 2020/12/15].
61. Butler MG. Genomic imprinting disorders in humans: A mini-review. *J Assist Reprod Genet*. 2009;26(9–10):477–86. doi: 10.1007/s10815-009-9353-3 [published Online First: 2009/10/22].
62. Green MP, Mouat F, Miles HL, et al. Phenotypic differences in children conceived from fresh and thawed embryos in in vitro fertilization compared with naturally conceived children. *Fertil Steril*. 2013;99(7):1898–904. doi: 10.1016/j.fertnstert.2013.02.009 [published Online First: 2013/03/12].
63. Lim D, Bowdin SC, Tee L, et al. Clinical and molecular genetic features of Beckwith-Wiedemann syndrome associated with assisted reproductive technologies. *Hum Reprod*. 2009;24(3):741–7. doi: 10.1093/humrep/den406 [published Online First: 2008/12/17].
64. Manipalviratn S, DeCherney A, Segars J. Imprinting disorders and assisted reproductive technology. *Fertil Steril*. 2009;91(2):305–15. doi: 10.1016/j.fertnstert.2009.01.002 [published Online First: 2009/02/10].
65. Lazaraviciute G, Kauser M, Bhattacharya S, et al. A systematic review and meta-analysis of DNA methylation levels and imprinting disorders in children conceived by IVF/ICSI compared with children conceived spontaneously. *Hum Reprod Update*. 2014;20(6):840–52. doi: 10.1093/humupd/dmu033 [published Online First: 2014/06/26].
66. Lazaraviciute G, Kauser M, Bhattacharya S, et al. A systematic review and meta-analysis of DNA methylation levels and imprinting disorders in children conceived by IVF/ICSI compared with children conceived spontaneously. *Hum Reprod Update*. 2015;21(4):555–7. doi: 10.1093/humupd/dmv017 [published Online First: 2015/04/24].
67. Hattori H, Hiura H, Kitamura A, et al. Association of four imprinting disorders and ART. *Clin Epigenetics*. 2019;11(1):21. doi: 10.1186/s13148-019-0623-3 [published Online First: 2019/02/09].
68. Novakovic B, Lewis S, Halliday J, et al. Assisted reproductive technologies are associated with limited epigenetic variation at birth that largely resolves by adulthood. *Nat Commun*. 2019;10(1):3922. doi: 10.1038/s41467-019-11929-9 [published Online First: 2019/09/04].
69. Halliday J, Oke K, Breheny S, et al. Beckwith-Wiedemann syndrome and IVF: A case-control study. *Am J Hum Genet*. 2004;75(3):526–8. doi: 10.1086/423902 [published Online First: 2004/07/31].
70. Mussa A, Molinatto C, Cerrato F, et al. Assisted reproductive techniques and risk of Beckwith-Wiedemann syndrome. *Pediatrics*. 2017;140(1) doi: 10.1542/peds.2016-4311 [published Online First: 2017/06/22].
71. Cortessis VK, Azadian M, Buxbaum J, et al. Comprehensive meta-analysis reveals association between multiple imprinting disorders and conception by assisted reproductive technology. *J Assist Reprod Genet*. 2018;35(6):943–52. doi: 10.1007/s10815-018-1173-x [published Online First: 2018/04/27].

72. Henningsen AA, Gissler M, Rasmussen S, et al. Imprinting disorders in children born after ART: A Nordic study from the CoNARTaS group. *Hum Reprod.* 2020;35(5):1178–84. doi: 10.1093/humrep/deaa039 [published Online First: 2020/05/13].
73. Young LE, Sinclair KD, Wilmut I. Large offspring syndrome in cattle and sheep. *Rev Reprod.* 1998;3(3):155–63. doi: 10.1530/ror.0.0030155 [published Online First: 1998/11/26].
74. Mol BWJ, Roberts CT, Thangaratinam S, et al. Pre-eclampsia. *Lancet.* 2016;387(10022):999–1011. doi: 10.1016/s0140-6736(15)00070-7 [published Online First: 2015/09/08].
75. Wang SF, Shu L, Sheng J, et al. Birth weight and risk of coronary heart disease in adults: A meta-analysis of prospective cohort studies. *J Dev Orig Health Dis.* 2014;5(6):408–19. doi: 10.1017/s2040174414000440 [published Online First: 2014/09/30].
76. Zhang B, Wei D, Legro RS, et al. Obstetric complications after frozen versus fresh embryo transfer in women with polycystic ovary syndrome: Results from a randomized trial. *Fertil Steril.* 2018;109(2):324–29. doi: 10.1016/j.fertnstert.2017.10.020 [published Online First: 2018/01/18].
77. Huang P, Wei L, Li X, et al. Modified hMG stimulated: An effective option in endometrial preparation for frozen-thawed embryo transfer in patients with normal menstrual cycles. *Gynecol Endocrinol.* 2018;34(9):772–74. doi: 10.1080/09513590.2018.1460342 [published Online First: 2018/04/21].
78. Mather AR, Dom AM, Thorburg LL. Low-dose aspirin in pregnancy: Who? when? how much? and why? *Curr Opin Obstet Gynecol.* 2021;33(2):65–71. doi: 10.1097/gco.0000000000000694 [published Online First: 2021/02/24].

6

Safety of assisted reproduction and fertility preservation in women with Turner syndrome

Kenny A. Rodriguez-Wallberg

Introduction

Turner syndrome is the most common chromosomal abnormality in women and a common cause of infertility due to early ovarian failure (1). The estimated prevalence is about 1/2500 live-born females (2). The Turner spectrum is wide and includes mosaicism karyotypes 45,X/46,XX that usually present with only minor phenotypic features. As a consequence, a large number of women presenting with a Turner genotype remain undiagnosed throughout life (3). It has been estimated that only about half of women presenting with a Turner genotype would be identified by clinical features that will support the clinical investigations, including a karyotype exam, to receiving a diagnosis (4). Most women with a Turner genotype are diagnosed in early childhood or adolescence and a minority beyond adult age. In some cases, adult women receive a diagnosis of Turner syndrome during an infertility workup. It has been established that most women with Turner syndrome are missing an entire sex chromosome, 20% have a mosaic karyotype (most commonly 45X, 46,XX), and 25% have a partial deletion of one X chromosome (5).

It is acknowledged that infertility is a major concern for women with Turner syndrome (6, 7), and although the clinical spectrum of Turner syndrome is wide, it may be expected that only a minority of the girls with a Turner genotype undergo spontaneous puberty development, and very few of them would maintain fertility at adult age. Hence, fertility preservation counseling is currently recommended for these girls at young age and their families, as reported by clinical programs of fertility preservation (8). However, pregnancies in women with Turner syndrome are also recognized as having an increased risk of complications, the rate of pregnancy loss is increased, and severe obstetric complications including aortic dissection and maternal death during pregnancy or postpartum have been reported as high as in 2% of the cases (9, 10).

In this chapter the safety of assisted reproductive technologies (ARTs) in women with Turner syndrome will be discussed, with special focus on the use of ART treatments to achieve pregnancy and the performance of fertility preservation.

Preconception counseling and pregnancy risks in women with Turner syndrome

Women with Turner syndrome may achieve pregnancy naturally, particularly if they present with mosaicisms. However, the rate of miscarriage on spontaneous pregnancies is reported as high as 48%, contrasting to that in the general population (8%–20%) (10). An increased frequency of fetal chromosomal abnormalities has been found as potentially explanatory of this excess risk, but also a compromised endometrial receptivity due to hypoestrogenism and a higher prevalence of autoimmune diseases, which is acknowledged in women with Turner syndrome (5).

Additional pregnancy complications that frequently occur in women with Turner syndrome include hypertensive disorders and preterm delivery, which are usually managed with appropriate antenatal care.

There is, however, a dangerous vascular complication in the form of aortic dissection that may account for maternal death during pregnancy and postpartum in about 2% of the cases (11–13). For this reason a complete cardiovascular investigation needs to be performed prior to preconception counseling, as pregnancy can only be recommended to women with Turner syndrome in the absence of any congenital heart or vessel disease (bicuspid aortic valve, coarctation of the aorta).

In many countries, programs for follow-up of women with Turner syndrome have been established. In Sweden, the national program for women and girls with Turner's syndrome is run by the multidisciplinary Swedish Turner Academy. The program recommends that irrespective of age, a thorough cardiac evaluation should be performed with echocardiography and/or magnetic resonance imaging (14). Cardiac examinations should be repeated every fifth year after transition to the adult clinic in order to follow the aortic root diameter. In the case of aorta dilation in relation to body surface area, blood pressure lowering is advised and a full cardiac investigation to evaluate indication for surgery. The congenital defects, including bicuspid aortic valve and coarctation of the aorta, as well as the aortic dilatation, are all strongly associated with future aortic dissection (15).

Studies of pregnancies reported in women with Tuner karyotype are scarce and of small sample size, and the data presented so far are heterogeneous. A previous retrospective study of morbidity and mortality after childbirth conducted in Sweden for a period of over 20 years found no mortality in a cohort of 124 women achieving live births. In that study the mode of conception was not recorded, and the study suggested that in the absence of cardiac anomalies diagnosed, pregnancy may develop uneventfully (16). Several reports of pregnancies in women with Turner syndrome in Sweden have been consistent on the absence of increased mortality, which seems to be dependent on the careful repeated cardiac evaluations before pregnancy induction/assistance following the health care guidelines of the Turner program (17). Similar data have been reported by Canadian researchers, including a population-based study reporting on 44 live births in women with Turner syndrome indicating no serious adverse events in the small population that achieved live birth (18), and a retrospective study across ten Canadian centers collecting 68 pregnancies in women with Turner syndrome, which found no increased cardiovascular events during pregnancy (19). A retrospective study of 156 women in the United Kingdom whereof 18 achieved live birth through natural conception and seven through oocyte donation reported no cases of severe vascular complications during pregnancy or postpartum; however, the aortic diameters increased during pregnancy in the cohort (10). Although these studies provide reassuring data, reports from other countries support a higher risk of death in women with Turner syndrome due to aortic dissection or rupture, owing to the increased cardiovascular demands of pregnancy, and the estimated maternal mortality rate is approximately 2% (11, 12, 20).

Assisted reproductive technologies in women with Turner syndrome

In line with international guidelines, medical assistance to achieve pregnancy should only be recommended to women with Turner syndrome in absence of congenital heart and/or vessel abnormalities (surgically corrected or not) or acquired aortic dilation (5, 14). In case of any of these anomalies, alternatives to become a parent should be presented as valid options, including gestational surrogacy with the woman's own or donated oocytes and adoption (20, 21).

If no contraindications to pregnancy are demonstrated, treatments with ART, including in vitro fertilization/intracytoplasmic sperm injection (IVF/ICSI) may be initiated. However, as the risk of aortic dissection has been acknowledged to be five times higher in multiple pregnancies than in singleton pregnancies (22), international Turner groups have clearly stated that multiple pregnancies must be avoided in women with Turner syndrome, and single embryo transfer must be the standard of practice. Women with Turner syndrome undergoing ART treatments with donor oocytes also have an increased risk of hypertensive disorders of pregnancy of up to 67% of cases (23), which is much higher than the already expected higher prevalence of hypertensive complications reported in healthy women undergoing IVF/ICSI using donor oocyte treatment in comparison to women who undergo similar treatments with autologous oocytes (24). In a previous retrospective matched study of 29 women with Turner syndrome undergoing 31 treatments using donor eggs (N = 31) vs. control women with ovarian insufficiency for other

Safety in women with Turner syndrome 63

causes undergoing similar treatments (N = 31), a significantly lower pregnancy rate and a higher rate of early pregnancy loss were observed in the group with a Turner syndrome diagnosis. Of seven pregnancies achieved (22.5%), only one was ongoing and one live birth was achieved (1/31, 3.2%) in the Turner group, in comparison with ten pregnancies achieved (32.2%) with an ongoing pregnancy rate of 22.5% (7/31) in the control group (25). Standard endometrial preparation using 6 mg estradiol valerate PO daily resulted in appropriate endometrial thickness, which was similar in both study groups, and all women of this study received a single fresh cleavage-stage embryo for transfer without difficulties for embryo transfer reported (25).

Fertility preservation in women and girls with Turner syndrome

Fertility counseling and recommendations for fertility preservation should be advised as earliest as a Turner diagnosis is confirmed (21). If the ovarian reserve markers currently clinically validated, such as the serum concentration of anti-Müllerian hormone (AMH), indicate a decline in the context of the age of the patient, fertility preservation methods may be presented to the patient and the family. For adult women and for teenagers postmenarche, methods including gonadotropin stimulation and transvaginal egg retrieval have been demonstrated as feasible (26).

In a large series of 1,254 women and girls undergoing fertility preservation at the Karolinska University Hospital in Sweden for either malignant or benign diagnoses, a Turner diagnosis was highly frequent in children as indication to fertility preservation, in comparison to as in adult women (Table 6.1) (8). In 90 cases oocytes or ovarian tissue from the patients have been cryopreserved in this cohort. Additionally, 13 mothers of girls presenting with confirmed ovarian insufficiency due to various diagnoses, including Turner syndrome, underwent ovarian stimulation and oocyte cryopreservation aiming at the future use of the oocytes by their daughters (8).

The use of cryopreservation of ovarian tissue has been reported as a frequent indication for fertility preservation for girls and women with Turner syndrome in programs for fertility preservation in the Nordic countries (Table 6.2) (27). In general, girls who present with spontaneous puberty and with serum concentrations of follicle-stimulating hormone (FSH) and AMH that are normal for age may be candidates for ovarian tissue cryopreservation early in postpubertal years, before the ovarian reserve is diminished (4, 5). The national Turner multidisciplinary program in Sweden

TABLE 6.1

Diagnoses Present in the Cohort of Women and Girls Referred for Fertility Preservation (FP) at Karolinska University Hospital between 1998 and 2018 for All Indications, Including Malignant Diseases and Benign Conditions

Table 1	Adult Women (≥18 yr) (N = 1076)	Girls (1–17 yr) (N = 178)	All patients (N = 1254)
Age – Mean ± SD (range)	30.0 ± 6.1 (18–43)	14.2 ± 2.8 (1–17)	27.8 ± 8.0 (1–43)
Malignant diseases	798 (74.1%)	54 (30.3%)	852 (67.9%)
Benign indications	**278 (25.8%)**	**124 (69.7%)**	**402 (32.1%)**
Genetic predisposition to POI	17	76	93
Turner syndrome	**16**	**74**	**90**
Galactosemia and other	1	2	3
Donation to a relative	13		13

Note: In this cohort 90 patients underwent FP for Turner syndrome out of 402 patients with a benign indication. Additionally, 13 mothers of girls presenting with ovarian insufficiency for various diagnoses, including Turner syndrome, underwent ovarian stimulation and oocyte cryopreservation.

Source: Reprinted with permission from Rodriguez-Wallberg et al., *Acta Obstet Gynecol Scand 2019* (Ref. 8).

Abbreviations: *POI* premature ovarian insufficiency, *SD* standard deviation.

TABLE 6.2

Clinical Characteristics of Patients Included in Fertility Preservation (FP) Programs That Practice Ovarian Tissue Cryopreservation (OTC) Since 1995 in the Nordic Countries

Center Practicing OTC	N of OTC Patients	Age Range (N)	Common Diagnosis in Adults	Common Diagnosis in Children	Size of Tissue Retrieved	Infection Screening (year initiated)	Complications Registered
Denmark							
Copenhagen University Hospital	822	18–38 (594) 13–17 (153) 0.6–12 (76)	Breast cancer, Hodgkin lymphoma, sarcoma	Hematological malignancies, sarcoma, SNC malignancy	Unilateral oophorectomy	Yes	None
Finland							
Kuopio University Hospital	5	18–30 (5)	Sarcoma, gynecological cancer	–	Unilateral oophorectomy	Yes (2007)	None
Oulu University Hospital	9	18–34 (9)	Hodgkin lymphoma, breast cancer, lymphoma	–	Ovarian biopsies	Yes (2008)	None
Tampere University Hospital	70	17–36 (63) 13–16 (7)	Hodgkin lymphoma, breast cancer, sarcoma	Hodgkin lymphoma, sarcoma	Ovarian biopsies	Yes (2003)	Minor (bleeding)
Turku University Hospital	5	24–32 (4) <12 (1)	Malignancy	Malignancy	Individualized from ovarian biopsies to unilateral oophorectomy	Yes (2002)	None
Norway							
Oslo University Hospital	164	18–36 (135) 10–17 (29)	Breast cancer, lymphoma, sarcoma	Lymphoma, sarcoma, hematological malignancies	Unilateral oophorectomy	Yes (2004)	None
Sweden							
Sahlgreska Univ Hospital, Gothenburg	35	18–43 (34) 15–17 (1)	Hodgkin lymphoma, breast cancer, gynecological cancer	Neuroblastoma, neural	Unilateral oophorectomy	Yes (2003)	Minor (bleeding)
Linköping University Hospital	24	17–35 (4) 3–13 (20)	Breast cancer, other	**Turner syndrome**	Ovarian biopsies	Yes (2002)	None
Uppsala University Hospital	25	18–38 (22) 12–16 (3)	Breast cancer, Hodgkin lymphoma, gynecological cancer	**Turner syndrome**, ovarian teratoma, vaginal cancer	Unilateral oophorectomy	Yes (2000)	None
Skåne University Hospital, Malmö	72	17–39 (69) <17 (3)	Breast cancer	Malignancies	Unilateral oophorectomy	Yes (2001)	None
Karolinska University Hospital, Stockholm	301	18–39 (188) 3–17 (113)	Breast cancer, lymphoma, sarcoma, gynecological cancer	Leukemia, cancer of the nervous system, **Turner syndrome**	Individualized from ovarian biopsies to unilateral oophorectomy	Yes (2000)	Minor (bleeding)
TOTAL CASES	**1,532**						

Notes: Age ranges, standard routines, and complications registered are presented. A diagnosis of Turner syndrome was among the most common diagnoses to perform OTC in pediatric patients at three of the Nordic FP centers.

thus currently recommends that adolescent girls who present with spontaneous start of puberty be referred for appropriate counseling on fertility preservation, and if possible, performance of fertility preservation should be individualized (4).

The efficacy of fertility preservation in women with Turner syndrome is yet to be demonstrated, as most of the patients reported having undergone those procedures are still very young (8, 26–28). At present, data on the use of cryopreserved oocytes from women with Turner syndrome are lacking, similarly to data on retransplantation of ovarian tissue that has been cryopreserved due to Turner syndrome as an indication. Cases and case series of mothers of daughters with Turner syndrome who are willing to freeze their own oocytes for future use by the daughter have so far been reported by two centers (8, 29), and no data are yet reported on the use of such oocytes. The option of freezing eggs to donate them to a relative may be available only in countries allowing the use of a known egg donor. Given that such intrafamilial donation comes with unique practical implications determined by different practice rules in different countries, careful additional ethical counseling is recommended for these cases by the current international Turner syndrome clinical practice guideline (5).

Conclusions

- Pregnancies in women with Turner syndrome are related to increased risks of pregnancy loss and obstetric complications.
- Women with a diagnosis of Turner syndrome considering pregnancy should be screened to evaluate cardiac malformations, including aorta root dilation, bicuspid aortic valve, and history of coarctation of the aorta. If any of these conditions are present, the pregnancy should be discouraged.
- Counseling of patients with Turner syndrome should include information about increased risks of fetal chromosome abnormalities. Prenatal genetic screening should be offered to women who are conceiving with their own oocytes.
- In cases of contraindication to pregnancy, gestational surrogacy and adoption should be recommended as favorable alternatives to pregnancy.
- Fertility preservation methods have been reported in women with Turner syndrome, but the efficacy of the methods is unknown.
- Data reported on pregnancies in women with a Turner karyotype are in general scarce.

REFERENCES

1. Bondy CA; Turner Syndrome Study Group. Care of girls and women with Turner syndrome: A guideline of the Turner Syndrome Study Group. *J Clin Endocrinol Metab.* 2007 Jan;92(1):10–25. doi: 10.1210/jc.2006-1374. Epub 2006 Oct 17. PMID: 17047017.
2. Nielsen J, Wohlert M. Chromosome abnormalities found among 34,910 newborn children: Results from a 13-year incidence study in Arhus, Denmark. *Hum Genet.* 1991 May;87(1):81–3. doi: 10.1007/BF01213097. PMID: 2037286.
3. Pasquino AM, Passeri F, Pucarelli I, Segni M, Municchi G. Spontaneous pubertal development in Turner's syndrome: Italian Study Group for Turner's syndrome. *J Clin Endocrinol Metab.* 1997 Jun;82(6):1810–13. doi: 10.1210/jcem.82.6.3970. PMID: 9177387.
4. Rodriguez-Wallberg KA, Landin-Wilhelmsen K, Swedish Turner Academy. The complexity of fertility preservation for women with Turner syndrome and the potential risks of pregnancy and cardiovascular complications. *Acta Obstet Gynecol Scand.* 2020 Dec;99(12):1577–8. doi: 10.1111/aogs.13999. PMID: 33226115; PMCID: PMC7756558.
5. Gravholt CH, Andersen NH, Conway GS, Dekkers OM, Geffner ME, Klein KO, Lin AE, Mauras N, Quigley CA, Rubin K, Sandberg DE, Sas TCJ, Silberbach M, Söderström-Anttila V, Stochholm K, van Alfen-van derVelden JA, Woelfle J, Backeljauw PF, International Turner Syndrome Consensus Group. Clinical practice guidelines for the care of girls and women with Turner syndrome: Proceedings from

the 2016 Cincinnati International Turner Syndrome Meeting. *Eur J Endocrinol.* 2017 Sep;177(3):G1–70. doi: 10.1530/EJE-17-0430. PMID: 28705803.
6. Sylvén L, Magnusson C, Hagenfeldt K, von Schoultz B. Life with Turner's syndrome: A psychosocial report from 22 middle-aged women. *Acta Endocrinol (Copenh).* 1993;129:188–94.
7. Sutton EJ, McInerney-Leo A, Bondy CA, Gollust SE, King D, Biesecker B. Turner syndrome: Four challenges across the lifespan. *Am J Med Genet A.* 2005 Dec 1;139A(2):57–66. doi: 10.1002/ajmg.a.30911. PMID: 16252273. PMCID: PMC2600710.
8. Rodriguez-Wallberg KA, Marklund A, Lundberg F, et al. A prospective study of women and girls undergoing fertility preservation due to oncologic and non-oncologic indications in Sweden: Trends in patients' choices and benefit of the chosen methods after long-term follow-up. *Acta Obstet Gynecol Scand.* 2019;98:604–15.
9. Practice Committee of American Society for Reproductive Medicine. Increased maternal cardiovascular mortality associated with pregnancy in women with Turner syndrome. *Fertil Steril.* 2012 Feb;97(2):282–4. doi: 10.1016/j.fertnstert.2011.11.049. Epub 2011 Dec 21. PMID: 22192347.
10. Calanchini M, Aye CYL, Orchard E, Baker K, Child T, Fabbri A, Mackillop L, Turner HE. Fertility issues and pregnancy outcomes in Turner syndrome. *Fertil Steril.* 2020 Jul;114(1):144–54. doi: 10.1016/j.fertnstert.2020.03.002. PMID: 32622407.
11. Karnis MF, Zimon AE, Lalwani SI, Timmreck LS, Klipstein S, Reindollar RH. Risk of death in pregnancy achieved through oocyte donation in patients with Turner syndrome: A national survey. *Fertil Steril.* 2003 Sep;80(3):498–501.
12. Chevalier N, Letur H, Lelannou D, Ohl J, Cornet D, Chalas-Boissonnas C, Frydman R, Catteau-Jonard S, Greck-Chassain T, Papaxanthos-Roche A, Dulucq MC, Couet ML, Cédrin-Durnerin I, Pouly JL, Fénichel P, French Study Group for Oocyte Donation. Materno-fetal cardiovascular complications in Turner syndrome after oocyte donation: Insufficient prepregnancy screening and pregnancy follow-up are associated with poor outcome. *J Clin Endocrinol Metab.* 2011 Feb;96(2):E260–7.
13. Bondy C. Pregnancy and cardiovascular risk for women with Turner syndrome. *Womens Health (Lond).* 2014 Jul;10(4):469–76. doi: 10.2217/whe.14.34. PMID: 25259906.
14. Landin-Wilhelmsen K. *The Swedish Turner Healthcare program (Vårdprogram vid Turners syndrom).* Available from: www.internetmedicin.se/page.aspx?id=6178.
15. Thunström S, Krantz E, Thunström E, Hanson C, Bryman I, Landin-Wilhelmsen K. Incidence of aortic dissection in Turner syndrome: A 23-year prospective cohort study. *Circulation.* 2019;139:2802–4.
16. Hagman A, Källén K, Bryman I, Landin-Wilhelmsen K, Barrenäs M-L, Wennerholm U-B. Morbidity and mortality after childbirth in women with Turner karyotype. *Human Reprod.* 2013;28:1961–73.
17. Bryman I, Sylvén L, Berntorp K, et al. Pregnancy rate and outcome in Swedish women with Turner syndrome. *Fertil Steril.* 2011;95:2507–10.
18. Ramage K, Grabowska K, Silversides C, Quan H, Metcalfe A. Maternal, pregnancy, and neonatal outcomes for women with Turner syndrome. *Birth Defects Res.* 2020 Aug;112(14):1067–73. doi: 10.1002/bdr2.1739. Epub 2020 Jun 11. PMID: 32524771.
19. Grewal J, Valente AM, Egbe AC, Wu FM, Krieger EV, Sybert VP, van Hagen IM, Beauchesne LM, Rodriguez FH, Broberg CS, John A, Bradley EA, Roos-Hesselink JW, AARCC Investigators. Cardiovascular outcomes of pregnancy in Turner syndrome. *Heart.* 2021 Jan;107(1):61–6. doi: 10.1136/heartjnl-2020-316719. Epub 2020 Jul 15. PMID: 32669396.
20. Karnis MF. Fertility, pregnancy, and medical management of Turner syndrome in the reproductive years. *Fertil Steril.* 2012 Oct;98(4):787–91. doi: 10.1016/j.fertnstert.2012.08.022. PMID: 23020910.
21. Oktay K, Bedoschi G, Berkowitz K, Bronson R, Kashani B, McGovern P, Pal L, Quinn G, Rubin K. Fertility preservation in women with Turner syndrome: A comprehensive review and practical guidelines. *J Pediatr Adolesc Gynecol.* 2016 Oct;29(5):409–16. doi: 10.1016/j.jpag.2015.10.011. Epub 2015 Oct 17. PMID: 26485320. PMCID: 5015771.
22. Hadnott TN, Gould HN, Gharib AM, Bondy CA. Outcomes of spontaneous and assisted pregnancies in Turner syndrome: The U.S. National Institutes of Health experience. *Fertil Steril.* 2011 Jun;95(7):2251–6. doi: 10.1016/j.fertnstert.2011.03.085. Epub 2011 Apr 15. PMID: 21496813; PMCID: PMC3130000.
23. Bodri D, Vernaeve V, Figueras F, Vidal R, Guillén JJ, Coll O. Oocyte donation in patients with Turner's syndrome: A successful technique but with an accompanying high risk of hypertensive disorders during pregnancy. *Hum Reprod.* 2006 Mar;21(3):829–32. doi: 10.1093/humrep/dei396. Epub 2005 Nov 25. PMID: 16311294.

24. Rodriguez-Wallberg KA, Berger AS, Fagerberg A, Olofsson JI, Scherman-Pukk C, Lindqvist PG, Nasiell J. Increased incidence of obstetric and perinatal complications in pregnancies achieved using donor oocytes and single embryo transfer in young and healthy women: A prospective hospital-based matched cohort study. *Gynecol Endocrinol.* 2019 Apr;35(4):314–19. doi: 10.1080/09513590.2018.1528577. Epub 2019 Jan 9. PMID: 30626251.
25. Bodri D, Guillén JJ, Schwenn K, Casadesus S, Vidal R, Coll O. Poor outcome in oocyte donation after elective transfer of a single cleavage-stage embryo in Turner syndrome patients. *Fertil Steril.* 2009 Apr;91(4 Suppl):1489–92. doi: 10.1016/j.fertnstert.2008.07.1762. Epub 2008 Sep 14. PMID: 18793776.
26. Oktay K, Rodriguez-Wallberg KA, Sahin G. Fertility preservation by ovarian stimulation and oocyte cryopreservation in a 14-year old adolescent with Turner syndrome mosaicism and impending premature ovarian failure. *Fert Steril.* 2010 Jul;94(2):753.e15–19.
27. Rodriguez-Wallberg KA, Tanbo T, Tinkanen H, et al. Ovarian tissue cryopreservation and transplantation among alternatives for fertility preservation in the Nordic countries: Compilation of 20 years of multicenter experience. *Acta Obstet Gynecol Scand.* 2016;95:1015–26.
28. Borgström B, Hreinsson J, Rasmussen C, et al. Fertility preservation in girls with Turner syndrome: Prognostic signs of the presence of ovarian follicles. *J Clin Endocrinol Metab.* 2009;94:74–80.
29. Gidoni YS, Takefman J, Holzer HE, Elizur SE, Son WY, Chian RC, Tan SL. Cryopreservation of a mother's oocytes for possible future use by her daughter with Turner syndrome: Case report. *Fertil Steril.* 2008 Nov;90(5):2008.e9–12. doi: 10.1016/j.fertnstert.2008.05.050. Epub 2008 Aug 9. PMID: 18692829.

7

Maternal and obstetric outcomes after oocyte cryopreservation

Alessandra Alteri and Valerio Pisaturo

Introduction

Cryopreservation of gametes and embryos represents an essential aspect of medically assisted reproduction (MAR). The proportion of cryopreserved oocyte or embryo transfer cycles compared with fresh cycles is growing in Europe (1). In 2012, the American Society of Reproductive Medicine (ASRM) stated that oocyte cryopreservation should no longer be considered an experimental strategy (2).

The widespread application of oocyte cryopreservation has not only increased safety and efficacy of MAR treatments but has also allowed fertility preservation. In particular, an efficient oocyte cryopreservation program is associated with various important advantages: (1) allowing fertility preservation for medical and non-medical indications; (2) enabling oocyte banking for donation and for managing low-responder patients; (3) postponing oocyte use in case of failure to obtain an adequate sperm sample on the day of oocyte retrieval; and (4) reducing the creation and freezing of supernumerary embryos due to religious and ethical concerns.

Slow-freezing and vitrification have been used as methods to freeze oocytes. Slow-freezing refers to carrying out the freezing procedure at a sufficiently slow rate for an adequate cellular dehydration, minimizing intracellular ice formation. On the other hand, vitrification allows the solidification of the cell(s) into a glass-like state without ice formation. Vitrification appears to be superior in terms of efficacy to slow-freezing for cryopreservation of human oocytes. Indeed, according to moderate-quality evidence, the introduction of vitrification has been associated with a substantial improvement of post-thaw cryosurvival rates of oocytes. On the other hand, the quality of the evidence demonstrating an advantage in favor of vitrification in terms of clinical pregnancy rates remains low (3).

It is well documented that MAR pregnancies may be characterized by maternal complications such as hypertensive disorders in pregnancy, placental complications such as placenta previa and third-trimester bleeding, and gestational diabetes with often an increased risk of preterm prelabor rupture of membranes. These complications are often associated with adverse neonatal outcomes (4).

Although thousands of children are born after oocyte cryopreservation and most of them after oocyte donation, little is known about maternal complications and perinatal outcome of infants born after autologous and donor oocyte cryopreservation. Moreover, in many studies, information regarding reasons for freezing of the woman's own oocytes, age at egg freezing, and cryopreservation method was not always available. In this context, it is paramount to understand the impact of the freezing technique on maternal and neonatal outcomes.

This chapter will focus on obstetric and perinatal outcomes of the oocyte cryopreservation procedure after slow-freezing or vitrification. Studies including data derived from both techniques will be discussed as well.

Obstetric and perinatal outcomes after oocyte cryopreservation by slow-freezing

The first children born after cryopreservation of oocytes were derived from eggs that had been frozen using slow-freezing. Few studies, mainly case reports, reported data on maternal and neonatal health (5). In particular, in most studies, the only information provided about children was the general "health status", while gestational age and birth weight were the only outcomes considered by very few studies.

Noyes and colleagues (2009) reviewed outcomes of more than 900 children born mainly with autologous oocytes cryopreserved by both slow-freezing and vitrification. In the case of slow-freezing, they found that the incidence of birth anomalies was similar between infants born from cryopreserved oocytes and those who were naturally conceived. (6).

A large observational study has analyzed obstetric and neonatal outcomes of pregnancies obtained from autologous fresh (N = 568) and slow frozen-thawed oocytes (N = 134), confirming no difference between the two strategies in the incidence of fetal and neonatal complications (7). In particular, no statistically significant differences related to congenital anomalies were observed between newborns from fresh and frozen oocytes (P = 0.499) (7). However, birth weight was significantly higher in singletons born after an embryo transfer from frozen oocytes (3231 ± 615 g) than born after an embryo transfer from fresh oocytes (3012 ± 659 g; P = 0.001) with similar gestational age at delivery between the two groups (38.4 ± 2.6 vs. 38.5 ± 2.7, respectively for frozen and fresh oocytes group, P = 0.747).

Despite the very limited available data, obstetric and neonatal outcomes derived from the slow-freezing strategy seem to be safe and reassuring.

Obstetric and perinatal outcomes after oocyte cryopreservation by vitrification

Few studies on maternal and neonatal outcomes after oocyte vitrification are similarly available. Preliminary findings from three different MAR centers considering only autologous vitrified oocytes showed that out of 165 pregnancies, all deliveries were beyond 34 weeks of gestation, and out of 200 healthy infants, no baby had a very low birth weight (LBW) (8).

As mentioned earlier, Noyes and colleagues (2009) found that no differences were reported in terms of congenital anomalies in children born from vitrified oocytes compared to naturally conceived infants (6).

The largest study to date was conducted by Cobo and co-workers, who analyzed babies born from vitrified oocytes (n= 1027) and fresh oocytes (n = 1224) (9). Adjusting for confounding factors, more invasive procedures such as chorionic villous sampling or amniocentesis (odds ratio [OR] = 2.12; 95% confidence interval [CI] 1.41–3.20) and a lower incidence of urinary tract infections (OR = 0.51; 95% CI 0.28–0.91) were reported to be associated with the vitrification group. On the other hand, no significant difference was observed between the two groups for rates of first-, second-, and third-trimester bleeding; anemia; gestational cholestasis; diabetes; pregnancy-induced hypertension; preterm premature rupture of membranes; preterm birth; LBW; birth malformations; admission to a neonatal intensive care unit; and puerperal problems. In addition, data on subgroups based on the woman's own and donated oocytes indicated there were no relevant differences between fresh and vitrified oocytes (9). These findings support the concept that oocyte vitrification does not adversely affect placentation, fetal development, and pregnancy progression.

While the studies cited earlier are related to the use of open devices for vitrification, reassuring data were obtained also for the closed system vitrification. It is well known that vitrification techniques are categorized as "open" or "closed" systems depending on the presence or not of a direct contact between the sample and liquid nitrogen during cryopreservation. While open systems allow direct contact between the sample and liquid nitrogen, allowing a higher cooling rate, the closed system consists of keeping the sample physically separated from liquid nitrogen during the cooling, storage, and warming procedure. This approach is considered safer, protecting the sample from potential microorganisms that might be present in the liquid nitrogen. A retrospective observational study analyzing obstetric and neonatal outcomes derived from closed system vitrification of donor oocytes showed that out of 112 pregnant women, 19.6% were affected by a hypertensive disorder, 4.5% had an abnormal placentation, 26.8% suffered hemorrhages during pregnancy, 2.7% were hospitalized for nausea and vomiting, 8.9% had a preterm labor, 11.6% were affected by gestational diabetes, and 3.6% had cholestasis (10). Moreover, no major adverse neonatal outcomes were observed. Considering that the oocyte donation program itself represents a significant risk factor for pregnancy complications, this study suggested that closed oocyte vitrification has no impact on obstetric and neonatal outcomes (10).

Oocyte cryopreservation has also emerged as an important strategy for female fertility preservation for both medical and non-medical indications (11, 12). Improvements in the oocyte cryopreservation strategy due to the introduction of vitrification have permitted facilities to offer fertility preservation to patients receiving gonadotoxic therapies for cancer or other medical diseases. Some studies have demonstrated the general safety of pregnancies achieved using autologous vitrified oocytes after chemotherapy. The same studies have provided reassurance about the perinatal outcomes of this strategy, with most of the deliveries at term with normal birth weight babies and no major or minor malformations (13, 14).

While the vitrification technique is generally applied on mature oocytes derived from controlled ovarian stimulation protocols, with the advent of in vitro maturation (IVM), cryopreservation of immature oocytes was proposed as a further option to preserve fertility in the case of female cancer. As a matter of fact, very few live births have been reported after IVM oocyte cryopreservation. Four pregnancies with live births were described after metaphase II oocyte vitrification of in vitro matured oocytes collected from human chorionic gonadotropin (hCG)–primed cycles (15). These preliminary data showed that pregnancies conceived after vitrification of in vivo or in vitro mature oocytes did not seem to be associated with adverse obstetric and perinatal outcomes (15). Very recently, the first birth achieved after cryopreservation of IVM oocytes using vitrification in a woman with breast cancer has been described, suggesting that IVM should be considered an efficient option in the strategy of female fertility preservation (16). Time is needed to collect data on obstetric and perinatal outcomes after cryopreservation of IVM oocytes for cancer patients.

Obstetric and perinatal outcomes after oocyte cryopreservation non-dependent on technical procedure

Some studies analyzed cryopreservation outcome without distinguishing the two freezing methods. Especially in studies based on MAR national registries, reasons for freezing of autologous oocytes, age at egg freezing, and method of cryopreservation (whether slow-freezing or vitrification) are not available.

Recently, a retrospective cohort study based on the Human Fertilisation and Embryology Authority (HFEA) database analyzed perinatal outcomes of singleton children born from frozen autologous or donor oocytes (17). No relevant differences between frozen own or frozen donor oocytes in terms of preterm birth (PTB) rates (adjusted OR 0.56, 95% CI 0.26–1.21) or in the incidence of macrosomia (adjusted OR 1.21, 95% CI 0.11–1.39) were reported. Infants born from frozen own oocytes showed a significantly lower risk of LBW compared to donor oocytes (adjusted OR 0.29, 95% CI 0.13–0.90). Moreover, babies from frozen embryos derived from fresh own oocytes showed a significant lower risk of LBW compared to fresh embryos derived from frozen donor oocytes. A plausible explanation could be a potentially reduced immune tolerance of the uterine environment to embryos derived from donor oocytes compared to own oocytes (18). On the other hand, the comparison between births following cycles with frozen donor oocytes and fresh donor oocytes showed no significant differences in PTB, LBW, or macrosomia rates, suggesting that freezing of oocytes may not adversely affect placentation (17).

The comparison in terms of perinatal outcomes between transfer of fresh embryos derived from cryopreserved oocytes and embryo transfer of cryopreserved embryos derived from fresh autologous oocytes represents another aspect to take into consideration. A retrospective single-center study showed no difference in mean gestational age at delivery, mean newborn birth weight, and preterm gestation rate in patients after transfer of fresh embryos from frozen own oocytes compared to transfer of frozen embryos from fresh own oocytes (19). On the other hand, comparing outcomes from the first cycle with frozen donor oocytes versus those from the first cycle with frozen embryos from own oocytes, a significantly higher risk of LBW babies with frozen donor oocytes was reported (adjusted OR 3.77, 95% CI 1.51–9.43). This would suggest that adverse perinatal outcomes may be more frequent in pregnancies following egg donation rather than for cryopreservation per se (17).

In the two studies cited, both the slow-freezing and vitrification methods were utilized for oocyte and embryo cryopreservation.

Still scarce data on the long term outcomes

Though oocyte cryopreservation is a well-established procedure, investigation of resulting obstetric and neonatal outcomes is still scarce. Data from systematic reviews and retrospective cohort studies are predominantly reassuring, suggesting that pregnancies obtained from embryo transfer derived from cryopreserved autologous oocytes are not associated with increased obstetric risks compared with those resulting from embryo transfer derived from fresh autologous oocytes, independently from the used technique.

It is important to point out that most of the data regarding pregnancy complications and adverse neonatal outcomes in children born after oocyte cryopreservation derive from oocyte donation programs. It is reasonable to think that different obstetric outcomes after autologous oocyte and donor oocyte cryopreservation might be observed. Since women use donor eggs in a shorter time interval than women who freeze oocytes for their own future, few studies on obstetric outcomes in pregnancies obtained from embryo transfer derived from autologous cryopreserved oocytes are available. Moreover, further reassuring evidence is derived from studies assessing the safety of oocyte vitrification in fertility preservation patients (14).

Conclusions

- Oocyte cryopreservation by both slow-freezing or vitrification does not appear to be associated with a higher risk of obstetric and perinatal harm. However, well-designed studies with larger sample size and follow-up studies are needed.
- Analyzing the current literature on maternal and offspring wellness using frozen oocytes shows that many shortcomings are evident, including:
  - Different indications for oocyte cryopreservation (oocyte donation program, fertility preservation and legal restrictions)
  - Different cryopreservation protocols and techniques
  - Limited access to obstetric and perinatal data
  - Lack of reporting of adverse events
- Based on these issues, a comparison of the results is difficult.

REFERENCES

1. European IVF-monitoring Consortium (EIM)‡ for the European Society of Human Reproduction and Embryology (ESHRE), Wyns C, Bergh C, Calhaz-Jorge C, De Geyter C, Kupka MS, Motrenko T, Rugescu I, Smeenk J, Tandler-Schneider A, Vidakovic S, Goossens V. ART in Europe, 2016: Results generated from European registries by ESHRE. *Hum Reprod Open.* 2020 Jul 31;2020(3):hoaa032.
2. Practice Committees of the American Society for Reproductive Medicine and the Society for Assisted Reproductive Technology. Mature oocyte cryopreservation: A guideline. *Fertil Steril.* 2013 Jan;99(1):37–43.

3. Rienzi L, Gracia C, Maggiulli R, LaBarbera AR, Kaser DJ, Ubaldi FM, Vanderpoel S, Racowsky C. Oocyte, embryo and blastocyst cryopreservation in ART: Systematic review and meta-analysis comparing slow-freezing versus vitrification to produce evidence for the development of global guidance. *Hum Reprod Update*. 2017 Mar 1;23(2):139–55.
4. Berntsen S, Söderström-Anttila V, Wennerholm UB, Laivuori H, Loft A, Oldereid NB, Romundstad LB, Bergh C, Pinborg A. The health of children conceived by ART: "The chicken or the egg?" *Hum Reprod Update*. 2019 Mar 1;25(2):137–58.
5. Wennerholm UB, Söderström-Anttila V, Bergh C, Aittomäki K, Hazekamp J, Nygren KG, Selbing A, Loft A. Children born after cryopreservation of embryos or oocytes: A systematic review of outcome data. *Hum Reprod*. 2009 Sep;24(9):2158–72.
6. Noyes N, Porcu E, Borini A. Over 900 oocyte cryopreservation babies born with no apparent increase in congenital anomalies. *Reprod Biomed Online*. 2009 Jun;18(6):769–76.
7. Levi Setti PE, Albani E, Morenghi E, Morreale G, Delle Piane L, Scaravelli G, Patrizio P. Comparative analysis of fetal and neonatal outcomes of pregnancies from fresh and cryopreserved/thawed oocytes in the same group of patients. *Fertil Steril*. 2013 Aug;100(2):396–401.
8. Chian RC, Huang JY, Tan SL, Lucena E, Saa A, Rojas A, Ruvalcaba Castellón LA, García Amador MI, Montoya Sarmiento JE. Obstetric and perinatal outcome in 200 infants conceived from vitrified oocytes. *Reprod Biomed Online*. 2008 May;16(5):608–10.
9. Cobo A, Serra V, Garrido N, Olmo I, Pellicer A, Remohí J. Obstetric and perinatal outcome of babies born from vitrified oocytes. *Fertil Steril*. 2014 Oct;102(4):1006–15.
10. De Munck N, Belva F, Van de Velde H, Verheyen G, Stoop D. Closed oocyte vitrification and storage in an oocyte donation programme: Obstetric and neonatal outcome. *Hum Reprod*. 2016 May;31(5):1024–33.
11. De Vos M, Smitz J, Woodruff TK. Fertility preservation in women with cancer. *Lancet*. 2014 Oct 4;384(9950):1302–10.
12. Alteri A, Pisaturo V, Nogueira D, D'Angelo A. Elective egg freezing without medical indications. *Acta Obstet Gynecol Scand*. 2019 May;98(5):647–52.
13. Garcia-Velasco JA, Domingo J, Cobo A, Martínez M, Carmona L, Pellicer A. Five years' experience using oocyte vitrification to preserve fertility for medical and nonmedical indications. *Fertil Steril*. 2013 Jun;99(7):1994–9.
14. Martinez M, Rabadan S, Domingo J, Cobo A, Pellicer A, Garcia-Velasco JA. Obstetric outcome after oocyte vitrification and warming for fertility preservation in women with cancer. *Reprod Biomed Online*. 2014 Dec;29(6):722–8.
15. Chian RC, Gilbert L, Huang JY, Demirtas E, Holzer H, Benjamin A, Buckett WM, Tulandi T, Tan SL. Live birth after vitrification of in vitro matured human oocytes. *Fertil Steril*. 2009 Feb;91(2):372–6.
16. Grynberg M, Mayeur Le Bras A, Hesters L, Gallot V, Frydman N. First birth achieved after fertility preservation using vitrification of in vitro matured oocytes in a woman with breast cancer. *Ann Oncol*. 2020 Apr;31(4):541–2.
17. Mascarenhas M, Mehlawat H, Kirubakaran R, Bhandari H, Choudhary M. Live birth and perinatal outcomes using cryopreserved oocytes: An analysis of the Human Fertilisation and Embryology Authority database from 2000 to 2016 using three clinical models. *Hum Reprod*. 2020 Dec 13:deaa343.
18. Mascarenhas M, Sunkara SK, Antonisamy B, Kamath MS. Higher risk of preterm birth and low birth weight following oocyte donation: A systematic review and meta-analysis. *Eur J Obstet Gynecol Reprod Biol*. 2017 Nov;218:60–7.
19. Ho JR, Woo I, Louie K, Salem W, Jabara SI, Bendikson KA, Paulson RJ, Chung K. A comparison of live birth rates and perinatal outcomes between cryopreserved oocytes and cryopreserved embryos. *J Assist Reprod Genet*. 2017 Oct;34(10):1359–66.

8

Perinatal complications in pregnancies achieved using donor oocytes

Roberto Matorras, Héctor Sainz, and Ana Matorras

Introduction

The first pregnancy obtained by oocyte donation (OD) was reported almost 40 years ago (68). Since then, the number of OD cycles is continuously increasing. In the last published European Society of Human Reproduction and Embryology (ESHRE) register there were 156,002 in vitro fertilization (IVF) cycles, 407,222 intracytoplasmic sperm injection (ICSI) cycles, and 73,927 OD cycles (12). OD is a very successful reproductive option. In the aforementioned ESHRE register (12), in OD cycles, the pregnancy rate (PR) per fresh embryo transfer (ET) was 49.4% and 43.6% per frozen oocyte ET, with the number of embryos transferred not being reported. The indications of OD are heterogenous, including advanced maternal age, primary and secondary ovarian insufficiency, inadequate ovarian response to stimulation, repeated IVF failures, diminished ovarian reserve, genetic diseases, previous chemotherapy/radiotherapy, and autoimmune diseases. The live birth rates following OD treatment depend on the age of the donor and are independent of the age of the recipient (38, 67).

Although there is agreement concerning the successful PRs, there is some concern regarding perinatal complications. Different studies have reported an increased rate of hypertensive disorders, gestational diabetes, cesarean sections, preterm delivery, and low birth weight, among other conditions.

It is difficult to ascertain the impact of OD per se from that of the causes that led to OD indication, such advanced age and known concomitant conditions (genetic disorder, immune diseases). In a recent work it has been shown that even in women <40 years OD pregnancies are associated with negative outcomes when compared with young IVF patients (53). However it could be speculated that some apparently healthy young women requiring OD would not be in as good a status to face pregnancy as their age-matched peers not needing OD.

First of all, there is a discrepancy concerning the definition of the most frequent OD indication, "advanced age". Older studies considered a pregnancy to be late if the mother was older than 35, while today late pregnancies are more likely to refer to pregnant women ≥40 years old, or even ≥45 years old (34). There is also a discrepancy regarding the upper age limit to receive OD. The Spanish Fertility Society advises against OD cycles when the recipient is aged ≥50, although each case must be evaluated individually (52), while the American Reproductive Medicine Society places the border at 55 (11). However, OD pregnancies have been reported even in women aged >60 years (8, 45, 45, 29,47, 63).

Methodological problems in assessing the impact of OD on pregnancy complications

A number of authors have reported impaired perinatal results in women/pregnancies obtained by OD. One of the main limitations of such comparisons is the definition of the control group. In the seven meta-analyses considered here (Table 8.1), there were remarkable differences concerning inclusion criteria, control group, and considered outcomes. From an ideal methodological point of view, the

DOI: 10.1201/9781003052524-8

best study would be a randomized study comparing pregnancies obtained by OD with pregnancies obtained by IVF/ICSI with autologous oocytes (AO) or even with natural pregnancies. However, since when clinically indicated (low ovarian reserve, advanced age), the PR with OD is so remarkably higher than that obtained by IVF/ICSI and natural intercourse, such a study will probably never be performed because of ethical reasons. Thus the comparisons are usually made using a control group of women of similar age getting pregnant by IVF/ICSI or natural intercourse. However, presumably women achieving pregnancy with their own oocytes are in a better medical situation and thus face pregnancy with a favorable status.

In different reports it has been stated that the mean age of women undergoing OD is around 41 years (24, 32), which is much higher than the mean age of women undergoing IVF with their own oocytes. It is well known that maternal age by itself is associated with an increased risk of miscarriage, hypertensive disorders, preterm delivery, diabetes, cesarean section, congenital abnormalities, perinatal mortality, and almost every obstetric complication (3, 6, 71). Moreover, when analyzing populations concerning advanced age, one should expect very different results in women close to 40 years old than those close to 60. For instance, one study focused on women >43 years old and found higher rates of hypertensive disorders in OD than in IVF than in those occurring naturally, but OD women were older than IVF women (34).

On the other hand, OD pregnancies all come from IVF, which by itself is associated with an increased risk of many of the aforementioned conditions (24). Moreover, in many of the OD reports there is a remarkable rate of multiple pregnancies, which also is by itself associated with many of the aforementioned conditions (28). In a study of OD pregnancies in recipients ≥45 years old, it was suggested that the high rate of multiple pregnancies (39.2%) was an important contributing factor to the high rate of perinatal complications (56). A higher rate of multiples has been reported in OD pregnancies compared with IVF pregnancies (34). Accordingly, there is an increased use of multifetal pregnancy reduction procedures in women ≥45 years (13). However, even in single pregnancies there is a consistently increased risk of negative obstetric/perinatal outcomes (53).

Reported studies include a mix of both fresh and frozen oocytes and fresh and frozen embryos. On the other hand, the source of donors can vary: "pure" donors (healthy young women with no known fertility problems) or "egg sharing" (donated surplus oocytes coming from women from infertile couples). Moreover, the influence of associated sperm donation is usually not considered. Another methodological limitation may be related to endometrial preparation. Finally, the majority of studies are not corrected by nulliparity, which is a well-known risk factor for many obstetric complications (37).

Obstetric and perinatal conditions

Placental characteristics

A number of immune-mediated placental abnormalities have been reported in OD pregnancies such as villitis of unknown etiology (49, 63), chronic deciduitis (18), increased perivillous fibrin (49), ischemic changes/infarctions (49), intervillous thrombi (49), injury in the chorionic plate (57), and intervillositis (57).

Immunological aspects

In OD pregnancies, the fetus is allogeneic to the mother, exposing her to foreign antigens and cells and generating an immunological paradox (55, 69). The relationship between the embryo/fetus and the mother in OD has been compared to the transplantation of a solid organ. However, it should be highlighted that in organ transplantation, the donors are screened to match with the recipients and a number of drugs are applied to reduce immune reaction. In organ transplantation, the degree of human leukocyte antigen (HLA) mismatches influences graft survival (43). In natural pregnancies, the highest number of HLA mismatches could be five, considering the five most immunogenic HLA antigens (HLA-A, -B, -C, -DR, and -DQ), while in OD pregnancies it could reach ten mismatches, and this could lead to a more intense maternal response (55). It has been suggested that in uncomplicated OD pregnancies a significantly higher level of HLA matching would be expected (33).

TABLE 8.1
Characteristics of the Meta-Analyses Reviewed

First Author	Year	Preterm Delivery (articles, n of OD, n of AO)	Low Birth Weight (articles, n of OD, n of AO)	Hypertensive Disorders	Cesarean Section	Inclusion Criteria	Control Group	Risk Assessment
		OD/AO (n)	OD/AO (n)	OD/AO (n)	OD/AO (n)			
Pecks	2011			NR/NR (11)		Singleton and multiples	All ART pregnancies and natural pregnancies	OR
Adams	2016	28,516/63,949 (13)	38,817/213,336 (15)			Singleton and multiples	IVF with AO	Risk ratio (RR)
Jeve	2016	1011/11651 (9)		970/10569 (11)	690/10283(6)	Fresh and frozen singleton and multiples	IVF with AO	OR
Masoudian	2016			2330/1996 (12) 1275/25,523 (13) (PE)		Singleton and multiples	All ART pregnancies and natural pregnancies	OR
Storgaard	2017	757/30,970 (4)	686/30,862 (3)	NR/NR (5)	NR/NR (12)	Singleton fresh and frozen	IVF with AO; natural pregnancies	aOR
Storgaard	2017					Multiple	IVF with AO	aOR
Mascarenhas	2017	19,885/188,498 (6)	19,784/187,964			Singleton, fresh ET	IVF with AO	OR
Moreno-Sepulveda	2019	46,671/301,381 (11)	55,852/286,150 (12)	2,466/52,254 (8) 2,459/52,296 (11) PE		Singleton	IVF with AO	OR

Abbreviations: *aOR* adjusted odds ratio, *ART* assisted reproductive techniques, *AO* autologous oocytes, *ET* embryo transfer, *IVF* in vitro fertilization, *NR* not reported, *OD* oocyte donation, *OR* odds ratio, *PE* preeclampsia.

Hypertensive disorders (Table 8.2)

Hypertensive disorders of pregnancy are a heterogeneous group of conditions that include gestational hypertension, preeclampsia, chronic hypertension, and preeclampsia superimposed on chronic hypertension. Hypertensive disorders account for a significant proportion of perinatal morbidity and mortality, representing nearly 10% of all maternal deaths in the United States (65). However, the impact of the different hypertensive disorders on pregnancy is not the same. Thus, the pregnancy outcomes of mild gestational hypertension are similar to those of the general population (5, 9). On the other hand, severe gestational hypertension and preeclampsia are significant causes of maternal and fetal mortality and morbidity worldwide (10, 31, 39).

Assisted reproductive technologies (ARTs) by themselves are associated with an increase of hypertensive disorders during pregnancy (66). Hypertensive disorders in OD pregnancies have been reported by many authors and reviewed in a number of meta-analyses. The following hypertensive disorders have been found to be significantly increased in OD cycles: preeclampsia, preeclampsia- eclampsia, and chronic hypertension.

The first meta-analysis considered (48) compared OD pregnancies with all ART pregnancies and natural pregnancies. The authors reported that the OR of hypertensive disorders in OD pregnancies was 2.57 (confidence interval [CI] = 1.91–3.47) when compared with IVF pregnancies and 6.60 (4.55–9.57) when compared with natural pregnancies. In another meta-analysis comparing fresh and frozen pregnancies (singleton and multiples) obtained by OD or IVF with AO, the risk of hypertensive disorders of pregnancy was increased in all OD pregnancies (odds ratio [OR] = 3.92, CI = 3.21–4.78) (22), both in singletons (OR = 3.63, CI = 2.92–4.51) and in twin pregnancies (OR = 3.64, CI = 2.57–5.16) (22). The OR of preeclampsia was 2.62 (CI = 1.75–3.93) (22). When the analysis was restricted to women >40 years old, the risk of hypertensive disorders remained increased in OD pregnancies (OR = 2.33, CI = 1.21–4.49) (22, 39). In a meta-analysis comparing OD with all ART pregnancies and natural pregnancies (singletons and multiples), the authors found that the OR of gestational hypertension was 3.00 (CI = 2.44–3.70) when compared with IVF pregnancies and 7.94 (CI = 1.73–36.36) when compared with natural pregnancies. Concerning preeclampsia, the OR were 2.54 (CI = 1.98–3.24) and 4.34 (CI = 3.10–6.06), respectively.

In another meta-analysis comparing OD pregnancies with IVF with AO and natural pregnancies, the adjusted OR (aOR) was 2.30 (CI = 1.60–3.32) for hypertensive disorders in singleton OD pregnancies when compared with singleton IVF pregnancies and 2.45 (CI = 1.53–3.93) in multiple OD pregnancies when compared with IVF multiple pregnancies (62). Concerning preeclampsia, the aOR was 2.11 (CI = 1.42–3.95) in singleton pregnancies, comparing OD pregnancies with IVF pregnancies. When singleton OD pregnancies were compared with singleton natural pregnancies, the aOR was 2.94 (CI = 2.29–3.76). Concerning multiple pregnancies, the aOR was 3.31 (1.61–6.90) when comparing OD pregnancies with IVF pregnancies (62). In the Moreno-Sepulveda and Checa meta-analysis (41), the risk of hypertensive disorders in OD compared with IVF and with AO was 2.63 (CI = 2.17–3.18) and 2.62 (CI = 1.93–3.55) when restricted to fresh ET. Regarding the risk of preeclampsia, the pooled OR was 2.64 (CI = 2.29–3.04), 3.17 (CI = 2.67–3.75) in fresh ET, and 1.75 (CI = 1.23–2.49) in frozen ET. Severe preeclampsia was also significantly increased, and the OR was 3.22 (CI = 2.30–4.49). Severe preeclampsia was also significantly increased in frozen ET (OR = 2.83, CI = 1.45–5.52). The risk of pregnancy-induced hypertension in a review of ten publications was also significantly increased (OR = 1.64, CI = 1.26–2.13).

In a meta-analysis with a different point of view, it was reported that whereas in IVF and ICSI the overall relative risk for hypertensive disorders were 1.43 (CI = 1.14–1.78) and 1.28 (CI = 1.12–1.47) when compared with natural pregnancies, in OD, the relative risk when compared with natural pregnancies was 4.13 (CI = 2.52–6.77) (66).

Gestational diabetes (Table 8.2)

Three meta-analyses have addressed this topic. Although the OR was similar in the three, in two studies there were no statistically significant differences (22, 62), but in one study there were (41). A meta-analysis involving seven studies revealed a similar rate of gestational diabetes in OD singleton pregnancies than

TABLE 8.2

Perinatal Complications Reported in the Considered Meta-Analyses

	Hypertensive Disorders	Preeclampsia	Gestational Diabetes	Cesarean Section	Postpartum Hemorrhage	Preterm Delivery	Early Preterm Delivery	Low Birth Rate	SGA	Intrauterine Death
Pecks	2.57 (1.91–3.47) 6.60 (4.55–9.57) vs. NP									
Adams						1.26 (1.23–1.30)		1.18 (1.14–1.22) 1.24 (1.15–1.35) for VLW		
Jeve (singletons)	3.63 (2.92–4.51)	2.62 (1.75–3.93)	1.25 (0.68–2.30)	2.71 (2.23–3.30)		1.34 (1.08–1.66)			1.81 (1.26–2.60) 1.44 (0.93–2.23)*	1.39 (0.32–6.15)
Jeve (multiples)	3.64 (2.572–5.16)									
Masoudian	3.00 (2.44–3.70) 7.94 (1.73–36.36)	2.54 (1.98–3.24) 4.34 (3.10–6.06) vs. NP								
Storgaard (singleton)	2.30 (1.60–3.32)	2.11 (1.42–3.15) 2.94 (2.29–3.70) vs. NP	1.33 (0.71–2.50)	2.20 (1.85–2.60) 2.38 (20.1–2.81) vs. NP	2.40 (1.49–3.88)	1.75 (1.39–2.20) 2.30 (1.09–4.87) vs. NP		1.53 (1.16–2.01) 1.94 (1.10–3.41) vs. NP	1.14 (0.83–1.56) 1.29 (0.91–1.92) vs. NP	
Storgaard (multiples)	2.45 (1.53–3.93)	3.31 (1.61–6.90) 1.33 (0.71–2.50)							0.97 (0.64–1.49)	
Mascarenhas						1.45 (1.20–1.77)	2.14 (1.40–3.25)	1.34 (1.12–1.60) 1.51 (1.17–1.95) (very VLW)		
Moreno-Sepulveda	2.63 (2.17–3.18) (fresh ET) 2.62 (1.93–3.55)	2.64 (2.29–3.04) (fresh ET) 3.17 (2.67–3.75) 1.75 (1.23–2.49) (frozen ET)		2.28 (2.14–2.42)		1.57 (1.33–1.86) 1.44 (1.20–1.74) (fresh ET) 1.96 (1.38–2.78) (frozen ET)	1.80 (1.51–2.15) 1.68 (1.10–2.59) (fresh ET) 2.93 (1.65–5.20) (frozen ET)	1.25 (1.20–1.30) 1.37 (1.22–1.54)	0.83 (0.78–0.98)	

* = With consistent definition.

Abbreviations: *NP* natural pregnancy, *VLW* very low weight.

in IVF or natural conception singleton pregnancies (aOR = 1.33, CI = 0.71–2.50) (62). Similarly another meta-analysis reviewing five studies also reported a similar rate of gestational diabetes when compared with IVF with AO (OR = 1.25, CI = 0.68–2.30) (22). However, in another meta-analysis involving seven studies, OD pregnancies were found to have an increased risk of gestational diabetes (OR = 1.27, CI 1.03–1.56) (41).

Cesarean section (Table 8.2)

The three meta-analyses considered revealed an increased risk of cesarean section in OD pregnancies (22, 41, 62). In a meta-analysis of 12 publications, the adjusted OR for OD vs. IVF singleton pregnancies was 2.20 (CI = 1.85–2.60) and 2.38 (CI = 20.1–2.81) vs. natural pregnancies (62). In a meta-analysis of six studies, the OR of cesarean section was significantly increased in OD pregnancies (OR = 2.71; CI = 2.23–3.30) (22). Similarly, in a meta-analysis of seven studies, OD pregnancies were associated with a significantly increased cesarean section rate (OR = 2.28, CI = 2.14–2.42) (41).

Postpartum hemorrhage and other hemorrhagic conditions

Placenta previa was found to have a similar rate in OD pregnancies and AO-IVF pregnancies (OR = 0.63, CI = 0.33–1.20). There were no differences regarding placental abruption rate either (OR = 1.15; CI = 0.52–2.53) (41). Two meta-analyses have addressed the issue of postpartum hemorrhage (41, 62). The first one reported an increased risk of postpartum hemorrhage in OD singleton pregnancies vs. IVF singleton pregnancies (aOR = 2.40; CI = 1.49–3.88) (62), and similar results were reported in the second meta-analysis (OR = 1.96, CI = 1.20–3.20) (41).

Preterm delivery (Table 8.2)

In a meta-analysis including 13 publications (28,516 OD/63,949 IVF with AO), an increased preterm delivery rate was reported, with a risk ratio of 1.26 (CI= 1.23–1.30) (2). A second meta-analysis including 11 publications (22) also reported a higher preterm delivery rate in OD pregnancies compared to IVF with AO pregnancies, with an OR of 1.34 (CI = 1.08–1.66). A meta-analysis including four studies comparing singleton preterm delivery in OD pregnancies (n = 757) vs. IVF with AO pregnancies (n = 30,970) resulted in a pooled estimated aOR of 1.75 (CI = 1.39–2.20) (62) and of 2.30 (CI = 1.09–4.87) when OD singleton pregnancies were compared with natural singleton pregnancies (62). One third meta-analysis including six publications that compared fresh ET results in OD and IVF with AO cycles reported a significantly increased risk of preterm delivery in OD with an OR of 1.45 (CI = 1.20–1.77) (38). The risk of early preterm delivery, reported in three publications, was also significantly increased, with a risk ratio (RR) of 2.14 (CI = 1.40–3.25) (38). Data on preterm birth after frozen ET were available for 150 OD and 7,350 IVF with AO from two studies. The risk of preterm delivery was not significantly different between OD and AO IVF pregnancies (OR = 1.42; CI = 0.67–3.01). However, the pooled data indicated a significantly higher early preterm birth risk for OD compared to IVF with AO pregnancies, with an OR of 3.23 (CI = 1.32–7.88).

In the fourth meta-analysis including 16 studies, the overall OR for preterm delivery was 1.57 (1.33–1.86) in OD pregnancies (41). The risk was increased in both fresh ET (OR = 1.44; CI = 1.20–1.74) and frozen ET (OR = 1.96; CI = 1.38–2.78). Concerning early preterm delivery, the meta-analysis of six studies revealed an overall OR of 1.80 (CI = 1.51–2.15) (41). The risk was increased in both fresh ET (OR = 1.68; CI = 1.10–2.59) and frozen ET (OR = 2.93; CI = 1.65–5.20) (41).

Low birth weight (Table 8.2)

The first meta-analysis considered reported an increased RR of low weight in OD when compared with IVF with AO pregnancies (RR = 1.18; CI = 1.14–1.22) and also of very low weight (RR = 1.24; 1.15–1.35) (2). A second meta-analysis concerning data from three studies including 686 OD and 30,862 AO IVF singleton pregnancies also showed an increased risk of low birth weight following OD pregnancies when compared with IVF with AO pregnancies (aOR = 1.53; 1.16–2.01) and when compared with natural pregnancies (aOR = 1.94, 1.10–3.41) (62). A meta-analysis including five publications that compared fresh ET results in OD and AO cycles reported a significantly increased risk of low birth weight in OD (OR = 1.34; CI = 1.20–1.77) (38). The risk of very low birth weight, reported in two publications, was also significantly increased (OR = 1.51; CI = 1.17–1.95) (38). In a meta-analysis involving 12 studies, the overall OR of low birth weight in OD pregnancies was 1.25 (CI = 1.20–1.30) (41). The OR of very low birth weight was also significantly increased (OR = 1.37; CI = 1.22–1.54). Data from three studies including 686 OD and 30,862 AO IVF singleton pregnancies showed an increased risk of low birth rate following OD pregnancies (OR 1.53, 95% CI 1.16–2.01) (41).

There are two meta-analyses providing split data for fresh and frozen ET. Regarding frozen ET, in one meta-analysis (four studies; n = 36,614 patients), an increase in low birth rate was observed in OD pregnancies vs. IVF with AO (OR = 1.83; CI = 1.45–2.30). In the other meta-analysis regarding frozen ET on 150 OD and 7,350 IVF with AO cycles, there were no significant differences in the risk of low birth rate (OR = 1.65; CI = 0.92–2.96) (38). However, there was a significantly higher risk of very low birth rate in OD compared to AO IVF pregnancies (OR = 3.30; CI = 1.21–9.01). When the meta-analysis was restricted to fresh ET (ten studies, 220,645 patients), OD was associated with an increased risk of low birth weight compared with IVF with AO (OR = 1.25; CI = 1.13–1.38.)

Small for gestational age

The majority of meta-analyses did not show an increased risk of small for gestational age (SGA) in OD pregnancies. In a meta-analysis reviewing six articles the OR for SGA in OD was 1.81(CI = 1.26–2.60), but the SGA definitions differed widely (22). When the meta-analysis was restricted to the four studies employing consistent SGA definitions, the OR was 1.44 (CI = 0.93–2.23) (22). In the Storgaard et al meta-analysis, concerning singletons, the aOR was 1.14 (CI = 0.83–1.56) when comparing OD with IVF pregnancies and 1.29 (CI = 0.91–1.92) when comparing OD with natural pregnancies (62). In another meta-analysis data could not be pooled because of the different definitions used (38). On the other hand, in one meta-analysis involving five studies, OD pregnancies were associated with a diminished risk of SGA (OR = 0.83; CI = 0.78–0.98) (41)

Genetic abnormalities in the offspring

In general the incidence of genetic abnormalities in the OD/embryo donation (ED) offspring are related with the age of the donor and not of the recipient. Thus, when OD/ED is applied in women of advanced age, the rate of chromosome disorders should be much lower than in the recipient age group. For instance, the reported risk of Down syndrome is 0.75% at 40 years, 1.5% at 42 years, and 3.6% at 48 years, when the reported rates at 30 and 34 years are 0.1% and 0.3%, respectively (42). Similarly, the percentage of pregnancies ending in miscarriages increases from 10% at the age of 20–25, to 12% at 25–30, to 18% at 30–35, to 23% at 35–40, to 50% a 40–45, and to 90% at ≥45 years (20). Moreover with the recent genetic tests applied to the male partner and the OD to detect recessive disorders (1, 15, 16), a number of rare diseases can be avoided. The OR for congenital defects has been assessed in one meta-analysis, reporting an OR of 0.89 (CI = 0–75–1.05) (2). Since usually women of an advanced age have partners of an advanced age, there is some concern regarding the impact of spermatozoa of an advanced age in the offspring. A number of diseases have been linked with advanced male age: chromosomal diseases, autism, and schizophrenia (14, 36, 40, 51, 59, 60). However, in most of the studies it was difficult to isolate the effect of advanced paternal age from advanced maternal age. In two small studies analyzing OD, chromosomal disorders in the offspring were similar when fathers were young or old (15, 46).

Intrauterine death

A meta-analysis (22) of two studies reported that the rate of intrauterine death was not significantly increased in OD pregnancies (RR = 1.39, CI 0.32–6.15).

Specific associated conditions

Some preexisting conditions are associated with an increased rate of complications during pregnancy, including severe maternal complications and even death. Several cases of maternal death have been reported in OD pregnancies in women with Turner syndrome (7, 19, 23). The maternal risk of death from rupture or dissection of the aorta in pregnancy in women with Turner syndrome may be 2% or higher (23).

Age-related maternal risks

Some events, fortunately, are very rare during pregnancy, but their potential consequences should not be forgotten. However, their uncommon frequency makes it difficult to study them in the setting of case-control studies. In a large series analyzing the medical and obstetric events present at the time of delivery among women aged ≥45 (n = 23,807) compared with women aged <35 (n = 10,768,536) from the Nationwide Inpatient Sample (years 2008–2010), some very severe complications were analyzed (17, 54). The following increased risks were observed: maternal death (OR = 9.90; CI = 5.60–15.98), transfusion (OR = 2.46; CI = 2.27–2.68), myocardial infarction (OR = 21.38; CI = 11.46–39.88), cardiac arrest (OR = 21.38; CI = 11.46–39.88), pulmonary embolism (OR = 5.01; CI = 3.47–7.23), deep vein thrombosis (OR = 4.38; CI = 3.26–5.89), acute renal failure (OR = 6.38; CI = 5.06–8.04). Although not all the cases reported as mother aged ≥45 come from OD, such data can give an approximate estimate of what would occur in OD pregnant women ≥45.

The case of embryo donation

Embryo donation cycles represent 2.3%–2.6% of frozen transfers (25). Their perinatal results have received much less attention than those of OD pregnancy. Some studies have reported only a small series of pregnancies (n < 25) (30, 61). It has been reported that 23.2% of singletons coming from embryo donation cycles are preterm (25). A similar rate of hypertensive disorders has been reported in women receiving donor embryos (i.e., donated egg and sperm) (aOR 2.0; 95% CI 1.25–3.17) than among those receiving OD (aOR = 2.0; CI = 1.25–3.17) (26).

Discussion

In a number of studies several perinatal complications have been reported as consistently increased in OD pregnancies. After controlling for multiplicity, the majority of the aforementioned increased risks persisted. Concerning the probably more important confounding factor, maternal age, few studies controlled for it. The increased risks of OD can be explained by three theories, not necessarily exclusive. The first one we would call "immunologic oocyte theory". In a healthy natural pregnancy, the maternal organism does not immunologically react against the oocyte (since it is fully maternal material). In AO pregnancies, the embryo shares with the mother at least 50% of histocompatibility antigens. Thus, the immune tolerance to the embryo/fetus during pregnancy should be easier to achieve than in OD pregnancies, where the antigen dissimilarity between the mother and the embryo/fetus can reach 100%. It has been shown that the incidence of hypertensive disorders is significantly higher if the oocyte donor is unrelated to the recipient compared with a related sibling donor (27). One of the mechanisms presumably involved in the pathogenesis of preeclampsia is precisely related with a failure in the immune tolerance mechanisms (35, 44). In agreement with this, changing the sperm source does not impair OD results. Thus, similar preeclampsia rates have been reported in OD cycles when donor sperm or partner sperm were used (50).

The second theory could be related to the "OD procedure". OD pregnancies differ in a number of aspects from IVF with AO and/or natural pregnancies: endometrial preparation, embryo freezing, estradiol levels during the cycle of oocyte pick-up, and gonadotropin administration (influencing the oocytes during ovarian stimulation, but not the uterus). It has been suggested that high estradiol levels during controlled ovarian stimulation can be associated with an increased risk of preeclampsia and low birth weight (21, 38). It has been reported that if >20 oocytes have been retrieved, there is an increased risk of preterm delivery and low birth weight (4, 38, 64).

The third theory could be called "maternal insufficiency". Pregnancy rates in OD recipients are very similar to those obtained in patients who are in the same age group as the donors. However, this does not apply to obstetric complications. As we previously said, maternal age by itself is a risk factor for almost all perinatal complications. Moreover, one can speculate that even after controlling for age, some recipient women undergoing OD could be in an inferior health status than those getting pregnant with their own oocytes. That would be the case of vascular, metabolic, immunological, and uterine problems, both known and undetectable. In agreement with this, in a study comparing the results obtained with embryos resulting from donated oocytes, the gestational carriers (mean age = 31) had significantly lower rates of prematurity compared to intended parent recipients (mean age = 41) (58). Similarly a study in mice suggested that abnormal placentation and decidualization in an older uterine environment is the cause of intrauterine growth restriction and congenital anomalies (70).

Regardless of all this, it has to be highlighted that current practice has remarkably improved and some of the aforementioned risks have decreased, such as those related to multiple pregnancies since the implementation of single embryo transfer (SET) in these patients. Similarly, those related to unknown cardiac problems can be improved with testing for heart diseases. For the moment it remains speculative if HLA matching the OD with the recipients could improve perinatal results. Before undergoing OD, women and their partners should be informed of the risks of OD. The message should be that in women <50, where a thorough medical evaluation has ruled out conditions that could impair pregnancy, if SET is performed, OD is a highly successful and safe alternative.

Conclusions

- Women undergoing OD, as indicated by a diagnosis of premature ovarian insufficiency, should be evaluated to rule out that the cause of ovarian insufficiency might increase the pregnancy risks.
- Women ≥45 years undergoing OD should undergo a medical evaluation in order to rule out conditions that could impair the pregnancy outcome, such as cardiovascular and metabolic disorders.
- OD should not be offered to women ≥50 years.
- Genetic tests to detect recessive disorders in oocyte donors and male partners should be offered.
- SET should be mandatory.
- Women/couples undergoing OD should be informed of the risks.
- In women <50, where a thorough medical evaluation has ruled out conditions that could impair pregnancy, if SET is performed, OD is a highly successful and safe alternative.

REFERENCES

1. Abulí A, Boada M, Rodríguez-Santiago B, Coroleu B, Veiga A, Armengol L, Barri PN, Pérez-Jurado LA, Estivill X. NGS-based assay for the identification of individuals carrying recessive genetic mutations in reproductive medicine. *Hum Mutat.* 2016;37:516–23.
2. Adams DH, Clark RA, Davies MJ, de Lacey S. A meta-analysis of neonatal health outcomes from oocyte donation. *J Dev Orig Health Dis.* 2015;1–16.
3. Al-Zirqi I, Vangen S, Forsen L, Stray-Pedersen B. Prevalence and risk factors of severe obstetric haemorrhage. *BJOG.* 2008;115:1265–72.
4. Baker VL, Brown MB, Luke B, Conrad KP. Association of number of retrieved oocytes with live birth rate and birth weight: An analysis of 231, 815 cycles of in vitro fertilization. *Fertil Steril.* 2015;103:931–8.
5. Barton JR, O'Brien JM, Bergauer NK, Jacques DL, Sibai BM. Mild gestational hypertension remote from term: Progression and outcome. *Am J Obstet Gynecol.* 2001;184:979–83.

6. Bianco A, Stone J, Lynch L, Lapinski R, Berkowitz G, Berkowitz RL. Pregnancy outcome at age 40 and older. *Obstet Gynecol.* 1996;87:917–22.
7. Boissonnas CC, Davy C, Bornes M, Arnaout L, Meune C, Tsatsatris V, Mignon A, Jouannet P. Careful cardiovascular screening and follow-up of women with Turner syndrome before and during pregnancy is necessary to prevent maternal mortality. *Fertil Steril.* 2009;91:929.e5–7.
8. Borini A, Bafaro G, Violini F, Bianchi L, Casadio V, Flamigni C. Pregnancies in postmenopausal women over 50 years old in an oocyte donation program. *Fertil Steril.* 1995;63:258–61.
9. Buchbinder A, Sibai BM, Caritis S, Macpherson C, Hauth J, Lindheimer MD, Klebanoff M, Vandorsten P, Landon M, Paul R, Miodovnik M, Meis P, Thurnau G, National Institute of Child Health and Human Development Network of Maternal-Fetal Medicine Units. Adverse perinatal outcomes are significantly higher in severe gestational hypertension than in mild preeclampsia. *Am J Obstet Gynecol.* 2002;186:66–71.
10. Chang J, Elam-Evans LD, Berg CJ, Herndon J, Flowers L, Seed KA, Syverson CJ. Pregnancy-related mortality surveillance-United States, 1991–1999. *MMWR Surveill Summ.* 2003;52:1–8.
11. Ethics Committee of the American Society for Reproductive Medicine. Oocyte or embryo donation to women of advanced reproductive age: An Ethics Committee opinion. *Fertil Steril.* 2016;106:e3–7.
12. European IVF-monitoring Consortium (EIM) for the European Society of Human Reproduction and Embryology (ESHRE), Wyns C, Bergh C, Calhaz-Jorge C, De Geyter C, Kupka MS, Motrenko T, Rugescu I, Smeenk J, Tandler-Schneider A, Vidakovic S, Goossens V. ART in Europe, 2016: Results generated from European registries by ESHRE. *Hum Reprod Open.* 2020;(3):hoaa032. doi: 10.1093/hropen/hoaa032.
13. Evans MI, Hume RF Jr, Polak S, Yaron Y, Drugan A, Diamond MP, Johnson MP. The geriatric gravida: Multifetal pregnancy reduction, donor eggs, and aggressive infertility treatments. *Am J Obstet Gynecol.* 1997;177:875–8.
14. Fisch H, Hyun G, Golden R, Hensle TW, Olsson CA, Liberson GL. The influence of paternal age on down syndrome. *J Urol.* 2003;169:2275–8.
15. Gallardo E, Simon C, Levy M, Guanes PP, Remohi J, Pellicer A. Effect of age on sperm fertility potential: Oocyte donation as a model. *Fertil Steril.* 1996;66:260–4.
16. Garrido N, Bosch E, Alamá P, Ruiz A. The time to prevent mendelian genetic diseases from donated or own gametes has come. *Fertil Steril.* 2015;104:833–5.
17. Grotegut CA, Chisholm CA, Johnson LN, Brown HL, Heine RP, James AH. Medical and obstetrical complications among pregnant women aged 45and older. *PLoS One.* 2014;9:e96237.
18. Gundogan F, Bianchi DW, Scherjon SA, Roberts DJ. Placental pathology in egg donor pregnancies. *Fertil Steril.* 2010;93:397–404.
19. Hagman A, Loft A, Wennerholm UB, Pinborg A, Bergh C, Aittomäki K, Nygren KG, Bente Romundstad L, Hazekamp J, Söderström-Anttila V. Obstetric and neonatal outcome after oocyte donation in 106 women with Turner syndrome: A Nordic cohort study. *Hum Reprod.* 2013;28:1598–609.
20. Heffner LJ. Advanced maternal age: How old is too old? *New Engl J Med.* 2004;351:1927–9.
21. Imudia AN, Awonuga AO, Doyle JO, Kaimal AJ, Wright DL, Toth TL, Styer AK. Peak serum estradiol level during controlled ovarian hyperstimulation is associated with increased risk of small for gestational age and preeclampsia in singleton pregnancies after in vitro fertilization. *Fertil Steril.* 2012;97:1374–9.
22. Jeve Y, Potdar N, Opoku A, Khare M. Donor oocyte conception and pregnancy complications: A systematic review and meta-analysis. *BJOG Int J Obstet Gynaecol.* 2016;123:1471–80.
23. Karnis MF, Zimon AE, Lalwani SI, Timmreck LS, Klipstein S, Reindollar RH. Risk of death in pregnancy achieved through oocyte donation in patients with Turner syndrome: A national survey. *Fertil Steril.* 2003;80:498–501.
24. Kawwass JF, Badell ML. Maternal and fetal risk associated with assisted reproductive technology. *Obstet Gynecol.* 2018;132:763–72.
25. Kawwass JF, Crawford S, Hipp HS, Boulet SL, Kissin DM, Jamieson DJ, National ART Surveillance System Group. Embryo donation: National trends and outcomes, 2000 through 2013. *Am J Obstet Gynecol.* 2016;215:747.e1–e5.
26. Kennedy AL, Stern CJ, Tong S, Hastie R, Agresta F, Walker SP, Brownfoot FC, MacLachlan V, Vollenhoven BJ, Lindquist AC. The incidence of hypertensive disorders of pregnancy following sperm donation in IVF: An Australian state-wide retrospective cohort study. *Hum Reprod.* 2019;34:2541–54.

27. Kim HSYK, Cha SH, Song IO, Kang IS. Obstetric outcomes after oocyte donation in patients with premature ovarian failure. Abstracts of the 21st Annual Meeting of the ESHRE, Copenhagen, Denmark: ESHRE; 2005. p. O-094.
28. Korb D, Schmitz T, Seco A, Le Ray C, Santulli P, Goffinet F, Deneux-Tharaux C. Increased risk of severe maternal morbidity in women with twin pregnancies resulting from oocyte donation. *Hum Reprod*. 2020;35:1922–32.
29. Kort DH, Gosselin J, Choi JM, Thornton MH, Cleary-Goldman J, Sauer MV. Pregnancy after age 50: Defining risks for mother and child. *Am J Perinatol*. 2012;29:245–50.
30. Kovacs GT, Breheny SA, Dear MJ. Embryo donation at an Australian university in-vitro fertilisation clinic: Issues and outcomes. *Med J Aust*. 2003;178:127–9.
31. Kuklina EV, Ayala C, Callaghan WM. Hypertensive disorders and severe obstetric morbidity in the United States. *Obstet Gynecol*. 2009;113:1299–306.
32. Kupka MS, Ferraretti AP, de Mouzon J, Erb K, D'Hooghe T, Castilla JA, Calhaz-Jorge C, De Geyter C, Goossens V, European IVF-Monitoring Consortium, for the European Society of Human Reproduction and Embryology. Assisted reproductive technology in Europe, 2010: Results generated from European registers by ESHRE. *Hum Reprod*. 2014;29:2099–113.
33. Lashley LE, van der Hoorn ML, Haasnoot GW, Roelen DL, Claas FH. Uncomplicated oocyte donation pregnancies are associated with a higher incidence of human leukocyte antigen alloantibodies. *Hum Immunol*. 2014;75:555–60.
34. Le Ray C, Scherier S, Anselem O, Marszalek A, Tsatsaris V, Cabrol D, Goffinet F. Association between oocyte donation and maternal and perinatal outcomes in women aged 43 years or older. *Hum Reprod*. 2012;27:896–901.
35. Levron Y, Dviri M, Segol I, Yerushalmi GM, Hourvitz A, Orvieto R, Mazaki-Tovi S, Yinon Y. The "immunologic theory" of preeclampsia revisited: A lesson from donor oocyte gestations. *Am J Obstet Gynecol*. 2014;211:383.e1–5.
36. Lowe X, Eskenazi B, Nelson DO, Kidd S, Alme A, Wyrobek AJ. Frequency of XY sperm increases with age in fathers of boys with Klinefelter syndrome. *Am J Hum Genet*. 2001;69:1046–54.
37. Macharey G, Gissler M, Ulander VM, Rahkonen L, Väisänen-Tommiska M, Nuutila M, Heinonen S. Risk factors associated with adverse perinatal outcome in planned vaginal breech labors at term: A retrospective population-based case-control study. *BMC Pregnancy Childbirth*. 2017;17;93.
38. Mascarenhas M, Sunkara SK, Antonisamy B, Kamath MS. Higher risk of preterm birth and low birth weight following oocyte donation: A systematic review and meta-analysis. *Eur J Obstet Gynecol Reprod Biol*. 2017 Nov;218:60–7.
39. Masoudian P, Nasr A, de Nanassy J, Fung-Kee-Fung K, Bainbridge SA, El Demellawy D. Oocyte donation pregnancies and the risk of preeclampsia or gestational hypertension: A systematic review and metaanalysis. *Am J Obstet Gynecol*. 2016;214:328–39.
40. McIntosh GC, Olshan AF, Baird PA. Paternal age and the risk of birth defects in offspring. *Epidemiology*. 1995 May;6(3):282–8. doi: 10.1097/00001648-199505000-00016.
41. Moreno-Sepulveda J, Checa MA. Risk of adverse perinatal outcomes after oocyte donation: A systematic review and meta-analysis. *J Assist Reprod Genet*. 2019;36:2017–37.
42. Newberger D. Down syndrome: Prenatal risk assessment and diagnosis. *Am Fam Physician*. 2000;62:825–32.
43. Opelz G, Döhler B. Effect of human leukocyte antigen compatibility on kidney graft survival: Comparative analysis of two decades. *Transplantation*. 2007;84:137–43.
44. Pados G, Camus M, Van SA, Bonduelle M, Devroey P. The evolution and outcome of pregnancies from oocyte donation. *Hum Reprod (Oxford, England)*. 1994;9:538–42.
45. Paulson RJ, Boostanfar R, Saadat P, Mor E, Tourgeman DE, Slater CC, Francis MM, Jain JK. Pregnancy in the sixth decade of life: Obstetric outcomes in women of advanced reproductive age. *JAMA*. 2002;288:2320–3.
46. Paulson RJ, Milligan RC, Sokol RZ. The lack of influence of age on male fertility. *Am J Obstet Gynecol*. 2001;184:818–22.
47. Paulson RJ, Thornton MH, Francis MM, Salvador HS. Successful pregnancy in a 63-year-old woman. *Fertil Steril*. 1997;67:949–51.

48. Pecks U, Maass N, Neulen J. Oocyte donation: A risk factor for pregnancy-induced hypertension: A meta-analysis and case series. *Dtsch Arztebl Int.* 2011;108:23–31.
49. Perni SC, Predanic M, Cho JE, Baergen RN. Placental pathology and pregnancy outcomes in donor and non-donor oocyte in vitro fertilization pregnancies. *J Perinat Med.* 2005;33:27–32.
50. Preaubert L, Vincent-Rohfritsch A, Santulli P, Gayet V, Goffinet F, Le Ray C. Outcomes of pregnancies achieved by double gamete donation: A comparison with pregnancies obtained by oocyte donation alone. *Eur J Obstet Gynecol Reprod Biol.* 2018;222:1–6.
51. Reichenberg A, Gross R, Weiser M, Bresnahan M, Silverman J, Harlap S, Rabinowitz J, Shulman C, Malaspina D, Lubin G, Knobler HY, Davidson M, Susser E. Advancing paternal age and autism. *Arch Gen Psychiatry.* 2006;63:1026–32.
52. Remohí J, Nadal FJ, Del Pozo D, Mendoza R, Boada M, Martínez F, Alberto JC, Palumbo A, Llacer J, Mashlab A. Donación de ovocitos. In: Matorras R, Hernández J, editors. *Estudio y tratamiento de la pareja estéril. Recomendaciones de la Sociedad Española de Fertilidad, con la colaboración de la Asociación para el Estudio de la Biología de la Reproducción, la Asociación Española de Andrología y la Sociedad Española de Contracepción.* Madrid: Adalia; 2007. pp. 349–60.
53. Rodriguez-Wallberg KA, Berger AS, Fagerberg A, Olofsson JI, Scherman-Pukk C, Lindqvist PG, Nasiell J. Increased incidence of obstetric and perinatal complications in pregnancies achieved using donor oocytes and single embryo transfer in young and healthy women: A prospective hospital-based matched cohort study. *Gynecol Endocrinol.* 2019;35:314–19.
54. Sauer MV. Reproduction at an advanced maternal age and maternal health. *Fertil Steril.* 2015;103:1136–4.
55. Savasi VM, Mandia L, Laoreti A, Cetin I. Maternal and fetal outcomes in oocyte donation pregnancies. *Hum Reprod Update.* 2016;22:620–33.
56. Sauer MV, Paulson RJ, Lobo RA. Oocyte donation to women of advanced reproductive age: Pregnancy results and obstetrical outcomes in patients 45 years and older. *Hum Reprod.* 1996;11:2540–3.
57. Schonkeren D, Swings G, Roberts D, Claas F, de Heer E, Scherjon S. Pregnancy close to the edge: An immunosuppressive infiltrate in the chorionic plate of placentas from un complicated egg cell donation. *PLoS One.* 2012;7:e32347.
58. Segal TR, Kim K, Mumford SL, Goldfarb JM, Weinerman RS. How much does the uterus matter? Perinatal outcomes are improved when donor oocyte embryos are transferred to gestational carriers compared to intended parent recipients. *Fertil Steril.* 2018;110:888–95.
59. Sharma R, Agarwal A, Rohra VK, Assidi M, Abu-Elmagd M, Turki RF. Effects of increased paternal age on sperm quality, reproductive outcome and associated epigenetic risks to offspring. *Reprod Biol Endocrinol.* 2015 Apr 19;13:35.
60. Sipos A, Rasmussen F, Harrison G, Tynelius P, Lewis G, Leon DA, Gunnell D. Paternal age and schizophrenia: A population based cohort study. *BMJ.* 2004;329:1070.
61. Söderström-Anttila V, Foudila T, Ripatti UR, Siegberg R. Embryo donation: Outcome and attitudes among embryo donors and recipients. *Hum Reprod.* 2001;16:1120.
62. Storgaard M, Loft A, Bergh C, Wennerholm UB, Söderström-Anttila V, Romundstad LB, Aittomaki K, Oldereid N, Forman J, Pinborg A. Obstetric and neonatal complications in pregnancies conceived after oocyte donation: A systematic review and meta-analysis. *BJOG.* 2017;124:561–72.
63. Styer AK, Parker HJ, Roberts DJ, Palmer-Toy D, Toth TL, Ecker JL. Placental villitis of unclear etiology during ovum donor in vitro fertilization pregnancy. *Am J Obstet Gynecol.* 2003;189:1184–6.
64. Sunkara SK, La Marca A, Seed PT, Khalaf Y. Increased risk of preterm birth and low birthweight with very high number of oocytes following IVF: An analysis of 65 868 singleton live birth outcomes. *Hum Reprod.* 2015;30:1473–80.
65. Sutton ALM, Harper LM, Tita ATN. Hypertensive disorders in pregnancy. *Obstet Gynecol Clin North Am.* 2018;45:333–47.
66. Thomopoulos C, Salamalekis G, Kintis K, Andrianopoulou I, Michalopoulou H, Skalis G, Archontakis S, Argyri O, Tsioufis C, Makris TK, Salamalekis E. Risk of hypertensive disorders in pregnancy following assisted reproductive technology: Overview and meta-analysis. *J Clin Hypertens (Greenwich).* 2017;19:173–83.
67. Toner JP, Grainger DA, Frazier LM. Clinical outcomes among recipients of donated eggs: An analysis of the U.S. national experience, 1996–1998. *Fertil Steril.* 2002;78:1038–45.
68. Trounson A, Leeton J, Besanko M, Wood C, Conti A. Pregnancy established in an infertile patient after transfer of a donated embryo fertilised in vitro. *Br Med J (Clin Res Ed).* 1983;286:835–8.

69. van der Hoorn ML, Lashley EE, Bianchi DW, Claas FH, Schonkeren CM, Scherjon SA. Clinical and immunologic aspects of egg donation pregnancies: A systematic review. *Hum Reprod Update.* 2010;16:704–12.
70. Woods L, Perez-Garcia V, Kieckbusch J, Wang X, DeMayo F, Colucci F, Hemberger M. Decidualisation and placentation defects are a major cause of age-related reproductive decline. *Nat Commun.* 2017;8:352.
71. Yogev Y, Melamed N, Bardin R, Tenenbaum-Gavish K, Ben-Shitrit G, Ben-Haroush A. Pregnancy outcome at extremely advanced maternal age. *Am J Obstet Gynecol.* 2010;203:558 e551–e557.

9

Obstetric risks and pregnancy outcomes specific to patients with very advanced maternal age (over 45)

Filipa Rafael, Marta Carvalho, and Samuel Santos-Ribeiro

The mid-90s was a time in which the world witnessed a progressive empowerment of women. This occurred not only with the expansion of readily accessible contraception but also due to the increasing social acceptance of a female-led decision to voluntary terminate an unwanted pregnancy. These changes in reproductive rights combined with a progressive shift in the behavior of modern-day society over time have led to a significant delay in the average age at which couples pursue parenthood for the first time. This change included not only an increase of better – and consequently more time-demanding – educational and career opportunities for women but also from repeated adjustments in the perceived role of men in family-related everyday living responsibilities (1). Moreover, prospective parents also seem to be relatively unaware of the age-dependent risk for infertility, which, at least in part, is due to a positively biased media coverage of pregnancies at extremely advanced ages (2). This lack of awareness has led to an inadvertent overestimation in couples of their true chances to conceive at older ages (Figure 9.1), both spontaneously and following assisted reproductive technology (ART), resulting in an increase in the number of women attempting their first pregnancy at the age of 40 or older (3).

Collectively, the changes in both age of first child-wish and the increased use of ART and oocyte donation have generalized pregnancy at advanced maternal age to an extent in which its definition (i.e., a pregnancy occurring at an age of 35 years old or above) has become trivial, leading to alternative subclassifications, including pregnancy at very advanced maternal age (i.e., at the age of 45 years old or above) (4). The frequency of pregnancies at this age have varied substantially worldwide, tripling over the span of 10 years in a cohort study performed in Spain, in which it accounted for 2.6% of all pregnancies (5). Conversely, between 2010 and 2018, a national survey using data from the United States concluded that pregnancies in this age group had only seen a very modest increase over time, representing between 0.7 and 0.9 birth per 1000 women (6).

At the age of 35, female fertility declines substantially, but this decrease becomes most evident as the woman reaches an age >40 years. Reports on the impact of a very advanced maternal age (>45 years) describe that the probability of a spontaneous conception achieving a live birth is below 3%, odds that do not seem to significantly improve following ART treatments when using autologous oocytes (7). From a cellular perspective, as maternal age increases, there is both an important depletion in ovarian reserve and a decline in ovarian functional potential. Regarding the latter, a decrease in "oocyte quality" is best represented by a higher incidence in mitochondrial dysfunction and chromosome segregation errors, ultimately leading to the production of embryos with a significantly compromised implantation potential. Interestingly, while chromosome segregation errors occur during both male and female gametogenesis, paternal errors seem to be eliminated through cellular checkpoint mechanisms, thus emphasizing that age-related aneuploidies are mostly of maternal origin (8). Overall, these important cellular modifications not only imply that a clinical pregnancy is more difficult to achieve as maternal age advances but also that there is a significant increase in the probability of having a miscarriage and molar pregnancies when conception does occur, ultimately leading to the loss of up to 90% of all pregnancies in women over 45 years old (9).

However, a decrease in ovarian function is not the only cause for hindered pregnancy outcomes as women age. Other potential factors include a decrease in coital frequency and a higher prevalence of diseases which impair fertility such as endometriosis, myomas, or tubal factor infertility (10).

DOI: 10.1201/9781003052524-9

Risks/outcomes for advanced-age patients 87

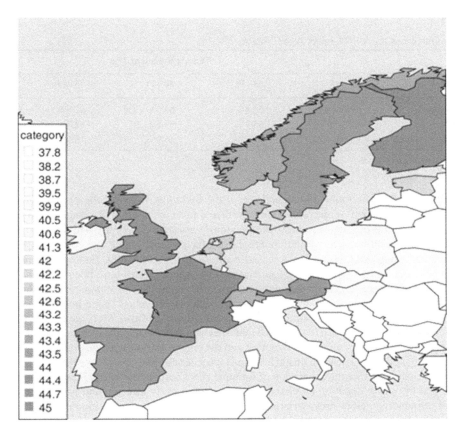

FIGURE 9.1 Reported age that a woman is too old to consider having more children, respondents aged 25–42 years old, selected European countries.

[From Mills et al. (3), with permission.]

Besides the lower ongoing pregnancy rates, advanced maternal age is also concomitantly associated with a higher risk of a variety of adverse fetal and maternal outcomes, including cesarean section delivery, preeclampsia, gestational diabetes, prematurity, and stillbirth (11, 12). Moreover, there is also an increased risk of several neurodevelopmental conditions such as cerebral palsy, impaired cognitive development, attention deficit hyperactivity or autism spectrum disorder, and growth or cardiovascular dysfunction, among other abnormalities (13, 14). Many of these long term health issues seem to not vary significantly between ART-derived pregnancies and spontaneously conceived children; however, this is mostly the case only when the analysis is restricted to singletons (14). That said, these risks are frequently unintentionally further exacerbated in ART-derived gestations, in which multiple embryos are transferred in an attempt to counteract the poor prognosis associated with this age group.

The extremely poor prognosis when using autologous oocytes has led maternal age to become the main indication for oocyte donation which, independently of the recipient age, can attain live birth rates higher than 50% per transfer (15, 16). In the last decades, oocyte donation has increasingly become a more accepted and effective strategy to treat female age-related infertility, leading to a sharp increase of pregnancies at advanced maternal age. This sudden surge in pregnancies at very advanced age stresses the need for a more comprehensive reflection and understanding among the medical community of the associated obstetric risks at an age when women, until recently, were seldomly expecting (2).

Despite the implantation rates in oocyte donation cycles being, at first glance, almost exclusively dependent on the age of the donor, uterine receptivity and adequate endometrial development can still potentially have a significant impact on pregnancy outcomes (Table 9.1). Specifically, while the value

TABLE 9.1

Pregnancy Outcomes for All Recipient Age Cohorts

	Female Recipient Age				
	≤34	35–39	40–44	45–49	≥50
Clinical pregnancy	64.9%	65.4%	64.7%	62.8%	59.9%
Live birth	56.7%	55.7%	55.8%	52.7%	48.6%
Miscarriage	16.0%	17.7%	16.9%	18.5%	19.0%

Source: Adapted from Yeh et al. (102).

of endometrial thickness remains unreconcilable in the literature, it is still the most commonly used prognostic tool for endometrial receptivity and considered to be essential in placentation. To that extent, inadequate endometrial development has been previously associated not only with a lower probability of achieving a live birth but also with an increased risk for placenta previa and compromised embryo/fetal growth following ART (17) and decreased birth weight z-scores (18). Endometrial proliferation appears to be dependent on reproductive age, and lower pregnancy rates have been reported below the 7-mm threshold, progressively increasing until 10 mm (19). Although a very thin endometrial thickness seems to be a seldomly reported event, the impact of such cut-off values might be more prominent in older women, considering that an endometrial thickness ≥8 mm in fresh ART cycles was found to be more difficult to achieve in women of advanced maternal age (20). Finally, the particularity of a complete immunogenetic dissimilarity between the mother and the embryo/fetus in oocyte donation cycles should not be neglected, and it may pose an obstacle against a successful pregnancy as well. More specifically, recent evidence suggests that the expression of immune checkpoint coinhibitory ligands by trophoblasts in the placenta of oocyte donation pregnancies can be significantly affected and potentially reflect the differential immunoregulatory processes in such pregnancies, possibly justifying the higher prevalence of several conditions, such as gestational hypertensive disorders (21).

Short term maternal and fetal risks

Profound anatomical, physiological, and biochemical adaptations occur to accommodate pregnancy. These astonishing changes begin soon after fertilization and continue throughout gestation. Most occur in response to physiological stimuli provided by the placenta and the fetus. These adaptations of normal pregnancy can be frequently misinterpreted as pathologic or unmask/worsen a preexisting disease, particularly in older women. For instance, changes in cardiac physiology include an increase in cardiac output, heart rate, left ventricular stroke workload, and mean arterial pressure and a decrease in systemic and pulmonary vascular resistance, as well as colloid osmotic pressure. Functional systolic heart murmurs, dyspnea, edema in the lower extremities, fatigue, exercise intolerance, and other clinical findings are also frequently present in normal pregnancies. These may confound the diagnosis of heart disease, which is more prevalent in older women. This is particularly concerning, since heart disease is now the leading cause of indirect maternal deaths, accounting for 20% of all cases (22). Cardiovascular diseases also account for a significant amount of maternal morbidity and are the leading cause of obstetric intensive care unit admissions. Regardless of the cause, the risk of maternal mortality in women over 40 years old is fivefold higher (46 versus 9 per 100,000 live births) then in women aged between 25 and 29 years old (23, 24). In a UK-based registry study of maternal deaths for older women, other risk factors associated with increased likelihood of death included inadequate use of antenatal care, medical comorbidities, previous complication of pregnancy, and maternal smoking during pregnancy (25).

During the later stages of pregnancy, preexisting and pregnancy-related hypertension frequently complicate pregnancies. Chronic hypertension is one of the most common serious complications encountered during pregnancy, particularly in older women. There is an increased rate of cardiovascular, cerebrovascular, and renal disease in hypertensive women, which can worsen during pregnancy, besides contributing to the risk of fetal loss. The incidence of preeclampsia is 5%–10% in women over the age of 40 and can be as high as 35% in women over 50 (26, 27). The use of ART is an important risk factor in large cohort studies (28), albeit potentially related at least in a large portion to other confounding factors (29). Furthermore, a recent study reported that the risk of hypertensive disorders in pregnancy seemed to be increased in frozen embryo transfers (in both autologous and donor oocyte cycles) and fresh donor oocyte embryo transfers, but not after autologous oocyte fresh embryo transfers (30). It has been postulated that this increased risk may be associated with the lack of corpus luteum in artificial transfer cycles (31–33). Recent publications on the physiopathology of preeclampsia indicate that the corpus luteum is the main source of hormonal production until placental formation and, apart from the secretion of estrogen and progesterone, the corpus luteum also produces important substances involved in maternal circulatory adaptation, such as relaxin (34). For this reason, natural cycles should be considered for endometrium preparation whenever feasible, particularly in older women or those most at risk to develop gestational hypertensive disorders (35, 36). Additionally, careful obstetric monitoring is also essential to reduce further morbidity and mortality related to these hypertensive disorders, including preterm birth, cesarean delivery, and small-for-gestational-age deliveries (37). It has been suggested that the use of aspirin in high-risk patients could reduce the risk of obstetric complications in hypertensive disorders of pregnancy, particularly in older women, although there is still conflicting data on the true benefit of this approach (38, 39).

Another common medical problem in this group of women is diabetes (both pregestational and gestational). The reported rate of pregestational diabetes in women between 35 and 44 years old is 5.4%, raising to 12% by the age of 50 (40). Pregestational diabetes contributes to a higher rate of congenital anomalies, perinatal mortality, and morbidity. The incidence of gestational diabetes in women over 40 varies between 7% and 12%, rising to 20% in women above 50 (26, 27, 41). A recent meta-analysis of over 120 million participants concluded that there is a linear relationship between maternal age and gestational diabetes risk, with an odds ratio of 4.86 (95% confidence interval between 3.78 and 6.24) for women over 40 when compared to women under 20 years (42). Major complications of gestational diabetes include macrosomia, dystocia, vaginal/rectal lacerations during delivery, neonatal hypoglycemia, and Erb's palsy.

Placental problems are also more prevalent in older women, namely placental abruption, which is associated with higher parity and hypertension, both risk factors that are more frequent in this age group. Moreover, age is also an independent risk factor for placenta previa, with a ten-fold increase in women over 40 (37).

The likelihood of labor dystocia and cesarean delivery are also increased (26, 37, 43, 44). Uterine dysfunction appears to increase steadily with age, particularly the length of the second stage (45). In a cohort study including over 78,000 singleton births, 36% of women between 45 and 49 years old (and 61% for women above 50) had their first cesarean delivery at that age (44). The reasons behind this spike might include an increased prevalence of other concomitant medical conditions, induction of labor, and a lower threshold for performing a cesarean delivery (46). Another recent study reports that elective cesarean deliveries were independently associated with maternal age above 50. In their multivariate analysis adjusted for previous cesarean delivery, preeclampsia, pregestational body mass index (BMI), and multiple gestation, the authors found an odds ratio for cesarean delivery in women above 50 (compared to women of 45–49 years) of 3.00 (95% confidence interval between 1.29 and 6.98) (47).

Not all adverse events occur only in the later stages of pregnancy. In fact, the increased likelihood of hindered outcomes is apparent immediately following conception. Specifically, older women face a higher risk of spontaneous abortion, with the majority of losses happening between 6 and 14 weeks of gestation (48). In a Scandinavian prospective register linkage study, women aged 45 years or above had a 74.7% risk of spontaneous abortion, regardless of the number of previous miscarriages or parity (49). When karyotyping of the products of conception was performed, it showed that most of these pregnancy losses were related to aneuploidy, the most common of which were autosomal trisomies. Likewise, there is an increased risk of molar pregnancy, particularly complete mole, which can be several hundred times greater after the age of 50 (50, 51).

The risk of congenital malformation also increases with female aging. In a population-based case-control study, cardiac defects, esophageal atresia, hypospadias, and craniosynostosis seem all to increase independently with maternal age (52). Advanced maternal age is also associated with a fourfold to eightfold increased risk of ectopic pregnancy when compared to younger women, which is the most important source of maternal mortality and morbidity in early pregnancy (53).

These short term maternal risks need to be addressed by the professionals that follow pregnancies of women of older age. To reduce these concerning risks, it is of utmost importance to adequately advise these patients in the preconception setting. High-risk populations should be screened for occult type 2 diabetes and microvascular or macrovascular complications, with an ophthalmologist consult, proteinuria assessment and an echocardiography. Breast cancer screening could also be offered over 45 years of age. Medication needs to be optimized and adapted for pregnancy. Advice regarding diet and regular physical activity should also be offered. Finally, when considering the use of ART, limiting multiple pregnancies is key in reducing the eventual risks (54). Moreover, recommendations for first-trimester management include early ultrasound to determine gestational location (to promptly exclude or actively treat ectopic pregnancy); non-invasive and/or invasive screening for chromosomal aberrations; and ultrasound screening for detection of fetal congenital anomalies, including, if needed, a fetal echocardiography. During the second trimester, efforts should be made to screen for gestational diabetes, hypertension and proteinuria, as well as to schedule ultrasound exams to assess placental location and fetal weight at 32, 34, and 36 weeks of gestation (54). Regarding timing of delivery, induction of labor at 39 weeks could contribute to decrease the risk of stillbirth. Despite the controversy, there is some evidence that advocates for planned vaginal delivery in the adequate setting (55).

Long term maternal risks

Pregnancy is frequently compared to a stress test because of the significant amount of adaptations that occurs in practically every organ system of the female body to accommodate the developing embryo/fetus. These substantial changes over the span of a 9-month period in a woman with very advanced maternal age carry not only an immediate maternal risk but may also have long term consequences. Moreover, the rise of ART in this age group has also led to an increase in the concern between the risk of exogenous gonadotropin use and long term female health. These fears are twofold, since infertile women with advanced maternal age frequently will have multiple other risk factors for cardiovascular disease (56) and cancer (57), but also since many cancers, namely those of the reproductive system, can be hormone-dependent (58).

Overall, despite the existence of multiple valid reasons for concern, the bulk of the long term data so far has assessed women above 35–40 years old as a single group, limiting the possibility to ascertain the true effect among those above 45 years old. For example, a recent registry analysis concluded that childbirth after the age of 40 was associated with an increased risk of cancer and other diseases in multiple organ systems in the 5 following years, a finding that was mostly associated with female age and, albeit to a lesser extent, the use of ART (59). Among the risks mentioned, cardiovascular disease was one of the most notable, which is further conflated with the fact that gestational hypertensive disorders (also more common in older pregnant women) are also associated with diseases such as chronic hypertension, heart failure, stroke, diabetes, and end-stage renal disease later in life (60). Among the other organ systems assessed, the authors also found that diseases of the blood and immune system, endocrine or metabolic disorders, sensory abnormalities (namely ear-related conditions), mental and behavioral issues, musculoskeletal and connective illnesses, and genitourinary disorders also occurred at an increased risk following a pregnancy at advanced age.

The risk of a future cancer is also a frequent concern with pregnancies occurring later in life, especially in women who performed ART. However, regarding at least (borderline) ovarian (61, 62), breast (63), and endometrial (64) cancers and melanoma (65), these concerns have been relatively assuaged for now by large registry analyses in which the potential effect of ovarian stimulation was untangled from the confounding factors involved in infertility itself (66–70), namely female-cause infertility, specifically endometriosis (71).

More globally, another longitudinal study found that women with their first pregnancy above 38 years old reported a lower degree of satisfaction, most prominently 3 years after birth (72). This stresses the importance of how much childrearing itself could be an important risk factor for disease, a conclusion also reached in another study associating the number of children fathered with coronary heart disease risk in the male counterparts (73). These difficulties may also be further exacerbated in women who are raising children alone at an advanced maternal age, with single parenting showing an increased risk in the incidence of mental and behavioral disorders in the 5 years following delivery (59).

Long term risks for the newborn

Although long term consequences for the newborn in this age group cannot be disregarded, the preceding literature on the topic remains rather limited. Still, advanced maternal age has been associated with an increased risk of low birth weight and preterm delivery, both of which may later increase the risk of death, morbidity, and long term disability. These disabilities include developmental disorders (e.g., cerebral palsy and blindness), respiratory problems, learning disabilities (e.g., lower IQ and lower academic achievement), and behavioral issues (e.g., attention deficit hyperactivity disorder). Reassuringly, most of the identified risk associations have comparable outcomes to naturally conceived children when the analysis is restricted to singleton pregnancies (74–76).

Despite an increasing effort to reduce this issue, women at advanced maternal age are still frequently conceiving twin pregnancies. In 2006, 20% of births in women aged 45–54 years were twins (77), which were associated with both a higher rate of naturally conceived twins and a higher use of ART in older women. Multiple births carry an increased risk of prematurity, as more than 12% of twins and 30% of triplets are born at under 32 weeks, compared with 2% of singleton pregnancies. The perinatal mortality rate is also significantly higher among twins (29.8 cases per 1000 pregnancies) and triplets (59.6 cases per 1000 cases pregnancies) when compared to that of singletons (6.0 cases per 1000 pregnancies) (74). Efforts in reducing twin pregnancy are key in preventing such perinatal outcomes. For these reasons, single embryo transfer is strongly recommended, particularly in treatments with donated oocytes, in which pregnancy rates are significantly higher.

Despite that, a higher risk of perinatal mortality following a pregnancy at advanced maternal age has also been reported in singleton pregnancies in most large studies, with relative risks ranging between 1.2 and 4.5 (78). This excess perinatal mortality in older women is present even after controlling for risk factors such as hypertension, diabetes, antepartum bleeding, smoking, and multiple gestation, and is most likely due to unexplained stillbirths. In pregnancies following oocyte donation, the capacity to conceive and deliver at term appears to be independent of uterine aging throughout the fifth decade of life (79, 80), although the preceding studies are limited to small sample sizes. The odds of stillbirth at term increased significantly with advancing maternal age (81), and some authors suggest that women over 40 years should be considered biologically "postterm" at 39 weeks' gestation, recommending that fetal monitoring be initiated at 38 weeks in this age group (74, 81). In a recent systematic review, newborns of women greater or equal to 45 years old compared with women with a maternal age of less than 45 were over 2-fold more likely to have a concerning 5-minute Apgar score (82).

Cerebral palsy (CP) is a symptom complex, rather than a specific disease. It is a range of non-progressive motor impairment syndromes secondary to lesions or anomalies of the brain arising in the early stages of its development. A significant increase in CP in near-term and term infants of mothers 35 years and older has also been shown (83–85). In this age group, CP tends to predominantly stem from antenatal factors, with prematurity playing a less important role in its development. Recently, genetic factors, including aberrant copy number variations, have also been posited as a possible cause, with around 1,700 genetic variations being more frequently found in the offspring of older mothers (86). Besides the considerable economic burden to society attributed to CP, it is known that caregivers of children with CP suffer from a substantial psychosocial burden (87). Nevertheless, there are no studies in this particular group of older aged caregivers.

Older maternal women may also find their offspring to be at a higher risk for autism spectrum disorders (88–90). In a 2012 metanalysis accruing data that included more than 8 million cases, the relative risk of autism increased monotonically with increasing maternal age and this association persisted even after adjusting for potential confounders such as paternal age (88). In contrast, older maternal age appears to exert a protective effect on offspring in terms of other behavioral and cognitive outcomes (91).

Specifically, a prospective birth cohort study found that increasing maternal age was associated with a decreased risk for both internalizing (e.g., anxious, depressed, somatic, or withdrawn) and externalizing (e.g., aggressive, delinquent) behaviors in offspring (92).

Several maternal factors were reported to increase the risk of type 1 diabetes in children, with higher maternal age (and, to a lesser extent, paternal age) at the time of delivery (93). A pooled analysis of 30 observational studies found a 5%–10% increase in childhood type 1 diabetes odds per 5-year increase in maternal age. The observed association between maternal age and diabetes could not be explained by birth order, birth weight, gestational age, cesarean section delivery, maternal diabetes, or breastfeeding. The mechanism behind the increased risk of childhood type 1 diabetes in children born to older mothers remains unclear. It is possible that maternal age is only a marker of some other factor more directly related to the risk of type 1 diabetes in children (94). One possibility is that maternal weight, which may increase with maternal age, could be involved, as a study found both maternal pre-pregnancy BMI and maternal weight gain during pregnancy to predict diabetes-associated islet autoimmunity in genetically susceptible children (95).

Childhood cancers have been suspected to arise from point mutations, and the relation to maternal age has been studied by several authors. In a population-based cohort study that included 4.3 million children, advanced maternal age was associated with early childhood cancers, particularly retinoblastoma and leukemia (96). A similar association, however, was not found for other cancers and in children up to the age of 18 years old (97). Besides leukemia, another study found an increased risk of intracranial and intraspinal embryonal brain tumors, germ cell tumors, and other malignant epithelial neoplasms and melanomas with advanced maternal age. These associations were fairly consistent in both categorical and continuous models (98).

Finally, maternal age at birth has been associated with an increased incidence of asthma, food allergy, and allergic rhinitis (99). The biologic mechanisms underlying most of these associations remain unknown. One mechanism by which maternal age could influence the health of offspring is through epigenetic modifications such as DNA methylation (100). Methylation at birth of the WNT signaling pathway, which regulates lung development and is associated with airway inflammation and remodeling in asthma, is associated with maternal age. This represents a possible mechanistic link between maternal age and risk of allergic disease (101).

Maternal age is inextricably connected with a complex system of physiological and psychosocial variables, and the challenge for future research is to better understand the relative influence of these variables on the relationship between offspring outcomes and maternal age.

Conclusions

- Reports on the impact of a very advanced maternal age describe a probability of a natural conception achieving a live birth of below 3%, odds which do not seem to improve significantly following ART treatments when using autologous oocytes.
- However, in the last decades, oocyte donation has increasingly become a more accepted and effective strategy to treat female age–related infertility, leading to a sharp increase of pregnancies at very advanced maternal age.
- This sudden surge stresses the need for a more comprehensive reflection and understanding among the medical community of the associated obstetric risks at an age when women, until recently, were seldom expecting.

REFERENCES

1. Schmidt L. Should men and women be encouraged to start childbearing at a younger age? *Expert Review of Obstetrics & Gynecology.* 2010;5(2):145–7.
2. Sauer MV. Reproduction at an advanced maternal age and maternal health. *Fertility and Sterility.* 2015;103(5):1136–43.

3. Mills M, Rindfuss RR, McDonald P, te Velde E, Reproduction E, Society Task F. Why do people postpone parenthood? Reasons and social policy incentives. *Human Reproduction Update.* 2011;17(6):848–60.
4. Jackson S, Hong C, Wang ET, Alexander C, Gregory KD, Pisarska MD. Pregnancy outcomes in very advanced maternal age pregnancies: The impact of assisted reproductive technology. *Fertility and Sterility.* 2015;103(1):76–80.
5. Claramonte Nieto M, Meler Barrabes E, Garcia Martínez S, Gutiérrez Prat M, Serra Zantop B. Impact of aging on obstetric outcomes: Defining advanced maternal age in Barcelona. *BMC Pregnancy and Childbirth.* 2019;19(1):342.
6. Martin JA, Hamilton BE, Osterman MJK, Driscoll AK. Births: Final data for 2018: National vital statistics reports: From the centers for disease control and prevention, national center for health statistics. *National Vital Statistics System.* 2019;68(13):1–47.
7. Sunkara SK, Rittenberg V, Raine-Fenning N, Bhattacharya S, Zamora J, Coomarasamy A. Association between the number of eggs and live birth in IVF treatment: An analysis of 400 135 treatment cycles. *Human Reproduction.* 2011;26(7):1768–74.
8. Vrooman LA, Nagaoka SI, Hassold TJ, Hunt PA. Evidence for paternal age-related alterations in meiotic chromosome dynamics in the mouse. *Genetics.* 2014;196(2):385–96.
9. Heffner LJ. Advanced maternal age: How old is too old? *New England Journal of Medicine.* 2004;351(19):1927–9.
10. Crawford NM, Steiner AZ. Age-related infertility. *Obstet Gynecol Clin North Am.* 2015;42(1):15–25.
11. Arya S, Mulla ZD, Plavsic SK. Outcomes of women delivering at very advanced maternal age. *Journal of Women's Health.* 2018;27(11):1378–84.
12. Berger BO, Wolfson C, Reid LD, Strobino DM. Adverse birth outcomes among women of advanced maternal age with and without health conditions in Maryland. *Women's Health Issues.* 2021;31(1):40–8.
13. Liu L, Gao J, He X, Cai Y, Wang L, Fan X. Association between assisted reproductive technology and the risk of autism spectrum disorders in the offspring: A meta-analysis. *Scientific Reports.* 2017;7:46207.
14. Bergh C, Wennerholm U-B. Long-term health of children conceived after assisted reproductive technology. *Upsala Journal of Medical Sciences.* 2020;125(2):152–7.
15. Savasi VM, Mandia L, Laoreti A, Cetin I. Maternal and fetal outcomes in oocyte donation pregnancies. *Human Reproduction Update.* 2016;22(5):620–33.
16. Berntsen S, Larsen EC, la Cour Freiesleben N, Pinborg A. Pregnancy outcomes following oocyte donation. *Best Practice & Research Clinical Obstetrics & Gynaecology.* 2020;70:81–91.
17. Rombauts L, Motteram C, Berkowitz E, Fernando S. Risk of placenta praevia is linked to endometrial thickness in a retrospective cohort study of 4537 singleton assisted reproduction technology births. *Human Reproduction.* 2014;29(12):2787–93.
18. Ribeiro VC, Santos-Ribeiro S, De Munck N, Drakopoulos P, Polyzos NP, Schutyser V, et al. Should we continue to measure endometrial thickness in modern-day medicine? The effect on live birth rates and birth weight. *Reproductive Biomedicine Online.* 2018;36(4):416–26.
19. Kasius A, Smit JG, Torrance HL, Eijkemans MJC, Mol BW, Opmeer BC, et al. Endometrial thickness and pregnancy rates after IVF: A systematic review and meta-analysis. *Human Reproduction Update.* 2014;20(4):530–41.
20. Liu KE, Hartman M, Hartman A, Luo ZC, Mahutte N. The impact of a thin endometrial lining on fresh and frozen-thaw IVF outcomes: An analysis of over 40 000 embryo transfers. *Human Reproduction (Oxford, England).* 2018;33(10):1883–8.
21. van 't Hof LJ, Dijkstra KL, van der Keur C, Eikmans M, Baelde HJ, Bos M, et al. Decreased expression of ligands of placental immune checkpoint inhibitors in uncomplicated and preeclamptic oocyte donation pregnancies. *Journal of Reproductive Immunology.* 2020;142:103194.
22. Simpson LL. Maternal cardiac disease: Update for the clinician. *Obstetrics and Gynecology.* 2012;119(2 Pt 1):345–59.
23. Chang J, Elam-Evans LD, Berg CJ, Herndon J, Flowers L, Seed KA, et al. Pregnancy-related mortality surveillance: United States, 1991–1999. *Morbidity and Mortality Weekly Report Surveillance Summaries.* 2003;52(2):1–8.
24. Callaghan WM, Berg CJ. Pregnancy-related mortality among women aged 35 years and older, United States, 1991–1997. *Obstetrics & Gynecology.* 2003;102(5, Part 1):1015–21.
25. McCall SJ, Nair M, Knight M. Factors associated with maternal mortality at advanced maternal age: A population-based case-control study. *BJOG: An International Journal of Obstetrics and Gynaecology.* 2017;124(8):1225–33.

26. Paulson RJ, Boostanfar R, Saadat P, Mor E, Tourgeman DE, Slater CC, et al. Pregnancy in the Sixth Decade of Life. *JAMA: The Journal of the American Medical Association.* 2002;288(18):2320.
27. Yogev Y, Melamed N, Bardin R, Tenenbaum-Gavish K, Ben-Shitrit G, Ben-Haroush A. Pregnancy outcome at extremely advanced maternal age. *American Journal of Obstetrics and Gynecology.* 2010;203(6):558.e1–e7.
28. Bartsch E, Medcalf KE, Park AL, Ray JG, High Risk of Pre-eclampsia Identification G. Clinical risk factors for pre-eclampsia determined in early pregnancy: Systematic review and meta-analysis of large cohort studies. *BMJ (Clinical Research Ed).* 2016;353:i1753-i.
29. Watanabe N, Fujiwara T, Suzuki T, Jwa SC, Taniguchi K, Yamanobe Y, et al. Is in vitro fertilization associated with preeclampsia? A propensity score matched study. *BMC Pregnancy and Childbirth.* 2014;14:69.
30. Luke B, Brown MB, Eisenberg ML, Callan C, Botting BJ, Pacey A, et al. In vitro fertilization and risk for hypertensive disorders of pregnancy: Associations with treatment parameters. *American Journal of Obstetrics and Gynecology.* 2020;222(4):350.e1–e13.
31. Wang Z, Liu H, Song H, Li X, Jiang J, Sheng Y, et al. Increased risk of pre-eclampsia after frozen-thawed embryo transfer in programming cycles. *Frontiers in Medicine.* 2020;7:104.
32. von Versen-Höynck F, Schaub AM, Chi Y-Y, Chiu K-H, Liu J, Lingis M, et al. Increased preeclampsia risk and reduced aortic compliance with in vitro fertilization cycles in the absence of a corpus luteum. *Hypertension (Dallas, Tex: 1979).* 2019;73(3):640–9.
33. Versen-Hoynck F, Chiu K-H, Chi Y-Y, Fleischmann RR, Zhang W, Winn VD, et al. Absence of the corpus luteum in early pregnancy increases the risk of preeclampsia. *Pregnancy Hypertension.* 2018; 13:S55.
34. Dall'Agnol H, García Velasco JA. Frozen embryo transfer and preeclampsia: Where is the link? *Curr Opin Obstet Gynecol.* 2020;32(3):213–18.
35. Rafael F, Robles GM, Navarro AM, Garrido N, Garcia-Velasco JA, Bosch E, et al. Similar perinatal outcomes in children born after fresh or frozen embryo transfer using donated oocytes. *Fertil Steril.* 2020;114(3):e108.
36. Asserhøj LL, Spangmose AL, Aaris Henningsen AK, Clausen TD, Ziebe S, Jensen RB, et al. Adverse obstetric and perinatal outcomes in 1,136 singleton pregnancies conceived after programmed Frozen Embryo Transfer (FET) compared with natural cycle FET. *Fertil Steril.* 2021;115(4):947–56.
37. Gilbert W. Childbearing beyond age 40: Pregnancy outcome in 24,032 cases. *Obstetrics & Gynecology.* 1999;93(1):9–14.
38. Atallah A, Lecarpentier E, Goffinet F, Doret-Dion M, Gaucherand P, Tsatsaris V. Aspirin for prevention of preeclampsia. *Drugs.* 2017;77(17):1819–31.
39. Askie LM, Duley L, Henderson-Smart DJ, Stewart LA. Antiplatelet agents for prevention of pre-eclampsia: A meta-analysis of individual patient data. *The Lancet.* 2007;369(9575):1791–8.
40. Kautzky-Willer A, Harreiter J, Pacini G. Sex and gender differences in risk, pathophysiology and complications of type 2 diabetes mellitus. *Endocr Rev.* 2016;37(3):278–316.
41. Cleary-Goldman J, Malone FD, Vidaver J, Ball RH, Nyberg DA, Comstock CH, et al. Impact of maternal age on obstetric outcome. *Obstetrics & Gynecology.* 2005;105(5, Part 1):983–90.
42. Li Y, Ren X, He L, Li J, Zhang S, Chen W. Maternal age and the risk of gestational diabetes mellitus: A systematic review and meta-analysis of over 120 million participants. *Diabetes Research and Clinical Practice.* 2020;162.
43. Waldenström U, Ekéus C. Risk of labor dystocia increases with maternal age irrespective of parity: A population-based register study. *Acta obstetricia et gynecologica Scandinavica.* 2017;96(9):1063–9.
44. Richards MK, Flanagan MR, Littman AJ, Burke AK, Callegari LS. Primary cesarean section and adverse delivery outcomes among women of very advanced maternal age. *Journal of Perinatology.* 2016;36(4):272–7.
45. Greenberg MB, Cheng YW, Sullivan M, Norton ME, Hopkins LM, Caughey AB. Does length of labor vary by maternal age? *American Journal of Obstetrics and Gynecology.* 2007;197(4):428.e1–e7.
46. Lin H-C, Xirasagar S. Maternal age and the likelihood of a maternal request for cesarean delivery: A 5-year population-based study. *American Journal of Obstetrics and Gynecology.* 2005;192(3):848–55.
47. Schwartz A, Many A, Shapira U, Rosenberg Friedman M, Yogev Y, Avnon T, et al. Perinatal outcomes of pregnancy in the fifth decade and beyond: A comparison of very advanced maternal age groups. *Scientific Reports.* 2020;10(1):1809.

48. Farr SL, Schieve LA, Jamieson DJ. Pregnancy loss among pregnancies conceived through assisted reproductive technology, United States, 1999–2002. *American Journal of Epidemiology*. 2007;165(12):1380–8.
49. Nybo Andersen AM, Wohlfahrt J, Christens P, Olsen J, Melbye M. Maternal age and fetal loss: Population based register linkage study. *BMJ (Clinical Research Ed)*. 2000;320(7251):1708–12.
50. Sebire NJ, Foskett M, Fisher RA, Rees H, Seckl M, Newlands E. Risk of partial and complete hydatidiform molar pregnancy in relation to maternal age. *BJOG: An International Journal of Obstetrics and Gynaecology*. 2002;109(1):99–102.
51. Gockley AA, Melamed A, Joseph NT, Clapp M, Sun SY, Goldstein DP, et al. The effect of adolescence and advanced maternal age on the incidence of complete and partial molar pregnancy. *Gynecol Oncol*. 2016;140(3):470–3.
52. Gill SK, Broussard C, Devine O, Green RF, Rasmussen SA, Reefhuis J, et al. Association between maternal age and birth defects of unknown etiology: United States, 1997–2007: Birth Defects Research Part A. *Clinical and Molecular Teratology*. 2012;94(12):1010–8.
53. Storeide O, Veholmen M, Eide M, Bergsjø P, Sandvei R. The incidence of ectopic pregnancy in Hordaland county, Norway 1976–1993. *Acta obstetricia et gynecologica Scandinavica*. 1997;76(4):345–9.
54. Attali E, Yogev Y. The impact of advanced maternal age on pregnancy outcome. *Best Practice & Research Clinical Obstetrics & Gynaecology*. 2021;70:2–9.
55. Lavecchia M, Sabbah M, Abenhaim HA. Effect of planned mode of delivery in women with advanced maternal age. *Maternal and Child Health Journal*. 2016;20(11):2318–27.
56. Park K, Wei J, Minissian M, Bairey Merz CN, Pepine CJ. Adverse pregnancy conditions, infertility, and future cardiovascular risk: Implications for mother and child. *Cardiovascular Drugs and Therapy/Sponsored by the International Society of Cardiovascular Pharmacotherapy*. 2015;29(4):391–401.
57. Casagrande JT, Louie EW, Pike MC, Roy S, Ross RK, Henderson BE. "Incessant ovulation" and ovarian cancer. *Lancet*. 1979;2(8135):170–3.
58. Kroener L, Dumesic D, Al-Safi Z. Use of fertility medications and cancer risk: A review and update. *Current Opinion in Obstetrics & Gynecology*. 2017;29(4):195–201.
59. Pettersson ML, Nedstrand E, Bladh M, Svanberg AS, Lampic C, Sydsjö G. Mothers who have given birth at an advanced age: Health status before and after childbirth. *Scientific Reports*. 2020;10(1):9739.
60. Ramlakhan KP, Johnson MR, Roos-Hesselink JW. Pregnancy and cardiovascular disease. *Nature Reviews Cardiology*. 2020;17(11):718–31.
61. Stewart LM, Holman CDAJ, Hart R, Bulsara MK, Preen DB, Finn JC. In vitro fertilization and breast cancer: Is there cause for concern? *Fertility and Sterility*. 2012;98(2):334–40.
62. van Leeuwen FE, Klip H, Mooij TM, van de Swaluw AM, Lambalk CB, Kortman M, et al. Risk of borderline and invasive ovarian tumours after ovarian stimulation for in vitro fertilization in a large Dutch cohort. *Human Reproduction*. 2011;26(12):3456–65.
63. Gennari A, Costa M, Puntoni M, Paleari L, De Censi A, Sormani MP, et al. Breast cancer incidence after hormonal treatments for infertility: Systematic review and meta-analysis of population-based studies. *Breast Cancer Research and Treatment*. 2015;150(2):405–13.
64. Kessous R, Davidson E, Meirovitz M, Sergienko R, Sheiner E. The risk of female malignancies after fertility treatments: A cohort study with 25-year follow-up. *Journal of Cancer Research and Clinical Oncology*. 2016;142(1):287–93.
65. Hannibal CG, Jensen A, Sharif H, Kjaer SK. Malignant melanoma risk after exposure to fertility drugs: Results from a large Danish cohort study. *Cancer Causes & Control*. 2008;19(7):759–65.
66. van den Belt-Dusebout AW, van Leeuwen FE, Burger CW. Breast cancer risk after ovarian stimulation for in vitro fertilization-reply. *JAMA*. 2016;316(16):1713.
67. Spaan M, van den Belt-Dusebout AW, Schaapveld M, Mooij TM, Burger CW, van Leeuwen FE, et al. Melanoma risk after ovarian stimulation for in vitro fertilization. *Human Reproduction*. 2015;30(5):1216–28.
68. Reigstad MM, Larsen IK, Myklebust TÅ, Robsahm TE, Oldereid NB, Omland AK, et al. Cancer risk among parous women following assisted reproductive technology. *Human Reproduction (Oxford, England)*. 2015;30(8):1952–63.
69. Luke B, Brown MB, Spector LG, Missmer SA, Leach RE, Williams M, et al. Cancer in women after assisted reproductive technology. *Fertility and Sterility*. 2015;104(5):1218–26.
70. Dayan N, Filion KB, Okano M, Kilmartin C, Reinblatt S, Landry T, et al. Cardiovascular risk following fertility therapy. *Journal of the American College of Cardiology*. 2017;70(10):1203–13.

71. Vassard D, Schmidt L, Glazer CH, Lyng Forman J, Kamper-Jørgensen M, Pinborg A. Assisted reproductive technology treatment and risk of ovarian cancer: A nationwide population-based cohort study. *Human Reproduction.* 2019;34(11):2290–6.
72. Aasheim V, Waldenström U, Rasmussen S, Espehaug B, Schytt E. Satisfaction with life during pregnancy and early motherhood in first-time mothers of advanced age: A population-based longitudinal study. *BMC Pregnancy and Childbirth.* 2014;14(1):86.
73. Peters SAE, Regitz-Zagrosek V. Pregnancy and risk of cardiovascular disease: Is the relationship due to childbearing or childrearing? *European Heart Journal.* 2017;38(19):1448–50.
74. Johnson JA, Tough S. No-271-delayed child-bearing. *Journal of Obstetrics and Gynaecology Canada: JOGC = Journal d'obstetrique et gynecologie du Canada: JOGC.* 2017;39(11):e500–e15.
75. McCormick MC, Richardson DK. Premature infants grow up. *New England Journal of Medicine.* 2002;346(3):197–8.
76. Hack M, Flannery DJ, Schluchter M, Cartar L, Borawski E, Klein N. Outcomes in young adulthood for very-low-birth-weight infants. *New England Journal of Medicine.* 2002;346(3):149–57.
77. Delbaere I, Verstraelen H, Goetgeluk S, Martens G, Derom C, De Bacquer D, et al. Perinatal outcome of twin pregnancies in women of advanced age. *Human Reproduction (Oxford, England).* 2008;23(9):2145–50.
78. Mutz-Dehbalaie I, Scheier M, Jerabek-Klestil S, Brantner C, Windbichler GH, Leitner H, et al. Perinatal mortality and advanced maternal age. *Gynecol Obstet Invest.* 2014;77(1):50–7.
79. Abdalla HI, Wren ME, Thomas A, Korea L. Age of the uterus does not affect pregnancy or implantation rates: A study of egg donation in women of different ages sharing oocytes from the same donor. *Human Reproduction (Oxford, England).* 1997;12(4):827–9.
80. Navot D, Drews MR, Bergh PA, Guzman I, Karstaedt A, Scott RT Jr, et al. Age-related decline in female fertility is not due to diminished capacity of the uterus to sustain embryo implantation. *Fertil Steril.* 1994;61(1):97–101.
81. Bahtiyar MO, Funai EF, Rosenberg V, Norwitz E, Lipkind H, Buhimschi C, et al. Stillbirth at term in women of advanced maternal age in the United States: When could the antenatal testing be initiated? *American Journal of Perinatology.* 2008;25(5):301–4.
82. Leader J, Bajwa A, Lanes A, Hua X, Rennicks White R, Rybak N, et al. The effect of very advanced maternal age on maternal and neonatal outcomes: A systematic review. *Journal of Obstetrics and Gynaecology Canada: JOGC = Journal d'obstetrique et gynecologie du Canada: JOGC.* 2018;40(9):1208–18.
83. Soleimani F, Vameghi R, Biglarian A. Antenatal and intrapartum risk factors for cerebral palsy in term and near-term newborns. *Archives of Iranian Medicine.* 2013;16(4):213–16.
84. Wu YW, Croen LA, Shah SJ, Newman TB, Najjar DV. Cerebral palsy in a term population: Risk factors and neuroimaging findings. *Pediatrics.* 2006;118(2):690–7.
85. Mcintyre S, Taitz D, Keogh J, Goldsmith S, Badawi N, Blair E. A systematic review of risk factors for cerebral palsy in children born at term in developed countries. *Developmental Medicine & Child Neurology.* 2013;55(6):499–508.
86. Schneider RE, Ng P, Zhang X, Andersen J, Buckley D, Fehlings D, et al. The association between maternal age and cerebral palsy risk factors. *Pediatric Neurology.* 2018;82:25–8.
87. Vadivelan K, Sekar P, Sruthi SS, Gopichandran V. Burden of caregivers of children with cerebral palsy: An intersectional analysis of gender, poverty, stigma, and public policy. *BMC Public Health.* 2020;20(1):645.
88. Sandin S, Hultman CM, Kolevzon A, Gross R, MacCabe JH, Reichenberg A. Advancing maternal age is associated with increasing risk for autism: A review and meta-analysis. *Journal of the American Academy of Child and Adolescent Psychiatry.* 2012;51(5):477–86.e1.
89. Grether JK, Anderson MC, Croen LA, Smith D, Windham GC. Risk of autism and increasing maternal and paternal age in a large north American population. *American Journal of Epidemiology.* 2009;170(9):1118–26.
90. Shelton JF, Tancredi DJ, Hertz-Picciotto I. Independent and dependent contributions of advanced maternal and paternal ages to autism risk. *Autism Research: Official Journal of the International Society for Autism Research.* 2010;3(1):30–9.
91. Tearne JE. Older maternal age and child behavioral and cognitive outcomes: A review of the literature. *Fertil Steril.* 2015;103(6):1381–91.

92. Tearne JE, Robinson M, Jacoby P, Li J, Newnham J, McLean N. Does late childbearing increase the risk for behavioural problems in children? A longitudinal cohort study. *Paediatric and Perinatal Epidemiology*. 2015;29(1):41–9.
93. Delli AJ, Lernmark Å. Chapter 39: Type 1 (insulin-dependent) diabetes mellitus: Etiology, pathogenesis, prediction, and prevention. In: Jameson JL, De Groot LJ, de Kretser DM, Giudice LC, Grossman AB, Melmed S, et al., editors. *Endocrinology: Adult and pediatric*. 7th ed. Philadelphia: W.B. Saunders; 2016. pp. 672–90.e5.
94. Cardwell CR, Stene LC, Joner G, Bulsara MK, Cinek O, Rosenbauer J, et al. Maternal age at birth and childhood type 1 diabetes: A pooled analysis of 30 observational studies. *Diabetes*. 2010;59(2):486–94.
95. Rasmussen T, Stene LC, Samuelsen SO, Cinek O, Wetlesen T, Torjesen PA, et al. Maternal BMI before pregnancy, maternal weight gain during pregnancy, and risk of persistent positivity for multiple diabetes-associated autoantibodies in children with the high-risk HLA genotype. *MIDIA Study*. 2009;32(10):1904–6.
96. Yip BH, Pawitan Y, Czene K. Parental age and risk of childhood cancers: A population-based cohort study from Sweden. *International Journal of Epidemiology*. 2006;35(6):1495–503.
97. Imterat M, Wainstock T, Sheiner E, Kapelushnik J, Walfisch A. 146: Advanced maternal age and the risk for long-term malignant morbidity in the offspring. *Am J Obstet Gynecol*. 2018;218:S102.
98. Contreras ZA, Hansen J, Ritz B, Olsen J, Yu F, Heck JE. Parental age and childhood cancer risk: A Danish population-based registry study. *Cancer Epidemiology*. 2017;49:202–15.
99. Lu HY, Chiu CW, Kao PH, Tsai ZT, Gau CC, Lee WF, et al. Association between maternal age at delivery and allergic rhinitis in schoolchildren: A population-based study. *World Allergy Organization Journal*. 2020;13(6):100127.
100. Markunas CA, Wilcox AJ, Xu Z, Joubert BR, Harlid S, Panduri V, et al. Maternal age at delivery is associated with an epigenetic signature in both newborns and adults. *PLoS One*. 2016;11(7):e0156361-e.
101. Holloway J, White C, Alzahrani A, Zhang H, Mansfield L, Arshad H, et al. Epigenome-wide association study of the effect of maternal age on offspring DNA methylation. *Journal of Allergy and Clinical Immunology*. 2018;141:AB279.
102. Yeh JS, Steward RG, Dude AM, Shah AA, Goldfarb JM, Muasher SJ. Pregnancy outcomes decline in recipients over age 44: An analysis of 27,959 fresh donor oocyte in vitro fertilization cycles from the Society for Assisted Reproductive Technology. *Fertility and Sterility*. 2014;101(5):1331–6.e1.

10

Obstetric, perinatal, and postnatal outcomes after PGT

Danilo Cimadomo, Letizia Papini, Nicoletta Barnocchi,
Laura Rienzi, and Filippo Maria Ubaldi

Introduction

According to the recent revision of the terminology used in assisted reproduction (1), the term preimplantation genetic testing (PGT) replaced the previously used terms preimplantation genetic diagnosis and screening (PGD and PGS). In the early 1990s, PGD was performed to identify embryos not affected from single gene defects, but soon its main application was testing chromosomal aneuploidies (at present preimplantation genetic testing for aneuploidies [PGT-A]) in advanced maternal age (AMA) women or patients suffering from repeated implantation failure (RIF), recurrent pregnancy loss (RPL), or severe male factor (SMF) (2). The sample to analyze was retrieved from a cleavage-stage embryo (i.e., a single blastomere) and submitted to fluorescent in situ hybridization (FISH) to visualize nine chromosomes. However, some limitations undermined the clinical value of this workflow, mainly the nature of the sample analyzed (i.e., a single cell from a precocious stage of preimplantation development) and the limited predictive power of the technique applied (3). The latter was soon replaced with more reliable comprehensive chromosome testing (CCT) approaches, like array comparative genomic hybridization (array-CGH), single nucleotide polymorphism array (SNP-array), quantitative polymerase chain reaction (qPCR), and next-generation sequencing (NGS). Conversely, the blastomere biopsy approach is still widely used worldwide, although two other strategies have been implemented clinically across the years, i.e., polar body biopsy and trophectoderm biopsy.

Any biopsy procedure is characterized by two steps: zona pellucida (ZP) opening and subsequent sample removal. ZP opening can be achieved mechanically (partial zona dissection) with a sharp micropipette, chemically through acidified Tyrode's medium, or via a laser beam (laser drilling). As introduced previously, the genetic material used for PGT can be of different origins: polar bodies from the oocyte and zygote, a blastomere from a cleavage-stage embryo, or five to ten trophectoderm cells from a blastocyst. The first approach is mainly adopted in countries where the biopsy cannot be performed after syngamy, although it is the most time-consuming approach and suffers from both technical and biological limitations due to the single-cell nature of the samples retrieved and the impossibility to assess paternal meiotic and mitotic errors possibly occurring postfertilization (4).

Some milestone papers compared the postbiopsy embryo developmental and implantation behavior between the two other approaches (5, 6), providing evidence that blastomere biopsy is detrimental for the embryo, while trophectoderm biopsy is not. Indeed, at present, trophectoderm biopsy combined with ZP opening, CCT, and vitrified-warmed transfer is the gold-standard workflow for PGT (4, 7). This approach is characterized by high reproducibility and reliability among experienced operators (8–10); still it involves further embryo manipulation if compared with conventional IVF. Therefore, many authors attempted to investigate whether an effect exists on obstetric, perinatal, and neonatal outcomes due to PGT. However, these studies are highly subject to biases because of (i) the heterogeneity of the biopsy strategies, indications to PGT, and/or transfer strategies; (ii) the fact that these outcomes are always secondary to the clinical ones (implantation, miscarriage, live birth); and (iii) the fact that the population of women involved is a subset of poor prognosis and AMA patients that can be hardly compared to the general in vitro fertilization (IVF) population or to women undergoing spontaneous conception. As a matter of fact, conflicting results were reported from the numerous studies comparing PGT pregnancies with conventional IVF or spontaneous conception, suggesting the need for an appropriate meta-analysis.

In a national multicenter study, Bay and colleagues (11) highlighted an increased prevalence of perinatal and neonatal risks in babies born after PGT conducted on cleavage-stage biopsies when compared to spontaneous conception and a higher prevalence of cesarean section and longer permanence in the neonatal intensive care unit (NICU) when compared to the conventional IVF group. Conversely, a meta-analysis by Hasson and colleagues (12) suggested that PGT-derived pregnancies involved similar obstetric, perinatal, and neonatal outcomes as conventional IVF. This evidence was supported also by the comprehensive systematic review and meta-analysis by Natsuaki and Dimler (13), who excluded an adverse effect of any biopsy approach adopted to PGT purposes on all obstetric, perinatal, and neonatal outcomes, including long term ones.

In this chapter, we summarized the evidence provided to date on this topic for each biopsy strategy adopted clinically for PGT purposes across the years. All the papers and inherent relevant information are summarized in Table 10.1.

Obstetric outcomes

Despite the increasing use of PGT, there has been very little examination of obstetric outcomes after its application, including placental complications (placental abruption, placenta previa, placenta accreta, manual lysis of the placenta, uterine revision), hypertensive disorders, preeclampsia, gestational diabetes, preterm premature rupture of membranes, postpartum hemorrhage, cesarean section delivery, induction of labor, and blood transfusion rate. Some concerns were moved in particular towards the use of trophectoderm biopsy, stating that this approach involved the removal of cells that will evolve as embryonic annexes, like the placenta itself.

Polar body biopsy

Polar bodies are waste products of maternal meiosis, and their removal from the oocyte and zygote can be performed with no impact on embryo development and implantation potential, as demonstrated by the European Society of Human Reproduction and Embryology (ESHRE) multicenter study published in 2018 (14). When it comes to pregnancy complications, few, but reassuring, data have been published.

The first work investigating obstetric outcomes after PGT performed through the sequential removal of both polar bodies for either single-gene disorders or aneuploidy testing dates back to 2000. The authors reported no significant detrimental effect on the first 102 children born after the application of this workflow at their center, with the exception of placenta previa, which showed a 4% prevalence with respect to the 0.4% reported after conventional IVF (15). More recently, Eldar-Geva and colleagues published a prospective follow-up cohort study comparing the obstetric outcomes of all PGT newborns after either polar body or blastomere biopsies versus both conventional IVF and spontaneous conception matched for maternal age, parity, and body mass index (16). Except for a higher adoption of cesarean section in singleton pregnancies after IVF with (28.5%) or without PGT (31.6%) with respect to spontaneous conception (11%), all other outcomes (e.g., prevalence of hypertension and gestational diabetes) were comparable in the three groups.

Blastomere biopsy

Blastomere biopsy is usually performed 72 hours post-insemination, when the embryo shows six to eight cells. As for polar body biopsy, only a few studies are available that investigated the prevalence of obstetric complications after blastomere biopsy.

Besides the already mentioned Eldar-Geva et al. study (16), another group investigated pregnancy and neonatal complications after blastomere biopsy. Here the authors compared two PGT workflows: cleavage-stage biopsy and fresh embryo transfer (CB-ET) (129 patients) and blastocyst-stage biopsy and

TABLE 10.1
Characteristics of the Studies Investigating the Potential Effects of PGT on Obstetric, Perinatal, and Postnatal Outcomes

Paper	Study Design	Sample Size	Biopsy Approach	Genetic Testing Technique	Obstetric Outcomes	Perinatal Outcomes	Postnatal Long Term Outcomes
Strom, 2000	Observational	102 PGT-derived newborns vs. IVF	PBs biopsy	FISH	Higher prevalence of placenta previa	No negative effect	—
Strom, 2000	Observational	109 PGT-derived newborns vs. IVF	PBs biopsy	FISH	—	No negative effect	—
Eldar-Geva, 2014	Follow-up of an observational study	245 PGT-derived newborns vs. 242 ICSI-derived newborns vs. 733 SC-derived newborns	PBs biopsy and blastomere biopsy	FISH, PCR, a-CGH, SNP-array	No effect	Gestational age and birth weight better in PGT-derived newborns (and SC) compared with ICSI-derived newborns Higher prevalence of LGA in PGT-derived singletons than SC-derived ones	
Bay, 2016	Observational with historical control	149 PGT-derived newborns vs. 36,115 IVF-derived newborns vs. 90,9624 SC-derived newborns	Blastomere biopsy	—	Higher prevalence of placenta previa, cesarean section, preterm birth in PGT- and IVF-derived vs. SC-derived conceptions Solely cesarean section was more prevalent in PGT-derived pregnancies vs. IVF-derived ones	Longer NICU permanence for PGT-derived newborns vs. IVF-derived ones	
Hasson, 2017	Observational	89 PGT-derived pregnancies vs. 166 ICSI-derived pregnancies	Blastomere biopsy	—	No negative effect	No negative effect	—
Heijlingers, 2018	Observational with historical control	366 PGT-derived newborns vs. EUROCAT	Blastomere biopsy	FISH or PCR		No negative effect	
Kuiper, 2018	Follow-up of a RCT	43 PGT-derived newborns vs. 56 IVF-derived newborns	Blastomere biopsy		—	—	No negative effect

Belva, 2018	Observational	87 PGT-derived newborns vs. 87 ICSI-derived newborns	Blastomere biopsy	–	–	–	No negative effect
Jing, 2016	Observational	317 PGT-derived newborns after 3 strategies: 129 CB-ET, 22 CB-FET, 166 BB-FET	Blastomere biopsy and TE biopsy	FISH or PCR	Higher prevalence of gestational diabetes, hypertension, and postpartum hemorrhage in BB-FET vs. CB-ET	Worse general neonatal outcomes with CB-ET vs. BB-FET	–
Natsuaki and Dimler, 2018	Meta-analysis	18 studies on PGT	Blastomere biopsy, TE biopsy	FISH, aCGH, CCT, NGS	–	–	No effect
Forman, 2014	Follow-up of a RCT	89 euploid SET vs. 86 untested DET	TE biopsy	qPCR	No negative effect	No negative effect	–
Zhang, 2019	Observational	177 PGT-derived newborns vs. 180 IVF-derived babies	TE biopsy	–	Higher prevalence of preeclampsia in PGT-derived pregnancies	No negative effect	–
Sacchi, 2019	Observational	370 PGT-derived pregnancies vs. 2,168 IVF-derived pregnancies	TE biopsy	qPCR	No negative effect	No negative effect	–

Abbreviations: *PGT*, preimplantation genetic testing; *ICSI*, intracytoplasmic sperm injection; *IVF*, in vitro fertilization; *SC*, spontaneous conception; *PBs*, polar bodies; *TE*, trophectoderm; *FISH*, fluorescence in situ hybridization; *PCR*, polymerase chain reaction; *aCGH*, array-comparative genomic hybridization; *SNP-array*, single nucleotide polymorphism array; *NGS*, next-generation sequencing; *qPCR*, quantitative-PCR; *LGA*, large for gestational age; *NICU*, neonatal intensive care unit; *CB-ET*, cleavage-stage biopsy and fresh embryo transfer; *CB-FET*, cleavage biopsy and frozen embryo transfer; *BB-FET*, blastocyst-stage biopsy and frozen embryo transfer; –, not reported; *SET*, single embryo transfer; *DET*, double embryo transfer.

frozen embryo transfer (BB-FET) (166 patients). Of note, while ZP opening was performed exclusively with the laser, different approaches were adopted for genetic testing (FISH, PCR, array-CGH, or SNP-array). They reported a higher prevalence of gestational hypertension and postpartum hemorrhage in the BB-FET group, while comparable results were shown for gestational diabetes, gestational anemia, placenta previa, and cesarean section (17). Possibly though, the differences are imputable to the different transfer strategy (frozen versus fresh) rather than to the different biopsy strategy (trophectoderm versus blastomere) (18). In 2016, Bay et al. published a study involving the multicentric obstetric and neonatal follow-up of pregnancies achieved after blastomere biopsy–based PGT, which were compared to conventional IVF-derived pregnancies and spontaneous conceptions. Both conventional IVF- and PGT-derived pregnancies resulted in a higher prevalence of placenta previa, cesarean section, and preterm birth when compared to spontaneous conception. When they were instead compared against each other, only the prevalence of cesarean section was different. Therefore, this study suggests no negative impact of the biopsy on the outcomes under investigation (11). In 2017, Hasson and colleagues compared the outcomes of singleton and twin pregnancies achieved after blastomere biopsy–based PGT and blastocyst fresh embryo transfer versus conventional IVF-derived pregnancies. No difference was reported in the two groups (12).

Trophectoderm biopsy

The trophectoderm biopsy approach has been gradually implemented in IVF from the end of the first decade of the 21st century, progressively replacing especially blastomere biopsy. The underlying reasons for this change are (i) the possibility to analyze more cells, (ii) the possibility to retrieve a sample from a section of the blastocyst that gives origin to the embryonic annexes and not to the embryo proper, (iii) the absence of a reported impact on embryo implantation potential, and (iv) the high positive and negative clinical predictive value when associated with CCT techniques (7).

In 2014, Forman and colleagues published the obstetric and perinatal follow-up outcomes of a randomized controlled trial published the former year that compared the clinical pregnancy and twin pregnancy rates in case of a single euploid rather than a double untested blastocyst transfer strategy. In the original study, these two strategies elicited similar clinical pregnancy rates with exclusively singletons when a single euploid blastocyst was transferred versus half twins when two untested blastocysts were instead transferred (19). Clearly, this in turn involved a significantly lower birth weight, higher preterm birth rates, and longer permanence in the NICU for the babies born with the latter strategy (20).

The previously mentioned paper published by Jing and colleagues in 2016 reported only a higher prevalence of gestational hypertension in the BB-FET group with respect to the CB-ET one (17), but all other outcomes were comparable.

At last, the recent observational cohort study by Zhang and colleagues compared 177 pregnancies achieved via IVF and trophectoderm biopsy–based PGT with 180 pregnancies achieved without PGT in the period 2011–2017 in their university-affiliated fertility center (21): no difference was unveiled, except for a higher prevalence of preeclampsia.

Perinatal and neonatal outcomes

Perinatal and neonatal outcomes include all the events occurring from the 28th gestational week until the 28th day after delivery, like preterm delivery (<37 weeks), early preterm delivery (<34 weeks), intrauterine growth restriction (IUGR; birth weight below the 10th percentile for gestational age), large for gestational age (LGA; birth weight above the 90th percentile), low birth weight (<2500 g), very low birth weight (<1500 g), birth defect, Apgar score at 5 minutes, NICU admission, jaundice, and morbidity (hypoglycemia, hypothermia, intraventricular hemorrhage, infection, sepsis, respiratory distress syndrome).

Polar body biopsy

In their study published in 2014 and already mentioned previously, Eldar-Geva et al. evaluated the perinatal outcomes of the three different populations of babies born between January 2005 and

December 2012 from age-, body mass index-, and parity-matched mothers, specifically 245 after polar body or blastomere biopsy–based PGT with mechanical ZP opening, 242 after conventional IVF, and 733 after spontaneous conception (16). PGT singleton newborns were comparable to babies conceived spontaneously, except for a higher prevalence of LGA. This prevalence was comparable to conventional IVF–derived newborns. This evidence complies with the reassuring data reported by Strom and colleagues in 2000 (22). Moreover, in Eldar-Geva and colleagues' study, the gestational age was longer and the birth weight higher in PGT- and SC-derived newborns compared with ICSI-derived ones. However, such a worse outcome in the latter arm of the study might be due to the assessment of only PGT-M cycles, and therefore possibly mostly fertile couples; infertility in the ICSI arm, instead, is an important confounder in the evaluation of gestational and perinatal outcomes, which might have biased the analysis.

Blastomere biopsy

In the same paper previously mentioned, Eldar-Geva and colleagues confirmed a higher gestational age and birth weight in the PGT-M group in case of blastomere biopsy application as well. Then, Bay et al.'s national multicenter report published in 2016 highlighted that the babies born in Denmark after PGT cycles entailing laser-assisted or acidified Tyrode's solution–based ZP opening and the biopsy of one or two blastomeres showed similar perinatal and neonatal risks compared to conventional IVF, except for a longer NICU admission (11). The results in both these groups were instead poorer when compared to babies conceived spontaneously; therefore, it is difficult to say which IVF procedure could be responsible for this or whether it is imputable to the poorer prognosis of the infertile women who undergoes IVF. In fact, the women in the PGT group were older and showed a 30% prevalence of twin pregnancy rather than 3% after spontaneous conception. Moreover, the sample size was too limited to draw any conclusion.

Jing et al. in their study (17) compared the data from 317 PGT babies clustered in three groups: CB-ET, CB-FET, and BB-FET. The mean gestational age was similar. Among twins, the median gestational age was lower in the CB-ET than in the BB-FET group, while the preterm birth prevalence was higher. The birth weight was lower in the CB-ET than in the BB-FET group. Again, it is difficult to assess whether the differences reported from this study are imputable to the stage of embryo transfer (ET) (cleavage versus blastocyst), the strategy of ET (fresh versus frozen), or the biopsy approach (blastomere versus trophectoderm).

Hasson and colleagues in their study also reported perinatal and neonatal outcomes (12). No difference emerged for preterm and early delivery, IUGR, low and very low birth weight, and malformations when comparing babies born after blastomere biopsy and blastocyst transfer with babies born from non-biopsied embryos transferred at the blastocyst stage.

In a recent report, Heijligers et al. showed the data from 439 pregnancies and 366 babies born from PGT cycles conducted between 1995 and 2014 in the Netherlands via laser-assisted ZP opening and the removal of one or two blastomeres analyzed then by FISH or PCR (23). The gestational weeks, birth weight, and prevalence of malformations were similar to conventional IVF–derived and spontaneously conceived babies. Therefore, also in this case, blastomere biopsy was deemed safe for the newborns. Of note, in this and in Hasson et al.'s studies, only PGT cycles for monogenic conditions (PGT-M) were examined to avoid the bias of AMA, RIF, or RPL conditions on the perinatal and neonatal outcomes.

Trophectoderm biopsy

Only a few recent studies exist on this topic. The observational cohort study by Zhang et al. published in 2019 described the perinatal and neonatal outcomes of 177 newborns obtained after PGT and compared to 180 conventional IVF–derived babies (21). No statistically significant differences emerged. In particular, the mean gestational age, prevalence of preterm birth, and average birth weight were all similar. In the same year, Sacchi et al. published another observational study analyzing perinatal and neonatal outcomes in PGT-A babies born after trophectoderm biopsy (24). Also, this group reported no increase in obstetric, perinatal, and neonatal risks with respect to the transfer of one to two cleavage-stage untested embryos or one untested blastocyst. This study reinforced the evidence already published by Forman

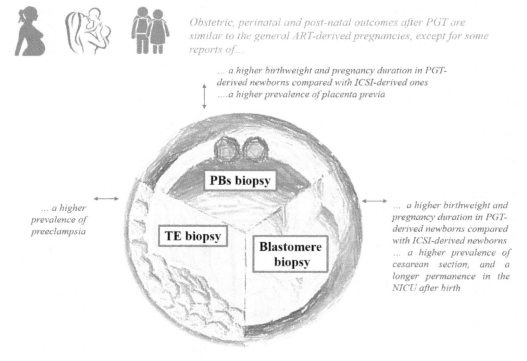

FIGURE 10.1 Summary of the obstetric, perinatal, and postnatal outcomes reported in the literature for the comparison between preimplantation genetic testing (PGT)–derived and general assisted reproduction technique (ART)–derived pregnancies and newborns.

Abbreviations: *PBs* polar bodies; *TE* trophectoderm; *LGA* large for gestational age, *NICU* neonatal intensive care unit.

and colleagues in 2014 (20): blastocyst-stage biopsy associated with single euploid blastocyst transfer represents a clinically effective strategy, which is also safe for the mother and the newborn.

Long term outcomes in children after PGT

It has been suggested that IVF babies, probably because of the intrinsic condition of infertility of their parents, might be exposed to less favorable neurodevelopmental and cardiometabolic outcomes. However, studies properly analyzing this issue in the absence of inherent biases are difficult to design. In turn, a potential long term impact of embryo biopsy on the babies born after PGT is yet undefined, although some studies attempted to provide some information on this topic.

In 2018, Kuiper et al. analyzed the neurodevelopment in a group of 9-year-old children born after PGT (25) during a randomized controlled trial. The data were compared to the conventional IVF–derived babies as part of the control group. In particular, the neurological optimality score, i.e., a sensitive measure of neurological condition (Touwen test), has been set as a primary outcome, while adverse neurological conditions, cognitive development, behavior, blood pressure, and anthropometrics were set as secondary ones. No significant differences were reported between the two groups. Overall these babies showed an increased prevalence of adverse neurological outcomes compared to the general population, as well as a higher mean blood pressure than expected. However, this evidence is in line with the literature focused on IVF-derived children (26).

In the same year, Belva and colleagues reported the data from a cohort study assessing the body composition (anthropometry) and blood pressure in a group of 6-year-old children conceived after IVF with (n = 87) or without (n = 87) blastomere biopsy for PGT-M or PGT-SR and blastocyst transfer (27). No difference was reported in the two groups. Of note, given that no PGT-A patient was included in this investigation, the study group is characterized from a population of patients not necessarily infertile because of AMA, RIF, or RPL indications.

Natsuaki and Dimler, in their meta-analysis (13), reinforced the evidence produced from Kuiper and Belva by stating that no anthropometric, psychomotor, neurological, cognitive, and behavioral issue has been reported to date related to any embryo biopsy approach.

Future perspectives

The novel avant-garde nature of non-invasive PGT (ni-PGT) represents an intriguing future perspective in terms of safety in this field (30). In fact, if performing chromosomal testing on the spent culture media after blastocyst culture, we might keep the embryo completely undisturbed. The evidence produced to date for embryo selection purposes is promising, although some concerns exist, especially related to the risk for maternal contamination and false-positive/-negative diagnoses. Non-selection studies and randomized controlled trials are currently in the pipeline, which will define the real clinical value of ni-PGT.

Conclusions

- Several studies and international consensuses outlined trophectoderm biopsy plus CCT as the current gold-standard workflow (28, 29).
- Nonetheless, even if in the hands of trained and skilled operators, more embryonic manipulations are required during PGT cycles than during conventional IVF ones.
- Consistent evidence exists to support the safety of both polar body and trophectoderm biopsy in terms of embryo implantation, and this is mirrored also by the reassuring obstetric, prenatal, neonatal, and long term postnatal developmental outcomes reported to date.
- PGT-derived outcomes are similar to ART-derived ones in general, except for the few pieces of evidence summarized in Figure 10.1.
- Systematic reviews and meta-analyses are required on this issue, especially for the most recent vitrified-warmed single euploid blastocyst transfer approach.

REFERENCES

1. Zegers-Hochschild F, Adamson GD, Dyer S, Racowsky C, de Mouzon J, Sokol R, et al. The international glossary on infertility and fertility care, 2017. *Fertil Steril.* 2017;108:393–406.
2. Coonen E, Rubio C, Christopikou D, Dimitriadou E, Gontar J, Goossens V, et al. ESHRE PGT Consortium good practice recommendations for the detection of structural and numerical chromosomal aberrations. *Hum Reprod Open.* 2020;2020:hoaa017.
3. Mastenbroek S, Twisk M, van der Veen F, Repping S. Preimplantation genetic screening: A systematic review and meta-analysis of RCTs. *Hum Reprod Update.* 2011;17:454–66.
4. Kokkali G, Coticchio G, Bronet F, Celebi C, Cimadomo D, Goossens V, et al. ESHRE PGT Consortium and SIG embryology good practice recommendations for polar body and embryo biopsy for PGT. *Hum Reprod Open.* 2020;2020:hoaa020.
5. Scott RT, Jr, Upham KM, Forman EJ, Zhao T, Treff NR. Cleavage-stage biopsy significantly impairs human embryonic implantation potential while blastocyst biopsy does not: A randomized and paired clinical trial. *Fertil Steril.* 2013;100:624–30.
6. Scott KL, Hong KH, Scott RT, Jr. Selecting the optimal time to perform biopsy for preimplantation genetic testing. *Fertil Steril.* 2013;100:608–14.

7. Cimadomo D, Rienzi L, Capalbo A, Rubio C, Innocenti F, Garcia-Pascual CM, et al. The dawn of the future: 30 years from the first biopsy of a human embryo: The detailed history of an ongoing revolution. *Hum Reprod Update.* 2020.
8. Capalbo A, Ubaldi FM, Cimadomo D, Maggiulli R, Patassini C, Dusi L, et al. Consistent and reproducible outcomes of blastocyst biopsy and aneuploidy screening across different biopsy practitioners: A multicentre study involving 2586 embryo biopsies. *Hum Reprod.* 2016;31:199–208.
9. Cimadomo D, Capalbo A, Levi-Setti PE, Soscia D, Orlando G, Albani E, et al. Associations of blastocyst features, trophectoderm biopsy and other laboratory practice with post-warming behavior and implantation. *Hum Reprod.* 2018;33:1992–2001.
10. Cimadomo D, Rienzi L, Romanelli V, Alviggi E, Levi-Setti PE, Albani E, et al. Inconclusive chromosomal assessment after blastocyst biopsy: Prevalence, causative factors and outcomes after re-biopsy and re-vitrification: A multicenter experience. *Hum Reprod.* 2018;33:1839–46.
11. Bay B, Ingerslev HJ, Lemmen JG, Degn B, Rasmussen IA, Kesmodel US. Preimplantation genetic diagnosis: A national multicenter obstetric and neonatal follow-up study. *Fertil Steril.* 2016;106:1363–9 e1.
12. Hasson J, Limoni D, Malcov M, Frumkin T, Amir H, Shavit T, et al. Obstetric and neonatal outcomes of pregnancies conceived after preimplantation genetic diagnosis: Cohort study and meta-analysis. *Reprod Biomed Online.* 2017;35:208–18.
13. Natsuaki MN, Dimler LM. Pregnancy and child developmental outcomes after preimplantation genetic screening: A meta-analytic and systematic review. *World J Pediatr.* 2018;14:555–69.
14. Verpoest W, Staessen C, Bossuyt PM, Goossens V, Altarescu G, Bonduelle M, et al. Preimplantation genetic testing for aneuploidy by microarray analysis of polar bodies in advanced maternal age: A randomized clinical trial. *Hum Reprod.* 2018;33:1767–76.
15. Strom CM, Strom S, Levine E, Ginsberg N, Barton J, Verlinsky Y. Obstetric outcomes in 102 pregnancies after preimplantation genetic diagnosis. *Am J Obstet Gynecol.* 2000;182:1629–32.
16. Eldar-Geva T, Srebnik N, Altarescu G, Varshaver I, Brooks B, Levy-Lahad E, et al. Neonatal outcome after preimplantation genetic diagnosis. *Fertil Steril.* 2014;102:1016–21.
17. Jing S, Luo K, He H, Lu C, Zhang S, Tan Y, et al. Obstetric and neonatal outcomes in blastocyst-stage biopsy with frozen embryo transfer and cleavage-stage biopsy with fresh embryo transfer after preimplantation genetic diagnosis/screening. *Fertil Steril.* 2016;106:105–12 e4.
18. Roque M, Haahr T, Geber S, Esteves SC, Humaidan P. Fresh versus elective frozen embryo transfer in IVF/ICSI cycles: A systematic review and meta-analysis of reproductive outcomes. *Hum Reprod Update.* 2019;25:2–14.19. Forman EJ, Hong KH, Ferry KM, Tao X, Taylor D, Levy B, et al. In vitro fertilization with single euploid blastocyst transfer: A randomized controlled trial. *Fertil Steril.* 2013;100:100–7 e1.
20. Forman EJ, Hong KH, Franasiak JM, Scott RT, Jr. Obstetrical and neonatal outcomes from the BEST Trial: Single embryo transfer with aneuploidy screening improves outcomes after in vitro fertilization without compromising delivery rates. *Am J Obstet Gynecol.* 2014;210:157 e1–6.
21. Zhang WY, von Versen-Hoynck F, Kapphahn KI, Fleischmann RR, Zhao Q, Baker VL. Maternal and neonatal outcomes associated with trophectoderm biopsy. *Fertil Steril.* 2019;112:283–90 e2.
22. Strom CM, Levin R, Strom S, Masciangelo C, Kuliev A, Verlinsky Y. Neonatal outcome of preimplantation genetic diagnosis by polar body removal: The first 109 infants. *Pediatrics.* 2000;106:650–3.
23. Heijligers M, van Montfoort A, Meijer-Hoogeveen M, Broekmans F, Bouman K, Homminga I, et al. Perinatal follow-up of children born after preimplantation genetic diagnosis between 1995 and 2014. *J Assist Reprod Genet.* 2018;35:1995–2002.
24. Sacchi L, Albani E, Cesana A, Smeraldi A, Parini V, Fabiani M, et al. Preimplantation genetic testing for aneuploidy improves clinical, gestational, and neonatal outcomes in advanced maternal age patients without compromising cumulative live-birth rate. *J Assist Reprod Genet.* 2019;36:2493–504.
25. Kuiper D, Bennema A, la Bastide-van Gemert S, Seggers J, Schendelaar P, Mastenbroek S, et al. Developmental outcome of 9-year-old children born after PGS: Follow-up of a randomized trial. *Hum Reprod.* 2018;33:147–55.
26. Guo XY, Liu XM, Jin L, Wang TT, Ullah K, Sheng JZ, et al. Cardiovascular and metabolic profiles of offspring conceived by assisted reproductive technologies: A systematic review and meta-analysis. *Fertil Steril.* 2017;107:622–31 e5.

27. Belva F, Roelants M, Kluijfhout S, Winter C, De Schrijver F, Desmyttere S, et al. Body composition and blood pressure in 6-year-old singletons born after pre-implantation genetic testing for monogenic and structural chromosomal aberrations: A matched cohort study. *Hum Reprod Open.* 2018;2018:hoy013.
28. Dahdouh EM, Balayla J, Garcia-Velasco JA. Comprehensive chromosome screening improves embryo selection: A meta-analysis. *Fertil Steril.* 2015;104:1503–12.
29. Chen M, Wei S, Hu J, Quan S. Can comprehensive chromosome screening technology improve IVF/ICSI outcomes? A meta-analysis. *PLoS One.* 2015;10:e0140779.
30. Leaver M, Wells D. Non-Invasive Preimplantation Genetic Testing (niPGT): The next revolution in reproductive genetics? *Hum Reprod Update.* 2020;26:16–42.

11

Multiple birth outcomes

A minimizing strategy for elective single embryo transfer

Zdravka Veleva

Introduction

In vitro fertilization (IVF) treatment and other assisted reproductive technologies (ARTs) comprising intracytoplasmic sperm injection (ICSI) and frozen-thawed embryo transfer (FET) have been increasing for the last 40 years. Significant scientific and technological breakthroughs have made ART treatment more effective than ever. This has led to improved embryo implantation rates and to the significant problem of multiple gestations after the transfer of more than one embryo.

The present chapter will provide an overview of the health problems to mothers and babies caused by multiple births after ART treatment, the history of embryo transfer, and the consequences of elective single embryo transfer (eSET) on multiple birth outcomes.

Multiple births after ART treatment

Natural gestation in the human is a singleton pregnancy. Among spontaneous gestations, dizygotic twins are observed in 12% of pregnancies (1), and monozygotic twins occur in 0.4% of pregnancies (according to Hellin's law). Rates of triplet and higher-order multiple pregnancies (quadruplet and even higher) (HOM) are even lower. In 2019, the Centers for Disease Control and Prevention (CDC) reported an overall twin rate of 32 per 1,000 live births and an overall triplet and HOM rate of 88/100,000 births (1). Because of the increased nutrient and metabolic requirements caused by the increased number of fetuses to carry, multiple gestations are characterized by premature births and restricted intrauterine growth, which determine higher morbidity and mortality for both mothers and babies. Multiple pregnancies after ART are further complicated by the underlying infertility causes as well as other factors, such as immunological conflict in case of donated oocytes or embryos.

History of multiple pregnancies in ART

In the early years of IVF practice, understanding of ovarian stimulation and embryo culture was in its initial phases, and consequently, treatment was characterized by very low chances of implantation into the uterus and subsequent live birth. This can be seen in the first annual reports of the Society for Assisted Reproductive Technologies (SART) that showed data for the year 1985 (2). In IVF, a median number of 2.8 embryos were transferred, with only 14.1% of cycles leading to clinical pregnancy (i.e., pregnancy with visible heartbeat at ultrasound examination). Of these pregnancies, only about half continued to live birth, and the overall live birth rate was only 7%.

The 1990s were characterized by improvement of embryo media cultures and increased knowledge about ovarian stimulation protocols. This is reflected in the report of SART for 1990 that showed the overall live birth rate after IVF had increased to 17% (3). However, during that time three to seven or even more embryos were routinely transferred, resulting in an overall multiple delivery rate of 22% (3).

This practice was typical in Europe as well and gave rise to the so-called "multiple birth epidemic" that was observed in the 1990s and the early 2000s. At its peak, there were up to 29% twin and 11.4% triplet and HOM in the United States (4), making the total number of multiple pregnancies over 40% in all.

In Europe, multiple birth rates followed a similar pattern. The first report of the European IVF Monitoring Programme (EIM) described treatment outcomes in 18 European countries for 1997 (5). The distribution of transfer of one, two, three, and four or more embryos was 11.5%, 35.9%, 38.4%, and 14.3%, respectively. Total multiple birth rates were 28.2%–29.6%, depending on fertilization technique. The percentage of HOM out of all births was 3.8% for IVF and 3.0% for ICSI; however there were significant variations per country, and the frequency of triplet deliveries ranged from 0.0% (Latvia) to 8.2% (Bulgaria). Data for 2002 for Europe, the United States, Australia and New Zealand, and individual Latin American and Middle East countries showed an overall twin delivery rate of 25.7% and an overall triplet delivery rate of 2.5% (6). However, the triplet delivery rate varied markedly, from 0.2% in Finland and Sweden, to >10% in Guatemala and the United Arab Emirates. The authors estimated that with up to 246,000 children born in 2002, of which half are from multiple pregnancies, the high rate of multiple pregnancies was already a significant problem. This is indicative of the high burden that multiple pregnancies caused to obstetric and neonatal units worldwide.

During the late 1990s and early 2000s, it became increasingly clear that implantation depends on the number of embryos transferred. Matorras and colleagues (7) calculated that in non-donor treatments, the implantation rate after single embryo transfer (SET) was 7.4%–11.1%. At least one gestational sac was visible in 7.9%–23.6% of cases after double embryo transfer (DET), in 16.4%–47.5% after triple embryo transfer (TET), and in 35.0%–44.0% after the transfer of five embryos. In their calculation, the proportion of multiple gestations also increased with relation to the number of embryos transferred, with up to 20% of multiple pregnancies after the transfer of four embryos.

The other essential factor that helps determine embryo implantation is embryo quality. First reports on embryo grading were published as early as in 1985 (8), but it took 15 years after this time to develop consistent grading criteria. Works by Fridström and colleagues (9) and Van Royen and colleagues (10) described criteria for cleavage-stage embryos on day 2 and 3. Gardner's criteria on blastocyst development (11) have also been increasingly used. Regardless of individual criteria listed and embryo development stage described, the transfer of a good-quality embryo is associated with higher chances of pregnancy and live birth rates but also with a higher chance of multiple pregnancies. This knowledge has allowed the possibility to decrease the number of embryos transferred in order to keep live birth rates unchanged but to diminish the number of gestational sacs developing.

Minimizing multiple births by elective single embryo transfer

The only logical way to ensure that ART patients have pregnancies and deliveries that are as close as possible to natural pregnancies is to ensure that the vast majority of these pregnancies are singleton ones by transferring only one embryo at a time. eSET is the practice in which more than one good-quality embryos are created after oocyte pickup but only one of them is transferred in the fresh cycle. All other good-quality embryos are cryopreserved for later use in FET. Embryos can also be transferred one by one in FET. In fact, FET was the first ART procedure that was developed with the aim of minimizing multiple pregnancies (12).

The first publication on eSET was in 1999: a study of Finnish women with contraindications for multiple pregnancy (13). Over the years, the practice has spread from Belgium (14) and Finland (15) to all other countries.

Following these developments, in Europe, the number of embryos transferred gradually decreased to two to three embryos, and in some countries it is currently close to one. The latest data available across countries are from the year 2016 (16). Figure 11.1 shows that transfer of only one embryo started in the early 2000s in both Europe and Australia and around 2005 in the United States. In 2016 already, Europe as a whole and the United States had a similar proportion of SETs, 42% and 40%, respectively, but this was less than half of the rate of SET in Australia. This difference can be explained by the considerable heterogeneity of practices in European countries and American clinics. The proportions of premature deliveries after ART in the three continents stratified by singleton, twin and triplet, or HOM status are shown in Figure 11.2. During the entire observation period 2002–2016, triplets and HOM were premature virtually always, twins 56%–72%, and singletons 10%–14%.

Overall health risks in ART multiple pregnancies and births

ART pregnancies start in a more unfavorable environment because of the underlying infertility problem and the years spent in identifying and treating it. Depending on the source, the mean age in IVF patients who had live births in Europe can vary between 33.1 years (17) and 34.2 years (18). This is considerably

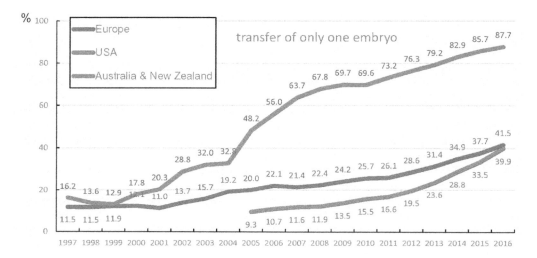

FIGURE 11.1a Proportion of single embryo transfers, transfers with two embryos, and transfers with three or more embryos in Europe, the United States, and Australia and New Zealand.

[Reproduced by permission from (16).]

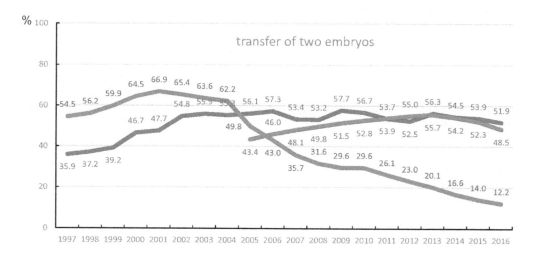

Figure 11.1b *(Continued)*

Multiple birth outcomes

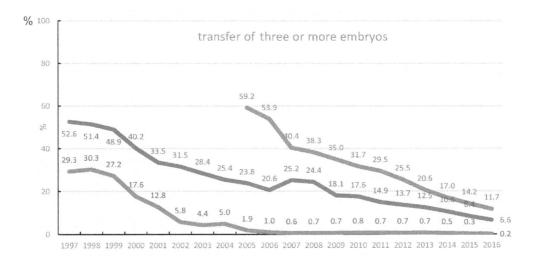

Figure 11.1c (*Continued*)

higher compared with the mean age in spontaneously conceived pregnancies: in the Finnish study, the mean age of the reference group with spontaneous pregnancies was only 30.0 years, and in the Danish analysis 30.5 years. In fact, female age is an important prognostic factor for pregnancy complications, and a higher maternal age is associated with higher risks of gestational diabetes, gestational hypertension, and cesarean delivery rates (19).

IVF/ICSI treatment has also been shown to increase the risk of adverse pregnancy outcomes, as seen in a meta-analysis comprising 2.5 million spontaneous and ART pregnancies (20). The risks with the highest relative ratios (RRs) were placenta previa (RR 3.71, 95% confidence interval [CI] 2.67–5.16), antepartum hemorrhage (RR 2.40, 95% CI 1.79–3.21), and oligohydramnios (RR 2.14, 95% CI 1.53–3.01). Among the various reasons for performing IVF/ICSI, endometriosis and polycystic ovary syndrome (PCOS) are the infertility diagnoses for which there are clear associations with an unfavorable pregnancy course. These are summarized in Table 11.1. Endometriosis appears to affect pregnancy outcome through several mechanisms. A thickening of the junctional zone may lead to abnormal remodeling of the spiral arteries and to a defective deep placentation. The abnormal inflammatory response and increased protease activity in endometriosis patients may predispose to preterm labor contractions and preterm rupture of membranes (21). In PCOS, the underlying pathological mechanism most probably is related to insulin resistance (22).

All of these factors explain why, compared to spontaneous multiple pregnancies, ART multiple pregnancies have elevated risks of age-related complications. Risks and odds ratios (ORs) or RRs from various studies are summarized in Table 11.2.

Chorionicity in ART multiple pregnancies

Most ART multiples are the result of the transfer of several embryos and therefore are multizygotic. By contrast, monozygotic twin pregnancies occur after a single embryo splits in two after transfer. Monozygotic twin pregnancies are characterized by much higher risks of premature delivery, growth discordance, and other types of perinatal morbidity and even mortality (31). This type of pregnancy has been difficult to study in large epidemiological trials because of the inconsistencies in zygosity recording, especially in triplet and HOM pregnancies. Recently, a meta-analysis evaluated data on monozygotic twins in IVF/ICSI that were collected from a total of 40 studies (32). The factor with the strongest

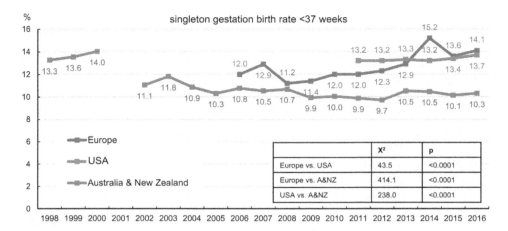

FIGURE 11.2a Changes in the proportion of premature deliveries (in singleton, twin, and triplet or higher grade) pregnancies after ART.

[Reproduced by permission from (16).]

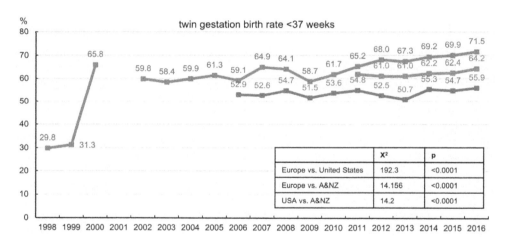

FIGURE 11.2b (*Continued*)

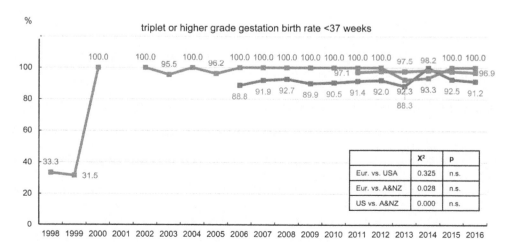

FIGURE 11.2c (*Continued*)

Multiple birth outcomes

TABLE 11.1

Pregnancy Risks in Certain Infertility Diagnoses

Parameter	OR (95% CI)
Endometriosis	
Gestational hypertension	1.14 (1.00–1.31)
Preeclampsia	1.19 (1.08–1.31)
Preterm birth	1.46 (1.26–1.69)
Placenta previa	2.99 (2.54–3.53)
Placental abruption	1.40 (1.12–1.76)
Cesarean section	1.49 (1.35–1.65)
Stillbirth	1.27 (1.07–1.51)
PCOS	
Miscarriage	1.41 (1.04–1.91)
Gestational diabetes mellitus	2.67 (1.43–4.98)
Pregnancy-induced hypertension	2.06 (1.45–2.91)
Preterm birth	1.60 (1.25–2.04)
LGA	2.10 (1.01–4.37)

Source: Modified from Refs. (21) and (22).

TABLE 11.2

Risks in ART Multiple Pregnancies and Births Compared to Spontaneous Multiple Pregnancies and Births

Parameter	OR or RR (95% confidence interval)	Study
Preeclampsia	Twin pregnancies OR 1.81 (1.50–2.17)	Reference 23
Preterm birth (<37 gw)	Twin pregnancies OR 1.83 (1.23–2.71)	Reference 24
	OR 1.05 (95% CI = 0.92–1.21)	Reference 17
Very preterm birth (<32 gw)	OR 1.11 (95% CI = 0.88–1.41)	Reference 17
Stillbirth	Dichorionic twin pregnancies: Risk similar at 37 gw. An additional 8.8 perinatal deaths per 1,000 pregnancies (95% CI 3.6 to 14.0/1,000) at 38 gw	Reference 25
	Monochorionic twin pregnancies: 36 gw vs. 34 gw: 2.5 per 1,000 perinatal deaths (−12.4 to 17.4/1,000)	
Specific congenital malformations	Chromosomal defects RR 1.36 (1.04–1.77). Urogenital defects RR 1.18 (1.03–1.36). Circulatory system malformations RR 1.22 (1.01–1.47).	Reference 26
Severe maternal morbidity	OR 2.5 (1.8–3.3). The risk of SMM was significantly higher with IVF-AO, for all-cause SMM (aOR = 2.0, 95% CI 1.5–2.7), for near misses (aOR = 1.9, 95% CI 1.3–2.8), and for intra/postpartum hemorrhages (aOR = 2.3, 95% CI 1.6–3.2). The risk of SMM was significantly higher with IVF-OD, for all-cause SMM (aOR = 18.6, 95% CI 4.4–78.5), for near misses (aOR = 18.1, 95% CI 4.0–82.3), for SMM due to hypertensive disorders (aOR = 16.7, 95% CI 3.3–85.4), and due to intra/postpartum hemorrhages (aOR = 18.0, 95% CI 4.2–77.8). Path analysis estimated that 21.6% (95% CI 10.1–33.0) of the risk associated with IVF-OD was mediated by multiple pregnancy and 49.6% (95% CI 24.0–75.1) of the SMM risk associated with IVF-AO	Reference 27
Severe acute maternal morbidity	IVF with autologous oocytes RR 1.3 (1.0–1.6) Oocyte donation RR 2.0 (1.4–2.8)	Reference 28
Hospital care utilization of IVF twins aged 2–7 years old	Overall OR 1.04 (0.96, 1.14) Surgical procedure: OR 1.37 (1.22, 1.51).	Reference 29
SGA Prematurity LBW NICU admission Perinatal mortality	SGA (OR = 1.27, 95% CI = 0.97–1.65) NICU 1.05 (1.01–1.09) PM 0.58 (0.44–0.77)	Reference 30

association with monozygotic twinning in IVF/ICSI was blastocyst transfer (OR 2.16, 95% CI 1.74–2.68). Young female age <35 years (OR 1.29; 95% CI 1.03–1.62), fertilization with IVF compared with ICSI (OR 1.19, 95% CI 1.04–1.35), and assisted hatching (OR 1.17, 95% CI 1.09–1.27) were among the other prognostic factors. The reasons why blastocyst transfer is associated with increased risk of monozygotic twins are not yet clearly understood. Until more evidence is available, the risks of monozygotic twinning have to be balanced with the good results from blastocyst transfer (33).

Conclusions

- Advances in IVF/ICSI have led to the introduction of eSET as the only effective strategy to minimize multiple pregnancies and births. This has allowed a clear drop in the number of mothers and offspring at risk.
- Considering the multitude of complications that characterize pregnancies after IVF/ICSI, treatment nowadays is safer for both mothers and children following the introduction of eSET.

REFERENCES

1. National Vital Statistics Reports, Vol. 70, No. 2, March 23, 2021. Available from: www.cdc.gov/nchs/data/nvsr/nvsr70/nvsr70-02-508.pdf.
2. Society for Assisted Reproductive Technology and the American Society for Reproductive Medicine. Assisted reproductive technology in the United States: 1998 results generated from the American Society for Reproductive Medicine/Society for Assisted Reproductive Technology Registry. *Fertil Steril*. 2002 Jan;77(1):18–31. doi: 10.1016/s0015-0282(01)02985-5.
3. Medical Research International. Society for Assisted Reproductive Technology (SART), The American Fertility Society. In Vitro Fertilization-Embryo Transfer (IVF-ET) in the United States: 1990 results from the IVF-ET Registry. *Fertil Steril*. 1992 Jan;57(1):15–24.
4. Jain T, Missmer SA, Hornstein MD. Trends in embryo-transfer practice and in outcomes of the use of assisted reproductive technology in the United States. *N Engl J Med*. 2004 Apr 15;350(16):1639–45. doi: 10.1056/NEJMsa032073. PMID: 15084696.
5. European IVF-Monitoring Programme (EIM), for the European Society of Human Reproduction and Embryology (ESHRE). Nygren KG, Andersen AN. Assisted reproductive technology in Europe, 1997. Results generated from European registers by ESHRE. *Hum Reprod*. 2001 Feb;16(2):384–91. doi: 10.1093/humrep/16.2.384. PMID: 11157839.
6. International Committee for Monitoring Assisted Reproductive Technology, de Mouzon J, Lancaster P, Nygren KG, Sullivan E, Zegers-Hochschild F, Mansour R, Ishihara O, Adamson D. World collaborative report on Assisted Reproductive Technology, 2002. *Hum Reprod*. 2009 Sep;24(9):2310–20. doi: 10.1093/humrep/dep098. Epub 2009 May 27. PMID: 19474459.
7. Matorras R, Matorras F, Mendoza R, Rodríguez M, Remohí J, Rodríguez-Escudero FJ, Simón C. The implantation of every embryo facilitates the chances of the remaining embryos to implant in an IVF programme: A mathematical model to predict pregnancy and multiple pregnancy rates. *Hum Reprod*. 2005 Oct;20(10):2923–31. doi: 10.1093/humrep/dei129. Epub 2005 Jul 21. PMID: 16037116.
8. Mohr LR, Trounson A, Freemann L. Deep-freezing and transfer of human embryos. *Vitro Fert Embryo Transf*. 1985 Mar;2(1):1–10. doi: 10.1007/BF01130825.
9. Fridström M, Carlström K, Sjöblom P, Hillensjö T. Effect of prednisolone on serum and follicular fluid androgen concentrations in women with polycystic ovary syndrome undergoing in-vitro fertilization. *Hum Reprod*. 1999 Jun;14(6):1440–4. doi: 10.1093/humrep/14.6.1440.
10. Van Royen E, Mangelschots K, Neubourg D, Valkenburg M, Meerssche M, Ryckaert G, et al. Characterization of a top quality embryo, a step towards single-embryo transfer. *Hum Reprod*. 1999;14: 2345–2349. doi: 10.1093/humrep/14.9.2345.
11. Gardner DK, Lane M, Stevens J, Schlenker T, Schoolcraft W. Blastocyst score affects implantation and pregnancy outcome: Towards a single blastocyst transfer. *Fertil Steril*. 2000;73:1155–8; doi: 10.1016/s0015-0282(00)00518-5.

12. Trounson A, Mohr L. Human pregnancy following cryopreservation, thawing and transfer of an eight-cell embryo. *Nature*. 1983 Oct 20–26;305(5936):707–9. doi: 10.1038/305707a0.
13. Vilska S, Tiitinen A, Hyden-Granskog C, Hovatta O. Elective transfer of one embryo results in an acceptable pregnancy rate and eliminates the risk of multiple birth. *Hum Reprod*. 1999;14:2392–5.
14. Gerris J, De Sutter P, De Neubourg D, Van Royen E, Vander Elst J, Mangelschots K, Vercruyssen M, Kok P, Elseviers M, Annemans L, et al. A real-life prospective health economic study of elective single embryo transfer versus two-embryo transfer in first IVF/ICSI cycles. *Hum Reprod*. 2004;19:917–23.
15. Martikainen H, Tiitinen A, Tomas C, Tapanainen J, Orava M, Tuomivaara L, Vilska S, Hyden-Granskog C, Hovatta O. One versus two embryo transfer after IVF and ICSI: A randomized study. *Hum Reprod*. 2001;16:1900–3.
16. De Geyter Ch, Wyns C, Calhaz-Jorge C, de Mouzon J, Ferraretti AP, Kupka M, Nyboe Andersen A, Nygren KG, Goossens V. 20 years of the European IVF-monitoring consortium registry: What have we learned? A comparison with registries from two other regions. *Human Reproduction*. 2020 Dec;35(12):2832–49. https://doi.org/10.1093/humrep/deaa250.
17. Pinborg A, Loft A, Rasmussen S, Schmidt L, Langhoff-Roos J, Greisen G, Nyboe Andersen A. Neonatal outcome in a Danish national cohort of 3438 IVF/ICSI and 10362 non-IVF/ICSI twins born in 1995–2000. *Hum Reprod*. 2004;19:435–41.
18. Pelkonen S, Koivunen R, Gissler M, Nuojua-Huttunen S, Suikkari A-M, Hyden-Granskog C, Martikainen H, Tiitinen A, Hartikainen A-L. Perinatal outcome of children born after frozen and fresh embryo transfer: The Finnish cohort study 1995–2006. *Hum Reprod*. 2010 Apr;25(4):914–23. doi: 10.1093/humrep/dep477. Epub 2010 Feb 2. PMID: 20124395.
19. Kahveci B, Melekoglu R, Evruke IC, Cetin C. The effect of advanced maternal age on perinatal outcomes in nulliparous singleton pregnancies. *BMC Pregnancy Childbirth*. 2018 Aug 22;18(1):343. doi: 10.1186/s12884-018-1984-x.
20. Qin J, Liu X, Sheng X, Wang H, Gao S. Assisted reproductive technology and the risk of pregnancy-related complications and adverse pregnancy outcomes in singleton pregnancies: A meta-analysis of cohort studies. *Fertil Steril*. 2016 Jan;105(1):73–85.e1–6. doi: 10.1016/j.fertnstert.2015.09.007. Epub 2015 Oct 9. PMID: 26453266.
21. Breintoft K, Pinnerup R, Henriksen TB, Rytter D, Uldbjerg N, Forman A, Arendt LH. Endometriosis and risk of adverse pregnancy outcome: A systematic review and meta-analysis. *J Clin Med*. 2021 Feb 9;10(4):667. doi: 10.3390/jcm10040667.
22. Sha T, Wang X, Cheng W, Yan Y. A meta-analysis of pregnancy-related outcomes and complications in women with polycystic ovary syndrome undergoing IVF. *Reprod Biomed Online*. 2019 Aug;39(2):281–93. doi: 10.1016/j.rbmo.2019.03.203. Epub 2019 Mar 29.
23. Okby R, Harlev A, Sacks KN, Sergienko R, Sheiner E. Preeclampsia acts differently in in vitro fertilization versus spontaneous twins. *Arch Gynecol Obstet*. 2018 Mar;297(3):653–8. doi: 10.1007/s00404-017-4635-y. Epub 2018 Jan 4. PMID: 29302809.
24. Saccone G, Zullo F, Roman A, Ward A, Maruotti G, Martinelli P, Berghella V. Risk of spontaneous preterm birth in IVF-conceived twin pregnancies. *J Matern Fetal Neonatal Med*. 2019 Feb;32(3):369–76. doi: 10.1080/14767058.2017.1378339. Epub 2017 Sep 21.
25. Cheong-See F, Schuit E, Arroyo-Manzano D, Khalil A, Barrett J, Joseph KS, Asztalos E, Hack K, Lewi L, Lim A, Liem S, Norman JE, Morrison J, Combs CA, Garite TJ, Maurel K, Serra V, Perales A, Rode L, Worda K, Nassar A, Aboulghar M, Rouse D, Thom E, Breathnach F, Nakayama S, Russo FM, Robinson JN, Dodd JM, Newman RB, Bhattacharya S, Tang S, Mol BW, Zamora J, Thilaganathan B, Thangaratinam S. Global Obstetrics Network (GONet) collaboration: Prospective risk of stillbirth and neonatal complications in twin pregnancies: Systematic review and meta-analysis. *BMJ*. 2016 Sep 6;354:i4353. doi: 10.1136/bmj.i4353.
26. Zheng Z, Chen L, Yang T, Yu H, Wang H, Qin J. Multiple pregnancies achieved with IVF/ICSI and risk of specific congenital malformations: A meta-analysis of cohort studies. *Reprod Biomed Online*. 2018 Apr;36(4):472–82. doi: 10.1016/j.rbmo.2018.01.009. Epub 2018 Jan 31.
27. Le Ray C, Pelage L, Seco A, Bouvier-Colle MH, Chantry AA, Deneux-Tharaux C, Epimoms Study Group. Risk of severe maternal morbidity associated with in vitro fertilisation: A population-based study. *BJOG*. 2019 Jul;126(8):1033–1041. doi: 10.1111/1471-0528.15668. Epub 2019 Mar 27. PMID: 30801948.
28. Korb D, Schmitz T, Seco A, Goffinet F, Deneux-Tharaux C, JUmeaux MODe d'Accouchement (JUMODA) study group and the Groupe de Recherche en Obstétrique et Gynécologie (GROG). Risk

factors and high-risk subgroups of severe acute maternal morbidity in twin pregnancy: A population-based study. *PLoS One*. 2020 Feb 28;15(2):e0229612. doi: 10.1371/journal.pone.0229612. eCollection 2020. PMID: 32109258.

29. Pinborg A, Loft A, Rasmussen S, Nyboe Andersen A. Hospital care utilization of IVF/ICSI twins followed until 2–7 years of age: A controlled Danish national cohort study. *Hum Reprod*. 2004 Nov;19(11):2529–36. doi: 10.1093/humrep/deh474. Epub 2004 Aug 19.

30. Helmerhorst FM, Perquin DA, Donker D, Keirse MJ. Perinatal outcome of singletons and twins after assisted conception: A systematic review of controlled studies. *BMJ*. 2004 Jan 31;328(7434):261. doi: 10.1136/bmj.37957.560278.EE. Epub 2004 Jan 23. PMID: 14742347.

31. Vaughan DA, Ruthazer R, Penzias AS, et al. Clustering of monozygotic twinning in IVF. *J Assist Reprod Genet*. 2016;33:19–26. https://doi.org/10.1007/s10815-015-0616-x.

32. Busnelli A, Dallagiovanna C, Reschini M, Paffoni A, Fedele L, Somigliana E. Risk factors for monozygotic twinning after in vitro fertilization: A systematic review and meta-analysis. *Fertil Steril*. 2019 Feb;111(2):302–17. doi: 10.1016/j.fertnstert.2018.10.025.

33. Glujovsky D, Farquhar C, Quinteiro Retamar AM, Alvarez Sedo CR, Blake D. Cleavage stage versus blastocyst stage embryo transfer in assisted reproductive technology. *Cochrane Database Syst Rev*. 2016 Jun 30;6:CD002118. doi: 10.1002/14651858.CD002118.pub5.

12

Obstetric outcomes after cancer treatment with or without assisted reproductive technologies

Giulia Maria Cillo and Arianna D'Angelo

Introduction: Impact of cancer treatment

It has been estimated that around 1 in 49 women under 40 years old develops cancer in the Western world. While overall cancer prevalence has increased, a significant improvement has been witnessed in the overall survival rate to the extent that 1 out of every 250–715 adults is becoming a cancer survivor.

Vast progress has been made in therapies used against cancer; however, these therapies, including chemotherapy and radiotherapy, still carry side effects which can reflect in temporary or permanent fertility loss. On the other hand, recent trends, such as delayed childbearing in Western societies, have resulted in an increasing number of women surviving cancer, who have not yet started creating their families and are willing to do so in the future.

Nowadays, thanks to innovative treatments, systematic screening programs, and an increased public awareness, most patients can expect to live a long life after cancer. Chemotherapy and radiotherapy regimens are more and more efficient to the point where for many malignancies affecting young women, survival rates can reach more than 80%–90%.

The operating mechanism of chemotherapeutic agents causes apoptotic damage in highly active replication cells. It is particularly pertinent that not only cancerous cells are affected but every cell with a significant turnover is damaged. Unfortunately, while damage to other highly dividing tissue can be reversed, damage to gonadal cells, whose number is fixed from fetal life, is considered irreversible.

Currently, iatrogenic infertility due to chemotherapy and radiotherapy is one of the main long term repercussions for women who survive cancer [1]. As such, young patients with new cancer diagnoses not only have to face the psychological distress given by the diagnosis itself but also have the concern associated with the future long term negative impact of treatments. It is estimated that up to 50% of young patients with a new diagnosis of breast cancer have a desire for pregnancy [2].

Chemotherapy and radiotherapy effects on gonadal function

Chemotherapy effects on gonadal function

Chemotherapy drugs cause repeated DNA alterations to tissue with high replication activity, resulting in impairment to basic cellular processes and cell proliferation. The subsequently induced DNA damage cannot be repaired, resulting in the death of the tumor cell, and it also leads to the death of germ cells in the gonadal tissue [1]. Gonadotoxic damages are age dependent, with susceptibility increasing with age, such that prepubertal girls are less susceptible [3]. Gonadotoxic effect clinically manifests with symptoms that range from menstrual irregularity to permanent amenorrhea. It is estimated that women who received chemotherapy have up to 38% less chance to conceive [4].

Since their development, chemotherapy drugs have been administered in combination in order to maximize their effect. However, this has made it difficult to determine the single impact of these therapies on the ovaries.

Gonadotoxicity effects vary with the different chemotherapy drugs. Cyclophosphamide and alkylating agents are well recognized to be highly toxic for the ovaries. In particular they act on depleting follicles, but they are also believed to create fibrosis and damage in the ovarian cortex and blood vessels (4). High doses of alkylating agents and high doses of radiotherapy used for bone marrow transplantation are associated with a higher risk of experiencing ovarian insufficiency (5).

Amenorrhea occurrence seems to be influenced by the type of neoplasm: patients with hematological cancer, and in particular Hodgkin lymphoma, seem to have a higher risk of premature ovarian failure after chemotherapy treatment (3). Fifty percent of women treated with MOPP, a regimen composed of nitrogen mustard, vincristine, procarbazine, and prednisone, experience permanent amenorrhea after treatment (1).

Fertility preservation options should be offered to all women of fertile age with future fertility desires (6). Established fertility preservation techniques include embryo and oocytes (mature and immature) cryopreservation, ovarian tissue cryopreservation, and gonadotropin-releasing hormone (GnRH) analog agonists. These techniques will be described in the following section. Most options can be performed in a 2-week time frame with no effect on the survival or recurrence rate. A recent study published in 2018 described 497 cancer patients who underwent counseling. Among them, 204 underwent ovarian stimulation, preserving their fertility. Importantly, no differences were found in recurrence or survival rate between the group who underwent fertility preservation and the one who did not (7).

Supporting data on safety and efficacy of fertility preservation were more recently published in another large study cohort study. A total of 1,275 women with a diagnosis of breast cancer were included in the cohort. Among them, 425 underwent fertility preservation, resulting in a significantly higher pregnancy rate after cancer. Reassuringly, the study shows similar survival rates compared to women who did not undergo fertility preservation (8).

The safety of hormonal stimulation in breast cancer patients has been reported in another large study. In particular, a cohort of women diagnosed with breast cancer between 1999 and 2013 were included in this study. No statistical differences in terms of overall survival rate or breast cancer recurrence were found in women who decided to undergo fertility preservation, with or without gonadotropin hormonal stimulation (9).

Effects of radiotherapy on gonadal function

The gonadal effects of radiotherapy have no correlation with the patient's age. However, intensity, dose, exposure time, and development stage of germinal cells are correlated with increased damage. Gonadotoxicity caused by radiotherapy is not correlated to cell turnover, and thus both the ovarian tissue and oocytes are susceptible to radiation damage. Radiotherapy can also induce damage to the uterine vascularization, altering its function, increasing myometrial fibrosis, and causing impairment in endometrial growth (3). Radiotherapy in the pelvic area is hence associated with irreversible damage and a high risk of premature ovarian insufficiency. Moreover, recent data suggest an increased risk of intrauterine growth restriction and fetal loss in cancer patients who receive pelvic radiotherapy at a prepubertal age, making elective single embryo transfer an important recommendation in this category of patients. Irradiation to the vagina can result in lubrication impairment and stenosis that can cause psychosexual and physical impairment to normal fertility (10).

Fertility preservation in the context of oncologic disease

Oncofertility counseling has only recently been introduced in the pathway for new cancer diagnosis. It is an interdisciplinary field where different specialists work together to provide the best care and support to cancer patients. Oncologists, gynecologists, reproductive biologists, research scientists, and patients should be included in the team to guarantee a multidisciplinary approach (11). This represents a crucial phase for cancer patients who are informed about the long term effects of chemotherapy and radiotherapy treatment on their future fertility (12).

The latest studies reveal that cancer patients who were not aware about future fertility impairment due to cancer treatment can reach as high a stress level as the one experienced in posttraumatic stress disorder (13, 14). Counseling should be considered standard of care and should be offered as soon as possible after the diagnosis and prior to the beginning of anticancer treatments. The consultation should provide information about the effects on fertility, on future pregnancy, and available fertility preservation options. Moreover, particular importance should be given to the menopausal symptoms and management to guarantee long term health and quality of life to women who experience chemotherapy- or radiotherapy-induced menopause. Cardiovascular, neurological, and bone function health are crucial in menopausal women, and possible concerns on these topics should be raised during the consultation. Contraception and sexuality should also be discussed during the oncofertility counseling (14).

Fertility preservation options

There are several options to preserve fertility for cancer patients. A counseling session should be offered to any woman with a new tumor diagnosis for the purpose of discussing her options and likelihood of success (15).

Oocyte and/or embryo cryopreservation

Cryopreservation of both oocytes and embryos are well-recognized procedures for preserving women's fertility. In younger patients without a partner, oocyte cryopreservation should be considered. Both oocyte and embryo cryopreservation require controlled ovarian stimulation (COH) followed by oocyte retrieval, when applicable, fertilization, and subsequent cryopreservation. The ovarian stimulation can be commenced at any point of the menstrual cycle, as the recent data show. This protocol, known as "random start", allows cancer patients to proceed with fertility preservation without delaying the commencement of chemotherapy (16). COH leads to an increase of estrogen blood levels. In breast cancer patients the COH protocol can be safely performed by administering letrozole in conjunction with the gonadotrophins; letrozole acts as an aromatase inhibitor to reduce the circulating estradiol levels, consequently reducing the risk of the potential cancer relapse or progression. Furthermore, letrozole use does not worsen the outcome of the in vitro fertilization process (17, 18). Supporting data have been recently published in a multicenter prospective study, where letrozole administration was compared to COH without letrozole administration. No significant difference was found in the number of embryos or oocytes suitable for cryopreservation between the two groups. It has also been suggested that to minimize the risk of ovarian hyperstimulation syndrome (OHSS), a GnRH analog (GnRHa) trigger should be preferred to human chorionic gonadotropin (hCG) in patients undergoing COH with letrozole. The same study also showed no difference in cryopreserved gametes between ordinary COH commencement and the random start protocol, supporting, once more, the latter as a valid and safe approach for cancer patients (19).

Immature oocyte or in vitro matured oocyte cryopreservation

Immature oocyte cryopreservation and in vitro matured oocyte cryopreservation are emerging strategies. These procedures allow specialists to retrieve oocytes with no to minimal stimulation. The immature oocytes, which in a normal ovarian stimulation are usually discarded, are matured in vitro or cryopreserved at the germinal stage (GV) or non-mature stage (MI) and subsequently matured before fertilization. Immature oocyte preservation has the advantage of reducing to almost zero the stimulation time and to prevent the estrogen level surge induced by the stimulation protocols (20). The average time from the first day of COH to oocyte collection is around 10 days. Immature oocyte collection or in vitro maturation procedures are particularly useful in cancer patients who cannot wait for their chemotherapy to commence. However, the techniques may also be beneficial in patients who underwent ovarian stimulation to maximize the number of oocytes or embryos cryopreserved. In fact, it is estimated that around 15%–20% of all the oocytes retrieved during an ovarian stimulation are immature (21).

Ovarian tissue cryopreservation

Ovarian tissue cryopreservation allows preservation of both reproductive and steroidogenic function by surgically retrieving ovarian tissue and subsequently cryopreserving the prepared cortex. The American Society for Reproductive Medicine has considered this an established procedure since 2019; however, many countries still consider it experimental (22). The opportunity to preserve fertility in prepubertal patients or patients without a partner and the possibility to start cancer therapies imminently after surgery are undeniable advantages of this procedure. The reimplant can then be performed orthotopically or heterotopically. Innovative approaches also include robotic technology and tissue scaffolding (23). A recent meta-analysis documents with this procedure a live birth rate as high as 57.5% and an endocrinological function resumption rate of 63.9% (24). A possible reason for concern is the risk of cancer recurrence when the ovarian tissue is retransplanted. The current advice is that the procedure be discussed with a multidisciplinary team and that it is not to be recommended in patients when the malignancy involves the ovary (15, 25).

GnRH analog agonists

GnRHa agonists have been proposed with the aim to reduce the chemotherapy gonadotoxicity by reducing ovarian turnover activity. GnRHa inhibits follicle recruitment by suppressing the pituitary follicle-stimulating hormone (FSH) secretion. The GnRHa drugs are supposed to be administered around 10 days prior to chemotherapy start due to transitory flare-up effects that run out in about 10 days. However, the efficacy of this is still controversial. Despite a recent meta-analysis revealing a lower incidence of chemotherapy-induced premature ovarian insufficiency (POI) and a higher pregnancy rate, the most recent guidelines (Table 12.1) suggest offering GnRHa to women who cannot use other proven fertility preservation methods (26).

Evaluation of recovery of ovarian function

Oncological patients' fertility assessment is a crucial part of oncofertility counseling, and it is also fundamental to evaluate fertility resumption after cancer treatment.

Menses resumption

Amenorrhea is defined by the absence of a menstrual cycle for three or more consecutive months, while oligomenorrhoea is defined by irregular menstrual cycles at intervals of more than 35 days. It is not unusual for cancer patients to experience amenorrhea or oligomenorrhea during cancer treatment. Ovarian function recovery after cancer therapy is defined in two ways: either with menstrual resumption and restoration of anti-Mullerian hormone (AMH) or FSH to baseline/expected level for age; alternatively, ovarian function can be defined as restored if pregnancy occurs (27).

Treatment-induced amenorrhea is commonly used in several studies to assess gonadotoxicity. However, amenorrhea does not always result in infertility; on the other hand, menses resumption does not imply ability to conceive. Moreover, women who experience regular menstruation after cancer treatments can still manifest premature menopause, resulting from the depletion of primordial follicle storage due to chemotherapy (2).

Anti-Müllerian hormone

AMH is a glycoprotein hormone produced by the primordial follicles' granulosa and by small antral follicles. The secretion starts with the growth of the first primordial follicle and continues until the follicles achieve the capacity to respond to FSH, when the follicles reach an average diameter of 3 or 4 mm. AMH is known to be an indirect marker of the quiescent primordial follicle storage in the ovary. Moreover, AMH serology concentration is not gonadotropin-dependent, resulting in consistent levels throughout

TABLE 12.1

Reproductive Options after Fertility Preservation for Cancer Patients

FP Option		Reproductive planning after cancer
No fertility preservation	If low impact of cancer on fertility	Natural pregnancy OR IVF
	If high impact of cancer on fertility	IVF with donor oocytes + partner/donor sperm OR other parenting options
Cryopreserved oocytes	If low impact of cancer on fertility	Natural pregnancy or IVF
	If high impact of cancer on fertility	IVF with cryopreserved oocytes + Partner sperm/donor sperm
	If insufficient number of cryopreserved oocytes	IVF with donor oocytes + partner/donor sperm
Cryopreserved ovarian tissue	If low impact of cancer on fertility	Natural pregnancy or IVF
	If high impact of cancer on fertility	OTT + natural pregnancy OR OTT + IVF (partner/donor sperm) OR OTT + IVM (partner/donor sperm)
Cryopreserved embryos (partner or donor sperm)	If low impact of cancer on fertility	Embryo transfer OR Natural pregnancy OR IVF with fresh oocytes
	If high impact of cancer on fertility	Embryo transfer
	If insufficient number of cryopreserved embryos	IVF with donor oocytes + partner/donor sperm OR donated embryos
	If new partner (and embryos with sperm of former partner)	IVF with Donor oocytes + current partner/donor sperm

Source: From Ref. 15, reproduced with permission.

Abbreviations: *FP*, fertility preservation; *IVF*, in vitro fertilization; *IVM*, in vitro maturation; *OTT*, ovarian tissue transplantation.

every phase of the menstrual cycle (28). AMH is hence considered a good ovarian reserve marker to evaluate fertility. Several studies have used AMH as a marker to assess the gonadotoxic effect of chemotherapy (29, 30). In fact, it has been shown that blood levels of AMH after treatment experience a consistent decrease and seem to remain low in women who do not resume ovarian function. Patients with an initial higher serologic level of AMH are shown to be the ones with a higher chance to regain normal ovarian function after the end of treatment (3). However, no consensus has been reached about AMH and its accuracy. One of the most recent studies published, in fact, suggests that AMH levels in younger patients do not significantly change before and after cancer treatment. A study by Li et al. concludes that AMH is a suitable predictor for ovarian damage in patients older than 35 years old (31).

Follicle-stimulating hormone

FSH is a glycoprotein hormone whose secretion is regulated by GnRH. Its main role is to induce follicle growth and maturation of the dominant follicle. Serology concentration fluctuates during the menstrual cycle, decreasing steadily to basal levels after ovulation. The hormone dosage, on average, on the third day of the menstrual cycle represents a good marker of ovarian reserve. In consideration of its characteristic, the conspicuous variations between menstrual cycles, and the lack of a standardized cut-off, many studies suggest that FSH only be considered as a screening test for counseling, rather than an ovarian reserve test to evaluate fertility (32).

Antral follicle count

Antral follicle count (AFC) is performed with a bidimensional or tridimensional transvaginal ultrasound, which allows the operator to recognize and count the number of follicles between 2 and 10 mm in the ovaries. AFC comes with several limitations: first of all, it is operator dependent. A follicle count more than 10 within the two ovaries is considered normal (33). An AFC lower than 10 seems more associated with subfertility (33). However, no consensus has been reached on the number of follicles that define normal, diminished, or poor reserve. AFC is considered to have a low threshold level to predict poor response or pregnancy (32).

Obstetric outcomes: Breast cancer

Breast cancer is the most frequent cancer in women worldwide. It has been estimated that 1.7 million women are diagnosed with breast cancer every year (27). It is mostly diagnosed in the 0–49 age group (41%), but also in the 50–69 (35%) and over 70 years old groups (22%) (34, 35). The disease holds a great geographic variability, with a higher rate in the most economically advanced countries. Modern technologies, scheduled screening, and new therapies are responsible for the progressive decrease in mortality rate (36). However, it has been suggested that breast cancer survivors may experience difficulties conceiving and have adverse obstetric outcomes, primarily due to the gonadotoxic effect of chemotherapy and the delay in conception to complete hormonal treatment (37).

Adverse obstetric outcomes such as preterm birth, low birth weight, cesarean section, intrauterine death, and fetal anomalies were the endpoint analyzed in a meta-analysis recently published. A total of 1,466 pregnant breast cancer survivors were compared to a control group composed of 6,912,485 pregnant women. The meta-analysis concluded that breast cancer survivors seem to have a higher risk of both preterm birth and low weight at birth. Increased risk was found in patients who had chemotherapy within 2 years before delivery. Moreover, fetal abnormalities seem to be higher in babies born to women with a breast cancer history. No clear cause has been established as of yet, but recent studies suggest it may be due to tamoxifen administration or the mutagenic effect of chemotherapy on germ cells (36). A higher rate of preterm labor has also been reported in a large study where 18,280 breast cancer survivors were compared to 91,400 controls. The study concluded that a history of breast cancer seemed to be associated with a higher risk of preterm labor (38).

Spontaneous pregnancy after breast cancer chemotherapy can be difficult to achieve. In fact, the usual treatment includes alkylating agents as well as anthracyclines and taxanes. Treatment-induced amenorrhea ranges between 40% and 60% after alkylating therapies in women younger than 40, but can reach more than 80% in older women. Anthracyclines and taxanes have an intermediate risk of inducing amenorrhea, especially when taxanes are associated with alkylating agents (39).

In consideration of these increased adverse obstetric outcomes, appropriate gynecological counseling should be offered to breast cancer survivors prior to conception.

Obstetric outcomes: Hematological cancer

Hematological cancers account for 17% of all cancers affecting premenopausal women (40). Over the last decades, survival rates for these malignancies have improved consistently, reaching more than 80%–90%, meaning that young women affected by these diseases may live a fairly long life cancer-free. However, the gonadotoxicity side effect of chemotherapy treatment leads the cancer survivors to having to deal with infertility and/or sterility (41).

Another study described 89 patients undergoing high chemotherapy doses followed by auto–stem cell transplantation for Hodgkin and non-Hodgkin lymphoma (42). Menstrual period resumption was recorded in 56 (63%) of them. The study suggests an increasing 11% risk of experiencing amenorrhea with each increasing year of age – only 4 out of 17 patients older than 30 resumed a regular menstrual cycle. The increasing risk of experiencing amenorrhea accounted for 13% with each chemotherapy cycle. Among the 89 patients considered in the study, 26 became pregnant. Three of them underwent assisted reproductive technology (ART) treatment to obtain their pregnancy. In particular, two of them had hormone-assisted ovulation, while only one patient needed in vitro fertilization. An older study published in 2011 reported reassuring pregnancy outcomes for 99 patients with lymphoma. All included patients who underwent chemotherapy and radiotherapy either alone or both together. One hundred and forty-five pregnancies were reported, resulting in 134 (91%) live births, 13 (9%) fetal losses, and no stillborn. These findings were quite similar to a normal population rate without cancer. Congenital abnormalities were also reported in another study: among the 134 live born children followed up in the study, 2 (1.4%) presented with congenital abnormalities such as gastroschisis and megaureter. Preterm delivery was experienced by nine women (9%) and three (3%) women had babies with low weight at birth (41). The most recent meta-analysis included 14 studies and a total of 744 hematological cancer survivors who received an allogenic or autologous hematopoietic stem cell transplantation. Among them, 59 underwent fertility preservation, with 22.7% (438) of the total treated patients conceiving and 7.5% (25) of them through ART techniques. Miscarriage rate was estimated around 10.4% with 361 (78%) live births documented (40).

Obstetric outcomes: Endometrial cancer

Endometrial cancer is most common in postmenopausal women, and the standard treatment usually involves a bilateral salpingo-oophorectomy and total hysterectomy. However, approximately 5.5% of cases affect women in their childbearing years. Fertility-sparing treatment can be considered in early cancer stages, especially for young women who have a future maternal desire. Conservative management includes treatment with progestin (local or oral) and frequent procedures such as dilation and curettage (D&C) and endometrial biopsies. These procedures have associated risks of endometritis, adhesions, and a thin endometrium lining.

Another retrospective study considered 98 women previously treated for endometrial cancer conservatively who were trying to conceive. Among them, 45 got pregnant but 68.4% needed fertility treatment such as intrauterine insemination, clomiphene administration, or in vitro fertilization/intracytoplasmic sperm injection (IVF/ICSI), accounting for 22.8%. The study concluded that factors directly associated with conception success are normal endometrial thickness, low number of D&C procedures, low age at attempting pregnancy, and recurrence (43).

Reproductive outcomes for women conservatively treated for complex atypical hyperplasia and an early stage of carcinoma have been reported in a systematic review. A total of 38 studies were considered and 315 women. Among them 36.2% (144) conceived at least once, resulting in 117 live births. However, the limit of this paper was to assess how many of these pregnancies were spontaneous, since not all the studies consistently reported whether these pregnancies were achieved via ART treatment (44).

Alternatively, the review published by Chao et al. considered endometrial cancer patients who received conservative treatment and conceived spontaneously or via ART. A total of 50 women were divided in two groups: 14 became pregnant after an IVF technique resulting in 23 live births, while 36 had an intrauterine insemination or spontaneously gave birth to a total of 54 babies. According to this review, the group who underwent ART techniques had higher rates of multiple pregnancies, preterm deliveries, and obstetric complications (45).

The spontaneous pregnancy rate accounted for 14.9% in the meta-analysis published in 2012 by Gallons et al. There were 451 endometrial cancer patients that had fertility-sparing treatment and who wanted to conceive were included; 142 underwent ART, and among them 56 had at least one live birth. Among the 309 who were assumed to have spontaneously attempted conception, 46 actually conceived (46).

Fertility sparing seems a feasible endometrial cancer treatment in selected patients. However, in order to avoid delaying their definitive total hysterectomy and salpingo-oophorectomy surgery, women should be advised to attempt conception as soon as it is deemed safe to do so. ART techniques should also be recommended to these women in order to increase their pregnancy success and minimize the continuous endometrial stimulation that increases recurrence or disease progression risk (47).

Obstetric outcomes: Ovarian cancer

Ovarian cancer is another common gynecological cancer, and it is estimated that approximately 12.5% of women affected are premenopausal. Fertility-sparing surgery involves sparing the uterus and the contralateral ovary and can be offered to women with early-stage ovarian cancer who wish to preserve future fertility. Obstetric outcomes of ovarian cancer patients have been reported in several studies. However, in most of them the sample included very few patients, making the results difficult to generalize to the normal population.

Moreover, two different retrospective studies were published with similar results. The first one considered 62 patients with invasive ovarian cancer who underwent conservative surgery. Of the 19 women who attempted conception, 15 become pregnant. Twenty-two live births and two miscarriages were recorded (48).

The second study considered 360 women with borderline ovarian tumors. One hundred and eighty-four underwent conservative surgical management, while 130 had radical surgery. Among the 184, 31 attempted conception and 27 conceived. At the last follow-up, 34 healthy live births, 32 singleton pregnancies and 1 twin pregnancy were documented (49). In both studies, all babies were reported as healthy with no congenital abnormalities.

Obstetric outcomes of epithelial ovarian cancer patients undergoing fertility-sparing surgery (n = 36) were described in a recent prospective study. These patients were compared to women with ovarian cancer undergoing radical surgery (n = 47). Results suggest that fertility-sparing surgery, in selected candidates is not associated with an increased disease recurrence rate, and obstetric outcomes were promising. Pregnancy and healthy live births were reported in nine (25%) ovarian cancer patients treated with fertility-sparing surgery (50).

The endpoints of an additional prospective study are reproductive and pregnancy outcomes in women with borderline ovarian malignancy. A total of 277 patients satisfy these criteria, and among them, 77% had fertility-sparing surgery, preserving their natural fertility. During the follow-up period a total of 62 healthy live births were recorded. No malformations were observed, and most of deliveries were at full term. Overall survival rate and recurrence in women undergoing fertility-sparing surgery were comparable to patients who had radical surgery (51).

Another retrospective analysis in 2018 included 105 women with malignant ovarian germ cell tumors. Forty-two of the 45 cancer survivors who attempted it experienced the pregnancy. Fifty-six healthy live babies were reported, with 96.4% delivered at term. Among the patients who conceived ten (17.4%) experienced a miscarriage (52).

The most recent systematic review concluded that fertility sparing is a feasible option for young women with future pregnancy desire. In terms of obstetric outcomes, of the 614 women with epithelial ovarian cancer, 307 tried to get pregnant and 242 (79%) conceived. Similarly, 66% of women with borderline ovarian tumor who were trying to conceive were successful. Fewer studies were available for non-epithelial ovarian cancer patients. Pregnancy rates in this case for women trying to conceive ranged between 65% and 95% (53).

Obstetric outcomes: Cervical cancer

Cervical cancer is the fourth most common malignancy often diagnosed in young women who still have uncompleted reproductive plans. Thanks to screening and the human papilloma virus vaccination, the cervical cancer incidence has seen a substantial decrease in the last decades, and the 5-year survival rate is up to 90%. According to the most recent guidelines in patients with childbearing desire and early cancer stage (IA and IB), fertility-sparing surgery can be offered (54). Fertility-sparing surgery for cervical cancer includes conization and trachelectomy procedures. A recent review reported an infertility rate after trachelectomy up to 30% with an overall pregnancy rate ranging between 30% and 79%; pregnancy was achieved in 53% of patients undergoing ART. Miscarriage risk seemed to be as high as the normal population, but patients with cervical cancer who had fertility-sparing surgery had an increased risk (26.6% in radical trachelectomy) of preterm delivery and second-trimester miscarriages (55).

A recent systematic review published in 2020 included 65 studies and 3,044 cervical cancer patients. After fertility-sparing surgery, 1,218 attempted conception and 1,047 conceived. Among these, 80% were spontaneous pregnancies, while 20% of patients obtained a pregnancy through ART. Women who underwent a radical trachelectomy seemed to have a lower live birth rate (63.4% versus 86.4%). The systematic review also agreed that fertility-sparing surgery is associated with a higher risk of preterm deliveries (56).

Obstetric outcomes: Other cancers

More than 50,000 people under 35 years old are diagnosed with cancer every year. Fertility preservation is estimated to be one of the predictors of emotional satisfaction for cancer survivors (57).

Obstetric outcomes: Colorectal cancer

Colorectal cancer represents the most common gastrointestinal cancer in the Western world. Incidence in patients younger than 40 years old is 3%–6%, but overall 48% of them are women.

Colorectal cancer surgery seems to have no effect on a patient's chance of getting pregnant or to carry the pregnancy full term. However, if surgery happens below the peritoneal reflection, this may have an impact on the ability to conceive. Unfortunately, there are no studies comparing different surgical approaches and fertility outcomes, but the main infertility cause in these patients seems to be due to the adhesions that might impair the reproductive organs' anatomy (58). In terms of chemotherapy, colorectal cancer is predominantly treated with 5-fluorouracil, which seems to have no or mild gonadotoxicity. Radiotherapy can also be required for colorectal cancer patients; dose, time of therapy, and irradiation field will determine the resulting ovarian damage (59). See Tables 12.2 and 12.3 for further information.

12.12 Conclusions

- The importance of a multidisciplinary approach to women in reproductive age with cancer is clear. Proper counseling should be offered to all patients with a new diagnosis of cancer, providing information about the risk of chemotherapy-induced POI.
- In the near future, progress of cancer treatments paired with increased public awareness will lead to a further increase in survival rates. This would result in an increasing number of women surviving cancer with a near-normal life expectancy and associated desires. Therefore, future challenges include allowing women to fullfil their desire for motherhood after cancer treatment, or if that is not possible, trying to minimize the negative impact infertility and/or sterility can have on the quality of life after cancer treatment.

TABLE 12.2
Overview of Data from Large Registers on Obstetrics Outcomes after Cancer

	(van der Kooi et al., 2018)	(Anderson et al., 2017)	(Madanat-Harjuoja et al., 2013)	(Fossa et al., 2005)	(Ji et al., 2016)
	Scotland	North Carolina	Finland	Norway	Sweden
Study group	10,271 nulliparous women diagnosed with cancer before the age of 40 years	21,716 women with a cancer diagnosis between ages 15 and 39 years	25,784 males and females	8,644 women after diagnosis in cancer patients aged 15–45	1,977 cancer survivors who had given birth before/after their cancer diagnosis
Control group	General population	General population	44,611 full and half-siblings of these patients		General population (without cancer)
Birth					
Antepartum hemorrhage	No difference (RR 1.13; 95% CI 0.86–1.50)				
Postpartum hemorrhage	Increased (RR 1.42; 95% CI 1.29–1.55)				
Operative or assisted delivery – elective	Increased (RR 1.59; 95% CI 1.35–1.88)	Increased (RR 1.08; 1.01–1.14)		Increased (OR 2.3; 95% CI 1.9–2.7)	
Operative or assisted delivery – emergency	Increased (RR 1.20; 95% CI 1.08–1.34)				
Perinatal Outcomes					
Small for gestational age	Decreased (RR 0.82; 95% CI 0.68–0.98)	No difference (PR 0.97; 0.85–1.11)			
Low Apgar score (<7)		No difference (PR 1.18; 0.87–1.61)			
Low birth weight	No difference (RR 1.15; 95% CI 0.94–1.39)	Increased (PR 1.59; 95% CI 1.38–1.83)		Increased (singletons) OR 2.5; 95% CI 2.0–3.2	
Preterm birth	Increased (RR 1.32; 95% CI 1.10–1.59)	Increased (PR 1.52; 95% CI 1.34%–1.71)		Increased (singletons) OR 2.8; 95% CI 2.3–3.4	
Early preterm birth		Increased (PR 2.03; 95% CI 1.62–2.55)			

Need for intensive care or neonatal monitoring	Increased (RR 1.03; 95% CI 0.90–119)	Increased (OR 1.90; 95% CI 1.65–2.19)
Perinatal death (<7 days after live birth)		No difference (OR 1.35; 95% CI 0.58–3.18)	No difference (OR 1.2; 95% CI 0.6–2.4)
National death (<28 days after live birth)		No difference (OR 1.40; 95% CI 0.46–4.24)	No difference (OR 1.13; 95% CI 0.80–1.60)
Early death (<1 year after birth)		No difference (OR 1.11; 95% CI 0.64–1.93)	
Stillbirth		No difference (OR 1.15; 95% CI 0.61–2.19)	No difference (OR 1.27; 95% CI 0.95–1.68)
Congenital abnormalities	No difference (RR 1.01; 95% CI 0.85–1.20)		No difference (OR 0.6; 95% CI 0.4–1.0)

Source: From Ref. 15, reproduced with permission.

Abbreviations: *PR* 3 ratio, *RR* relative risk, *OR* odds ratio, *CI* confidence interval.

TABLE 12.3

Overview of Specific Guidance for Types of Cancers

Disease	Treatment	Obstetric Risks	Recommendations for Care before Pregnancy	Recommendations for Care during/after Pregnancy
All cancers	(independent of treatment)	Cancer survivors are at increased risk of postpartum hemorrhage, cesarean section, and preterm birth	Preconception counseling	Appropriate obstetric monitoring
	Chemotherapy started <1 year before conception	Increased risk of preterm birth	Patients should be advised about these risks	
	Pelvic radiotherapy (field includes the uterus)	Increased risk of (possibly severe) pregnancy complications		Treat pregnancy as high risk in a center with advanced maternity services
Breast cancer	(Independent of treatment)	Increased risk of preterm birth and low birth weight	Pregnancy is safe	
	If chemotherapy started <1 year before conception	Increased risk of preterm birth	Patients should be advised about these risks	
	With adjuvant therapies	Risks unclear	Stop tamoxifen for at least 3 months before attempting pregnancy	
Endometrial cancer	Fertility-sparing surgery	Increased risk of obstetric complications + possible recurrence awaiting definitive treatment (Hx)	Inform patients that better outcomes are seen when conception occurs soon after documented tumor regression	High-risk pregnancy patients are to be monitored by an oncologist due to the risk of relapse
	Pelvic radiotherapy (field includes the uterus)	Risk of (possibly severe) pregnancy complications		Treat pregnancy as high risk in center with advanced maternity services
Ovarian cancer	Fertility-sparing surgery	No evidence		Follow general advice for cancer survivors
Cervical cancer	Radical trachelectomy	Risk of pregnancy loss and preterm birth		Treat pregnancy as high risk in a center with advanced maternity services
	Pelvic radiotherapy (field included the uterus)	Risk of (possibly severe) pregnancy complications		Treat pregnancy as high risk in a center with advanced maternity services

Source: From Ref. 15, reproduced with permission.

Abbreviation: *Hx* hysterectomy.

REFERENCES

1. Blumenfeld Z. Chemotherapy and fertility. *Best Pract Res Clin Obstet Gynaecol*. 2012 Jun 1;26(3):379–90.
2. Lambertini M, Goldrat O, Clatot F, Demeestere I, Awada A. Controversies about fertility and pregnancy issues in young breast cancer patients: Current state of the art. *Curr Opin Oncol*. 2017 Jul;29(4):243–52.
3. Cosgrove CM, Salani R. Ovarian effects of radiation and cytotoxic chemotherapy damage. *Best Pract Res Clin Obstet Gynaecol*. 2019 Feb 1;55:37–48.
4. Ovarian damage from chemotherapy and current approaches to its protection [Internet]. [cited 2020 Oct 1]. Available from: www.ncbi.nlm.nih.gov/pmc/articles/PMC6847836/
5. Meirow D. Reproduction post-chemotherapy in young cancer patients. *Mol Cell Endocrinol*. 2000 Nov 27;169(1):123–31.

6. Anazodo A, Laws P, Logan S, Saunders C, Travaglia J, Gerstl B, et al. How can we improve oncofertility care for patients? A systematic scoping review of current international practice and models of care. *Hum Reprod Update.* 2019 Mar 1;25(2):159–79.
7. Moravek MB, Confino R, Smith KN, Kazer RR, Klock SC, Lawson AK, et al. Long-term outcomes in cancer patients who did or did not pursue fertility preservation. *Fertil Steril.* 2018;109(2):349–55.
8. Marklund A, Lundberg FE, Eloranta S, Hedayati E, Pettersson K, Rodriguez-Wallberg KA. Reproductive outcomes after breast cancer in women with vs without fertility preservation. *JAMA Oncol.* 2021 Jan;7(1):1–6.
9. Rodriguez-Wallberg KA, Eloranta S, Krawiec K, Lissmats A, Bergh J, Liljegren A. Safety of fertility preservation in breast cancer patients in a register-based matched cohort study. *Breast Cancer Res Treat.* 2018;167(3):761–9.
10. Gunasheela D, Gunasheela S. Strategies for fertility preservation in young patients with cancer: A comprehensive approach. *Indian J Surg Oncol.* 2014 Mar;5(1):17–29.
11. Salama M, Anazodo A, Woodruff TK. Preserving fertility in female patients with hematological malignancies: A multidisciplinary oncofertility approach. *Ann Oncol.* 2019 Nov 1;30(11):1760–75.
12. Lange S, Tait D, Matthews M. Oncofertility: An emerging discipline in obstetrics and gynecology. *Obstet Gynecol Surv.* 2013 Aug;68(8):582–93.
13. Levine JM, Kelvin JF, Quinn GP, Gracia CR. Infertility in reproductive-age female cancer survivors. *Cancer.* 2015;121(10):1532–9.
14. Woodruff TK, Smith K, Gradishar W. Oncologists' role in patient fertility care: A call to action. *JAMA Oncol.* 2016 Feb 1;2(2):171–2.
15. The ESHRE Guideline Group on Female Fertility Preservation, ESHRE guideline: Female fertility preservation. *Human Reproduction Open.* 2020 [cited 2020 Dec 23];2020(4):hoaa052. https://doi.org/10.1093/hropen/hoaa052. Full guideline available via www.eshre.eu/Guidelines-and-Legal/Guidelines/Female-fertility-preservation.
16. Cakmak H, Rosen MP. Random-start ovarian stimulation in patients with cancer. *Curr Opin Obstet Gynecol.* 2015 Jun;27(3):215–21.
17. Oktay K, Hourvitz A, Sahin G, Oktem O, Safro B, Cil A, et al. Letrozole reduces estrogen and gonadotropin exposure in women with breast cancer undergoing ovarian stimulation before chemotherapy. *J Clin Endocrinol Metab.* 2006 Oct;91(10):3885–90.
18. Taylan E, Oktay K. Fertility preservation in gynecologic cancers. *Gynecol Oncol.* 2019 Dec 1;155(3):522–9.
19. Marklund A, Eloranta S, Wikander I, Kitlinski ML, Lood M, Nedstrand E, et al. Efficacy and safety of controlled ovarian stimulation using GnRH antagonist protocols for emergency fertility preservation in young women with breast cancer: A prospective nationwide Swedish multicenter study. *Hum Reprod.* 2020 Apr 28;35(4):929–38.
20. Fadini R, Dal Canto M, Mignini Renzini M, Milani R, Fruscio R, Cantù MG, et al. Embryo transfer following in vitro maturation and cryopreservation of oocytes recovered from antral follicles during conservative surgery for ovarian cancer. *J Assist Reprod Genet.* 2012 Aug;29(8):779–81.
21. Oktay K, Buyuk E, Rodriguez-Wallberg KA, Sahin G. In vitro maturation improves oocyte or embryo cryopreservation outcome in breast cancer patients undergoing ovarian stimulation for fertility preservation. *Reprod Biomed Online.* 2010 May;20(5):634–8.
22. Practice Committee of the American Society for Reproductive Medicine. Electronic address: asrm@asrm.org. Fertility preservation in patients undergoing gonadotoxic therapy or gonadectomy: A committee opinion. *Fertil Steril.* 2019 Dec;112(6):1022–33.
23. Oktay K, Taylan E, Kawahara T, Cillo GM. Robot-assisted orthotopic and heterotopic ovarian tissue transplantation techniques: Surgical advances since our first success in 2000. *Fertil Steril.* 2019 Mar;111(3):604–6.
24. Pacheco F, Oktay K. Current success and efficiency of autologous ovarian transplantation: A meta-analysis. *Reprod Sci Thousand Oaks Calif.* 2017;24(8):1111–20.
25. Ovarian tissue cryopreservation for fertility preservation: Clinical and research perspectives | Human Reproduction Open | Oxford Academic [Internet]. [cited 2020 Dec 24]. Available from: https://academic.oup.com/hropen/article/2017/1/hox001/3092402.
26. Lambertini M, Moore HCF, Leonard RCF, Loibl S, Munster P, Bruzzone M, et al. Gonadotropin-releasing hormone agonists during chemotherapy for preservation of ovarian function and fertility in premenopausal patients with early breast cancer: A systematic review and meta-analysis of individual patient-level data. *J Clin Oncol Off J Am Soc Clin Oncol.* 2018;36(19):1981–90.

27. Silva C, Ribeiro Rama AC, Reis Soares S, Moura-Ramos M, Almeida-Santos T. Adverse reproductive health outcomes in a cohort of young women with breast cancer exposed to systemic treatments. *J Ovarian Res* [Internet]. 2019 Oct 31 [cited 2020 Oct 1];12. Available from: www.ncbi.nlm.nih.gov/pmc/articles/PMC6824094/
28. Weenen C, Laven JSE, Von Bergh ARM, Cranfield M, Groome NP, Visser JA, et al. Anti-Müllerian hormone expression pattern in the human ovary: Potential implications for initial and cyclic follicle recruitment. *Mol Hum Reprod.* 2004 Feb;10(2):77–83.
29. Peigné M, Decanter C. Serum AMH level as a marker of acute and long-term effects of chemotherapy on the ovarian follicular content: A systematic review. *Reprod Biol Endocrinol RBE.* 2014 Mar 26;12:26.
30. Krawczuk-Rybak M, Leszczynska E, Poznanska M, Zelazowska-Rutkowska B, Wysocka J. Anti-Müllerian hormone as a sensitive marker of ovarian function in young cancer survivors [Internet]. Vol. 2013, *International Journal of Endocrinology.* Hindawi; 2013 [cited 2020 Dec 24]. p. e125080. Available from: www.hindawi.com/journals/ije/2013/125080/.
31. Li X, Liu S, Ma L, Chen X, Weng H, Huang R, et al. Can Anti-Müllerian hormone be a reliable biomarker for assessing ovarian function in women postchemotherapy? [Internet]. Vol. 12, *Cancer Management and Research.* Dove Press; 2020 [cited 2020 Oct 1]. p. 8171–81. Available from: www.dovepress.com/can-anti-muumlllerian-hormone-be-a-reliable-biomarker-for-assessing-ov-peer-reviewed-fulltext-article-CMAR.
32. Broekmans FJ, Kwee J, Hendriks DJ, Mol BW, Lambalk CB. A systematic review of tests predicting ovarian reserve and IVF outcome. *Hum Reprod Update.* 2006 Dec 1;12(6):685–718.
33. Agarwal A, Verma A, Agarwal S, Shukla RC, Jain M, Srivastava A. Antral follicle count in normal (fertility-proven) and infertile Indian women. *Indian J Radiol Imaging.* 2014;24(3):297–302.
34. Cancer Statistics Review, 1975–2014 – SEER Statistics [Internet]. *SEER.* [cited 2020 Dec 29]. Available from: https://seer.cancer.gov/archive/csr/1975_2014/.
35. Sgroi V, Bassanelli M, Roberto M, Iannicelli E, Porrini R, Pellegrini P, et al. Complete response in advanced breast cancer patient treated with a combination of capecitabine, oral vinorelbine and dasatinib. *Exp Hematol Oncol.* 2018 Jan 24;7(1):2.
36. D'Ambrosio V, Vena F, Di Mascio D, Faralli I, Musacchio L, Boccherini C, et al. Obstetrical outcomes in women with history of breast cancer: A systematic review and meta-analysis. *Breast Cancer Res Treat.* 2019 Dec 1;178(3):485–92.
37. Langagergaard V, Gislum M, Skriver MV, Nørgård B, Lash TL, Rothman KJ, et al. Birth outcome in women with breast cancer. *Br J Cancer.* 2006 Jan 16;94(1):142–6.
38. Lee HM, Kim BW, Park S, Park S, Lee JE, Choi YJ, et al. Childbirth in young Korean women with previously treated breast cancer: The SMARTSHIP study. *Breast Cancer Res Treat.* 2019 Jul 1;176(2):419–27.
39. Shah NM, Scott DM, Kandagatla P, Moravek MB, Cobain EF, Burness ML, et al. Young women with breast cancer: Fertility preservation options and management of pregnancy-associated breast cancer. *Ann Surg Oncol.* 2019 May;26(5):1214–24.
40. Gerstl B, Sullivan E, Koch J, Wand H, Ives A, Mitchell R, et al. Reproductive outcomes following a stem cell transplant for a haematological malignancy in female cancer survivors: A systematic review and meta-analysis. *Support Care Cancer.* 2019 Dec 1;27(12):4451–60.
41. De Sanctis V, Filippone FR, Alfò M, Muni R, Cavalieri E, Pulsoni A, et al. Impact of different treatment approaches on pregnancy outcomes in 99 women treated for Hodgkin lymphoma. *Int J Radiat Oncol Biol Phys.* 2012 Nov 1;84(3):755–61.
42. Akhtar S, Youssef I, Soudy H, Elhassan TAM, Rauf SM, Maghfoor I. Prevalence of menstrual cycles and outcome of 50 pregnancies after high-dose chemotherapy and auto-SCT in non-Hodgkin and Hodgkin lymphoma patients younger than 40 years. *Bone Marrow Transplant.* 2015 Dec;50(12):1551–6.
43. Inoue O, Hamatani T, Susumu N, Yamagami W, Ogawa S, Takemoto T, et al. Factors affecting pregnancy outcomes in young women treated with fertility-preserving therapy for well-differentiated endometrial cancer or atypical endometrial hyperplasia. *Reprod Biol Endocrinol RBE* [Internet]. 2016 Jan 15 [cited 2020 Sep 30]; 14. Available from: www.ncbi.nlm.nih.gov/pmc/articles/PMC4714532/.
44. Gunderson CC, Fader AN, Carson KA, Bristow RE. Oncologic and reproductive outcomes with progestin therapy in women with endometrial hyperplasia and grade 1 Adenocarcinoma: A systematic review. *Gynecol Oncol.* 2012 May 1;125(2):477–82.

45. Chao A-S, Chao A, Wang C-J, Lai C-H, Wang H-S. Obstetric outcomes of pregnancy after conservative treatment of endometrial cancer: Case series and literature review. *Taiwan J Obstet Gynecol*. 2011 Mar 1;50(1):62–6.
46. Gallos ID, Yap J, Rajkhowa M, Luesley DM, Coomarasamy A, Gupta JK. Regression, relapse, and live birth rates with fertility-sparing therapy for endometrial cancer and atypical complex endometrial hyperplasia: A systematic review and metaanalysis. *Am J Obstet Gynecol*. 2012 Oct;207(4):266.e1–e12.
47. Floyd JL, Campbell S, Rauh-Hain JA, Woodard T. Fertility preservation in women with early-stage gynecologic cancer: Optimizing oncologic and reproductive outcomes. *Int J Gynecol Cancer*. 2020 Jun 19;ijgc-2020-001328.
48. Park J-Y, Kim D-Y, Suh D-S, Kim J-H, Kim Y-M, Kim Y-T, et al. Outcomes of fertility-sparing surgery for invasive epithelial ovarian cancer: Oncologic safety and reproductive outcomes. *Gynecol Oncol*. 2008 Sep 1;110(3):345–53.
49. Park J-Y, Kim D-Y, Kim J-H, Kim Y-M, Kim Y-T, Nam J-H. Surgical management of borderline ovarian tumors: The role of fertility-sparing surgery. *Gynecol Oncol*. 2009 Apr;113(1):75–82.
50. Johansen G, Dahm-Kähler P, Staf C, Flöter Rådestad A, Rodriguez-Wallberg KA. A Swedish Nationwide prospective study of oncological and reproductive outcome following fertility-sparing surgery for treatment of early stage epithelial ovarian cancer in young women. *BMC Cancer*. 2020 Oct 19;20(1):1009.
51. Reproductive and obstetrical outcomes with the overall survival of fertile-age women treated with fertility-sparing surgery for borderline ovarian tumors in Sweden: A prospective nationwide population-based study. *Fertility and Sterility* [Internet]. [cited 2021 Apr 23]. Available from: www.fertstert.org/article/S0015-0282(20)30696-8/fulltext.
52. Tamauchi S, Kajiyama H, Yoshihara M, Ikeda Y, Yoshikawa N, Nishino K, et al. Reproductive outcomes of 105 malignant ovarian germ cell tumor survivors: A multicenter study. *Am J Obstet Gynecol*. 2018 Oct;219(4):385.e1–e7.
53. Bercow A, Nitecki R, Brady PC, Rauh-Hain JA. Outcomes after fertility-sparing surgery for women with ovarian cancer: A systematic review of the literature. *J Minim Invasive Gynecol* [Internet]. 2020 Aug 26 [cited 2020 Sep 30];0(0). Available from: www.jmig.org/article/S1553-4650(20)30407-6/abstract
54. Revised FIGO staging for carcinoma of the cervix uteri – Bhatla – 2019 – International Journal of Gynecology & Obstetrics – Wiley Online Library [Internet]. [cited 2020 Oct 1]. Available from: https://obgyn.onlinelibrary.wiley.com/doi/full/10.1002/ijgo.12749.
55. Šimják P, Cibula D, Pařízek A, Sláma J. Management of pregnancy after fertility-sparing surgery for cervical cancer. *Acta Obstet Gynecol Scand*. 2020;99(7):830–8.
56. Nezhat C, Roman RA, Rambhatla A, Nezhat F. Reproductive and oncologic outcomes after fertility-sparing surgery for early stage cervical cancer: A systematic review. *Fertil Steril*. 2020 Apr 1;113(4):685–703.
57. Knopman JM, Papadopoulos EB, Grifo JA, Fino ME, Noyes N. Surviving childhood and reproductive-age malignancy: Effects on fertility and future parenthood. *Lancet Oncol*. 2010 May 1;11(5):490–8.
58. Bhardwaj R, Parker MC. Impact of adhesions in colorectal surgery. *Colorectal Dis*. 2007;9(s2):45–53.
59. Spanos CP, Mamopoulos A, Tsapas A, Syrakos T, Kiskinis D. Female fertility and colorectal cancer. *Int J Colorectal Dis*. 2008 May 6;23(8):735.

13

An overview of ART and the risks of childhood cancer

Julian Gardiner and Alastair Sutcliffe

Possible mechanisms linking ART and childhood cancer

Introduction

There are a number of ways in which assisted reproductive technology (ART) procedures may lead to the children so conceived being at greater risk of health problems, including cancer. First, in most cases there is the underlying subfertility of the parents, which may be associated with poorer-quality ova and sperm than when natural conceptions occur. Second, there are the potential effects on the development of the embryo, which may be associated with exposure to higher-than-natural levels of hormones, with the physical manipulation of gametes and embryos and with exposure to an environment outside of the body, including exposure to culture media. These factors may affect the developing embryo, including potential epigenetic changes.

Epigenetics and imprinting

Epigenetics changes are heritable changes that do not affect the DNA sequence. These changes most commonly affect the way in which genes are expressed through genetic imprinting, a mechanism that causes genes to be expressed differently depending on which parent they are inherited from. Genetic imprinting occurs through DNA methylation and histone methylation, the latter affecting the histone protein core around which the DNA is wrapped.

Certain cancer cells have been found to exhibit hypomethylation as compared to their non-cancerous counterparts (1). Cancer cells may also exhibit hypermethylation of CpG islands (2), specific regions of the genome with a high frequency of CpG sites where a cytosine nucleotide is followed by a guanine nucleotide in the linear sequence of bases. Aberrant methylation of CpG islands has been found in retinoblastoma cells (3), glioma cells (4), and acute lymphatic leukemia cancer cells (5). This errant methylation of CpG islands in cancer cells is associated with the inactivation of tumor suppressor genes (6). Galetzka et al. reported a case of monozygotic twins, one of whom developed leukemia; the affected twin had a higher level of methylation of a tumor suppressor gene (7).

The increased risk of Beckwith-Wiedemann syndrome in ART-conceived children provides evidence that gene imprinting differs between ART-conceived and naturally conceived children (8–12). This raises the possibility that there may be more widespread epigenetic changes in ART-conceived children with health effects that are not yet fully recognized (13). Animal studies have found evidence of aberrant imprinting of maternal genes in ART-conceived embryos (14). Aberrant imprinting of maternal genes has also been found in ART-conceived children (15). Nelissen et al found evidence of hypomethylation of CpG sites in placental tissue from ART-conceived pregnancies (16).

The evidence for an association between ART conception and changes in genetic imprinting, considered alongside the aberrant gene imprinting known to be found in cancer cells, provides a putative mechanism that may link ART conception with an increased risk of childhood cancer.

Designing studies of cancer in ART-conceived children

Case studies

The earliest studies of ART treatments and childhood cancer were cases studies in which cancer was reported in an ART-conceived child or a small group of children. Although such studies are useful sources of hypotheses to be tested further, they do not in themselves provide evidence of a causal link between ART treatment and cancer.

Comparison with population cancer rates or with a control group

There are many possible designs for studies of cancer in ART-conceived children. An important distinction is between those studies in which the rate of cancer in a sample of ART children is compared with population rates and those studies in which cancer rates in ART children are compared with those in a control group of naturally conceived children. Using population rates has the advantage that data only need to be collected for the ART-conceived children. The main disadvantage of studies of this type is that their ability to control for covariates is limited. Studies using a control group have the potential to control for covariates, but it is necessary also to collect data on a sample of naturally conceived children; in order to maximize statistical power, this group should ideally be considerably larger than the ART-conceived group. This is most readily achieved using a linkage study design.

Linkage studies

Linkage data studies differ from traditional medical studies in that the data used are not collected for the specific purpose of scientific research. Instead, data collected for administrative purposes by hospitals or government agencies are used by researchers, subject to appropriate ethics approval and data anonymization. Linkage studies present specific challenges, such as ensuring a consistent definition of an exposure and data completeness, and the reliability of this approach has been questioned (17, 18). However, properly conducted linkage studies offer a valid research method (19), which has the potential to make available for analysis larger samples of subjects than is practicable using any other approach. Without the potential to use administrative data, the analysis of rare conditions, such as childhood cancer, would be severely limited.

Even for cancer, it is necessary to have a country with a middle to large sized population, such as the UK (20) or the United States (21), and good data recording. Where possible, it is advantageous to combine data from different countries using ICD-10 and ICD-11 codes (planned collaboration between the teams of Professor B. Luke, Michigan State University, and Professor A. Sutcliffe, University College London, personal communication September 2020).

Controlling for covariates

Confounders

When comparing the risks of a disease in two groups, it is important to be aware of the danger of confounding: that is, in addition to the difference between the groups in which we are interested, there may be some other variable that differs between the groups and so obscures the effect we wish to measure. In randomized clinical trials, the randomization of patients to treatment and control groups effectively removes the risk of confounding. Observational studies do not have this robustness to confounding; it is therefore necessary to identify and control for potential confounders.

When studying ART-conceived children, an important potential confounder is parental age. Couples who conceive using ART tend to be older on average than couples who conceive naturally. Unless parental age is controlled for, effects that are associated with parental age may falsely be attributed to ART treatment.

Mediators

A mediator is a variable that acts as an intermediary between the exposure being studied and the outcome. Mediators should usually not be controlled for, as doing so may cause the effect of the exposure on the outcome to be underestimated. For example, ART conception may have an influence on birth weight, which may in turn influence children's risk of cancer. Since birth weight may be part of the causal path linking ART conception and cancer risk, this variable may be a mediator and should not be controlled for in models of cancer risk in ART-conceived children.

An overview of the results of studies of cancer in ART-conceived children

Early case studies

In 1982, Melamed et al. reported a case of hepatoblastoma in a child born to a mother who had been treated with ovulation-inducing medication (22). Another study suggested a possible link between ovulation-inducing medication and four cases of neuroblastoma (23). Other case studies have suggested possible links between ART conception and cancers including hepatoblastoma (24), retinoblastoma (25), leukemia (26), and brain tumors (27). Although these studies could not in themselves prove a connection between ART conception and childhood cancer, the need for further studies was clear.

Medium-sized studies with negative results

Between 1998 and 2017 a series of studies were carried out with samples of between 2,500 and 10,000 ART-conceived children. These studies took place in the UK (28), Australia (29), the Netherlands (30), Sweden (31), Denmark (32), and Israel (33). The studies are summarized in Table 13.1. All the studies found no excess risk of all cancers among the ART-conceived children.

Because of the rarity of childhood cancer, even though these studies have many thousands of exposed children, their power to detect an elevated risk of cancer associated with ART conception is limited. In order for a study with around 10,000 ART-conceived children to detect an increased cancer risk, the risk of cancer among ART children would need to be around twice that in naturally conceived children (34). Thus, the conclusion of these studies that there was no evidence of increased risk of cancer among ART-conceived children is not sufficient to demonstrate that there is in fact no excess risk of childhood cancer among these children. It does, however, set a bound on the magnitude of this excess risk, specifically

TABLE 13.1

Summary of Results of Medium-Sized Studies of Cancer Risk in ART-Conceived Children

Reference	Location	Birth Years of Children	Sample Size	Number of Cancers in the ART Group	Comparison With	Risk of All Cancers
Doyle 1998 (28)	UK	1978–1991	2,507	2	Population rates	No excess risk
Bruinsma 2000 (29)	Victoria, Australia	1979–1995	5,249	6	Population rates	No excess risk
Klip 2001 (30)	Netherlands	1980–1995	9,484	7	Naturally conceived children	No excess risk
Ericson 2002 (31)	Sweden	1984–1997	9,056	11	Naturally conceived children	No excess risk
Lidegaard 2005 (32)	Denmark	1995–2001	6,052	0	Naturally conceived children	No excess risk
Lerner-Geva 2017 (33)	Israel	1997–2004	9,042	21	Naturally conceived children	No excess risk

The sample size is the number of ART-conceived children included in the study.

ART and the risks of childhood cancer 135

that if there is an increased risk of cancer in ART-conceived children as compared to their naturally conceived peers, then this increase in risk is not more than a factor of around 2.

Larger studies with mixed results

In the years since 2010 a number of larger studies have been undertaken with sample sizes of between 25,000 and 275,000. These studies were conducted in Sweden (35), the UK (20), Scandinavia (36), Norway (37), Israel (38), the Netherlands (39), and the United States (21). An overview is given in Table 13.2. Of these seven studies, five found no excess risk of all childhood cancers in ART-conceived children.

The study of Scandinavian children by Sundh et al. includes the Danish sample studied by Kallen, but with a longer follow-up time. Arguably, the negative result from the Sundh study therefore supersedes the association between ART conception and cancer risk found by Kallen.

The study of ART children in the United States by Spector et al. (21) has a sample size of 275,000, which is some two and half times larger than the next largest study, namely the UK study by Williams et al., with a sample size of 106,000 (20). This is the largest study of childhood cancer in ART-conceived children conducted to date, and a number of specialists in the field have confirmed that this study is methodologically sound (40), so the fact that this study finds a link between ART conception and the risk of all childhood cancers carries particular weight. This study also controls for a variety of potential confounding factors, including maternal age, maternal education, child's sex, plurality of birth (single/multiple), and maternal ethnicity. Birth weight and gestational age were not adjusted for, as these may be mediating factors, i.e., variables on the causal path between the exposure (ART conception) and the outcome (childhood cancer).

The hazard ratio for the increased risk of all cancers in ART-conceived children was 1.17 with a 95% confidence internal of 1.00–1.36. It is notable that the elevation in the risk of cancer among the ART children is small and that, even in this very large study, the effect only just reaches statistical significance. We may conclude that there is probably a link between ART conception and a slight elevation in childhood cancer risk, but until this result is replicated in a study of similar or larger size, this conclusion must remain tentative.

It should also be noted that the comparison group consists of naturally conceived children, most of whom will not have subfertile parents. Thus, this study is not able to demonstrate to what extent the

TABLE 13.2

Summary of Results of Larger Studies of Cancer Risk in ART-Conceived Children

Reference	Location	Birth Years of Children	Sample Size	Number of Cancers in the ART Group	Comparison With	Risk of All Cancers
Kallen 2010 (35)	Sweden	1982–2005	26,692	53	Naturally conceived children	Elevated risk in ART children
Williams 2013 (20)	UK	1992–2008	106,013	108	Population rates	No excess risk
Sundh 2014 (36)	Scandinavia	1982–2007	91,796	181	Naturally conceived children	No excess risk
Reigstad 2016 (37)	Norway	1984–2011	25,782	51	Naturally conceived children	No excess risk
Gilboa 2019 (38)	Israel	1999–2016	64,317	85	Naturally conceived children	No excess risk
Spaan 2019 (39)	Netherlands	1980–2001	24,269	93	Population rates and naturally conceived children of subfertile couples	No excess risk
Spector 2019 (21)	USA	2004–2013	275,686	321	Naturally conceived children	Elevated risk in ART children

The sample size is the number of ART-conceived children included in the study.

elevated cancer risk in ART-conceived children is caused by the ART treatment itself and to what extent it is attributable to parental subfertility.

Reviews and meta-analyses

A number of reviews and meta-analyses have been conducted with the aim of resolving the conflicting results of the existing studies of childhood cancer in ART-conceived children. However, the reviews published to date have not included the recent study by Spector et al. (21). As this is by far the largest study yet published, this makes the currently available reviews somewhat out of date.

The most comprehensive meta-analysis currently available was published in 2019 by Wang et al. (41). The combined result found from a meta-analysis of 12 cohort studies of ART and childhood cancer was a relative risk associated with ART/fertility treatment of 1.16 with a 95% confidence interval of 1.01–1.32. This result is strikingly similar to that of Spector et al. (21), and it may be that continuing research will confirm a modest increase in cancer risk of around this magnitude. Note that, as with Spector's result, it is not possible to determine how much of this excess risk is attributable to ART treatment and how much to parental subfertility.

Risk of specific cancers

There is evidence that the small increase in the risk of all cancers in ART-conceived children is driven mostly by certain specific cancer types.

A matched case-control study of 104 children with neuroblastoma published in 1987 found an elevated risk of this type of cancer to be associated with maternal exposure to sex hormones, either within 3 months prior to pregnancy or during pregnancy (42). A large Dutch study has found an increased risk of retinoblastoma among ART-conceived children (25, 43). The small increase in the risk of all cancers in ART children found by Spector et al. was specifically driven by an increase in the rate of hepatic tumors in ART-conceived children (21).

In a 2013 meta-analyses, ART-conceived children were found to be at increased risk of leukemia, neuroblastomas, and retinoblastomas (44). In a more recent meta-analysis by Wang et al. ART-conceived children were shown to have an increased risk of leukemia and hepatic tumors (41). Both these meta-analyses also reported an increased risk of all cancers among ART-conceived children.

In some other studies, no increase in overall cancer risk has been found to be associated with ART conception, but increased risks of specific childhood cancers have been observed. For example, Kallen et al. reported an increased risk of Langhorne histiocytosis in ART-conceived children (45), Sundh et al. found an increased risk of central nervous system cancers and epithelial neoplasms (36), Reigstad et al. found an increased risk of Hodgkin lymphoma (37), and Lerner-Geva et al. found an increased risk of retinoblastoma and renal tumors (33). In these instances, where no overall increase in cancer risk has been observed, the reported results for increased risk of specific cancer types should be regarded with some caution due to the testing of simultaneous statistical hypotheses.

When a single statistical hypothesis is tested, the test is devised so that if there is in fact no association between the exposure and the outcome (e.g., ART conception and childhood cancer), then the probability of a false-positive conclusion is no more than 5%. If five simultaneous hypothesis tests are carried out (e.g., simultaneous tests for the risks of five different types of cancer), then the probability of a false-positive conclusion rises to 23%, unless the hypothesis test is corrected for multiple testing, which is often not carried out in practice. As the number of hypotheses tested increases, the risk of a false-positive conclusion rises.

Thus, the possibility cannot be excluded that some of the increased risks found for specific cancers in ART-conceived children in studies that did not find an overall association between cancer and ART conception may be false positives resulting from the testing of a number of simultaneous hypotheses. For example, in the study by Sundh et al. (36) associations were found between ART conception and an increased risk of two specific cancer types. However, 12 different types of cancer were tested for an association with ART conception; this multiple testing means that the positive results found should be regarded with caution.

However, the increased risks of neuroblastoma, retinoblastoma, leukemia, and hepatic tumors in ART-conceived children have been confirmed by a number of studies and may now be considered to be fairly well established, although the extent to which the risk factor may be parental subfertility rather than ART treatment is still unclear.

Risks associated with specific ART methods

Most studies that have considered the risk of childhood cancer associated with ART conception have examined the risk associated with all ART conceptions, without distinguishing between the different ART methods that are in use. This approach is necessary because childhood cancer is rare and the possible increase in risk associated with ART conception is at the limits of what can be detected with the sample sizes that have been used to date. Nevertheless, there is great interest in whether the different ART procedures that have been developed over the years do differ in the long term prognosis for the children so conceived. In particular, there are questions as to whether newer ART methods such as intracytoplasmic sperm injection (ICSI) and frozen embryo transfer (FET) may carry additional risks compared to earlier in vitro fertilization (IVF) procedures.

A number of studies have examined the effects of specific ART methods as secondary hypotheses after the main hypotheses of "any effect of ART conception on childhood cancer" has been tested. As with testing for risks of specific types of childhood cancer, the potential dangers of false-positive conclusions from testing multiple hypotheses should be borne in mind.

Williams et al. found no increase in childhood cancer risk associated with the use of ICSI (46). In a study of ART in Denmark, an increased risk of childhood cancer was found among 3,356 children conceived using FET (47). However, this result was not replicated in the much larger study by Spector et al. (21), and should be regarded with caution. Spector et al. also found no difference in cancer risk between children conceived by ICSI and other ART children or between donor egg and autologous egg ART.

In conclusion, there is currently no clear evidence of differences in childhood cancer risk associated with the use of different ART methods.

Future research

In order to determine beyond a reasonable doubt whether or not there is in fact an increased cancer risk in ART-conceived children, it will be necessary to study larger samples than have been available so far. This will only be possible by combining national linkage studies through international collaboration. It is desirable that the children of subfertile couples are studied in addition to ART-conceived children and the naturally conceived children of fertile couples so that the effects of subfertility and ART treatment on childhood cancer risk can be separated.

The CREATE study is an ongoing international linkage study that is investigating cancer risk by combining cohorts of ART-conceived children from Australia, the UK, and Scandinavia, with a resulting sample size of approximately 400,000 children, larger than any study conducted to date. Results are expected in 2023 (Professor Claire Vajdic, UNSW Sydney, personal communication September 2020).

It is also desirable that future research should examine whether there is any increased risk of cancers in adulthood among those conceived using ART. Since the widespread use of ART began only in the 1990s, this question has not been accessible to research until very recently.

Conclusions

- The balance of evidence is that there is a slightly elevated risk of childhood cancer in children conceived through ART as compared to naturally conceived children.
- The best estimates currently available suggest that the risk of cancer in ART-conceived children is elevated by around 16%–17% as compared to the cancer risk in naturally conceived children (21, 41).

- It is probable that much of this elevated risk is attributable to the underlying subfertility of the parents of ART-conceived children and not to the ART procedures themselves.
- There is clearer evidence for an increased risk of certain types of cancer in ART-conceived children, specifically neuroblastoma, retinoblastoma, leukemia, and hepatic tumors.
- There is little evidence for any difference in childhood cancer risk between conventional IVF treatment and the more recently introduced ICSI and FET procedures.
- A fuller understanding of the health of ART-conceived children will only come from large-scale international studies where the controls include the naturally conceived children of both fertile and subfertile parents.

REFERENCES

1. Feinberg AP, Vogelstein B. Hypomethylation distinguishes genes of some human cancers from their normal counterparts. *Nature*. 1983;301(5895):89–92.
2. Esteller M. Epigenetic gene silencing in cancer: The DNA hypermethylome. *Human Molecular Genetics*. 2007;16:R50–R9.
3. Cohen Y, Merhavi-Shoharn E, Avraharn RB, Frenkel S, Pe'er J, Goldenberg-Cohen N. Hypermethylation of CpG island loci of multiple tumor suppressor genes in retinoblastoma. *Exp Eye Res*. 2008;86(2):201–6.
4. Otsuka S, Maegawa S, Takamura A, Kamitani H, Watanabe T, Oshimura M, et al. Aberrant promoter methylation and expression of the imprinted PEG3 gene in glioma. *P Jpn Acad B-Phys*. 2009;85(4):157–65.
5. Garcia-Manero G, Yang H, Kuang SQ, O'Brien S, Thomas D, Kantarjian H. Epigenetics of Acute Lymphocytic Leukemia. *Semin Hematol*. 2009;46(1):24–32.
6. Herman JG, Merlo A, Mao L, Lapidus RG, Issa JPJ, Davidson NE, et al. Inactivation of the Cdkn2/P16/Mts1 gene is frequently associated with aberrant DNA methylation in all common human cancers. *Cancer Res*. 1995;55(20):4525–30.
7. Galetzka D, Hansmann T, El Hajj N, Weis E, Irmscher B, Ludwig M, et al. Monozygotic twins discordant for constitutive BRCA1 promoter methylation, childhood cancer and secondary cancer. *Epigenetics*. 2012;7(1):47–54.
8. Gosden R, Trasler J, Lucifero D, Faddy M. Rare congenital disorders, imprinted genes, and assisted reproductive technology. *Lancet*. 2003;361(9373):1975–7.
9. Sutcliffe AG, Peters CJ, Bowdin S, Temple K, Reardon W, Wilson L, et al. Assisted reproductive therapies and imprinting disorders: A preliminary British survey. *Hum Reprod*. 2006;21(4):1009–11.
10. Halliday J, Oke K, Breheny S, Algar E, D JA. Beckwith-Wiedemann syndrome and IVF: A case-control study. *Am J Hum Genet*. 2004;75(3):526–8.
11. Maher ER, Brueton LA, Bowdin SC, Luharia A, Cooper W, Cole TR, et al. Beckwith-Wiedemann syndrome and Assisted Reproduction Technology (ART). *J Med Genet*. 2003;40(1):62–4.
12. DeBaun MR, Niemitz EL, Feinberg AP. Association of in vitro fertilization with Beckwith-Wiedemann syndrome and epigenetic alterations of LIT1 and H19. *Am J Hum Genet*. 2003;72(1):156–60.
13. Maher ER, Afnan M, Barratt CL. Epigenetic risks related to assisted reproductive technologies: Epigenetics, imprinting, ART and icebergs? *Hum Reprod*. 2003;18(12):2508–11.
14. Li T, Vu TH, Ulaner GA, Littman E, Ling JQ, Chen HL, et al. IVF results in de novo DNA methylation and histone methylation at an Igf2-H19 imprinting epigenetic switch. *Mol Hum Reprod*. 2005;11(9):631–40.
15. Gomes MV, Huber J, Ferriani RA, Amaral Neto AM, Ramos ES. Abnormal methylation at the KvDMR1 imprinting control region in clinically normal children conceived by assisted reproductive technologies. *Mol Hum Reprod*. 2009;15(8):471–7.
16. Nelissen EC, Dumoulin JC, Daunay A, Evers JL, Tost J, van Montfoort AP. Placentas from pregnancies conceived by IVF/ICSI have a reduced DNA methylation level at the H19 and MEST differentially methylated regions. *Hum Reprod*. 2013;28(4):1117–26.
17. Evers JLH, Sharpe RM, Somigliana E, Williams AC. The war on error. *Hum Reprod*. 2015;30(8):1747–8.
18. Grimes DA. Epidemiologic research with administrative databases: Red herrings, false alarms and pseudo-epidemics. *Hum Reprod*. 2015;30(8):1749–52.

19. Hansen M, de Klerk N, Stewart L, Bower C, Milne E. Linked data research: A valuable tool in the ART field. *Hum Reprod.* 2015;30(12):2956–7.
20. Williams CL, Bunch KJ, Stiller CA, Murphy MF, Botting BJ, Wallace WH, et al. Cancer risk among children born after assisted conception. *N Engl J Med.* 2013;369(19):1819–27.
21. Spector LG, Brown MB, Wantman E, Letterie GS, Toner JP, Doody K, et al. Association of in vitro fertilization with childhood cancer in the United States. *Jama Pediatr.* 2019;173(6).
22. Melamed I, Bujanover Y, Hammer J, Spirer Z. Hepatoblastoma in an infant born to a mother after hormonal treatment for sterility. *N Engl J Med.* 1982;307(13):820.
23. Mandel M, Toren A, Rechavi G, Dor J, Ben-Bassat I, Neumann Y. Hormonal treatment in pregnancy: A possible risk factor for neuroblastoma. *Med Pediatr Oncol.* 1994;23(2):133–5.
24. Toren A, Sharon N, Mandel M, Neumann Y, Kenet G, Kaplinsky C, et al. Two embryonal cancers after in vitro fertilization. *Cancer.* 1995;76(11):2372–4.
25. Moll AC, Imhof SM, Cruysberg JR, Schouten-van Meeteren AY, Boers M, van Leeuwen FE. Incidence of retinoblastoma in children born after in-vitro fertilisation. *Lancet.* 2003;361(9354):309–10.
26. Odone-Filho V, Cristofani LM, Bonassa EA, Braga PE, Eluf-Neto J. In vitro fertilization and childhood cancer. *J Pediatr Hematol Oncol.* 2002;24(5):421–2.
27. Rizk T, Nabbout R, Koussa S, Akatcherian C. Congenital brain tumor in a neonate conceived by in vitro fertilization. *Childs Nerv Syst.* 2000;16(8):501–2.
28. Doyle P, Bunch KJ, Beral V, Draper GJ. Cancer incidence in children conceived with assisted reproduction technology. *Lancet.* 1998;352(9126):452–3.
29. Bruinsma F, Venn A, Lancaster P, Speirs A, Healy D. Incidence of cancer in children born after in-vitro fertilization. *Hum Reprod.* 2000;15(3):604–7.
30. Klip H, Burger CW, de Kraker J, van Leeuwen FE, group OM-p. Risk of cancer in the offspring of women who underwent ovarian stimulation for IVF. *Hum Reprod.* 2001;16(11):2451–8.
31. Bergh T, Ericson A, Hillensjo T, Nygren KG, Wennerholm UB. Deliveries and children born after in-vitro fertilisation in Sweden 1982–95: A retrospective cohort study. *Lancet.* 1999;354(9190):1579–85.
32. Lidegaard O, Pinborg A, Andersen AN. Imprinting diseases and IVF: Danish National IVF cohort study. *Hum Reprod.* 2005;20(4):950–4.
33. Lerner-Geva L, Boyko V, Ehrlich S, Mashiach S, Hourvitz A, Haas J, et al. Possible risk for cancer among children born following assisted reproductive technology in Israel. *Pediatr Blood Cancer.* 2017;64(4).
34. Breslow NE, Day NE. *Statistical methods in cancer research: Volume II – the design and analysis of cohort studies.* Oxford: Oxford University Press; 1987.
35. Kallen B, Finnstrom O, Lindam A, Nilsson E, Nygren KG, Olausson PO. Cancer risk in children and young adults conceived by in vitro fertilization. *Pediatrics.* 2010;126(2):270–6.
36. Sundh KJ, Henningsen AK, Kallen K, Bergh C, Romundstad LB, Gissler M, et al. Cancer in children and young adults born after assisted reproductive technology: A Nordic cohort study from the Committee of Nordic ART and Safety (CoNARTaS). *Hum Reprod.* 2014;29(9):2050–7.
37. Reigstad MM, Larsen IK, Myklebust TA, Robsahm TE, Oldereid NB, Brinton LA, et al. Risk of cancer in children conceived by assisted reproductive technology. *Pediatrics.* 2016;137(3):e20152061.
38. Gilboa D, Koren G, Barer Y, Katz R, Rotem R, Lunenfeld E, et al. Assisted reproductive technology and the risk of pediatric cancer: A population based study and a systematic review and meta analysis. *Cancer Epidemiol.* 2019;63.
39. Spaan M, van den Belt-Dusebout AW, van den Heuvel-Eibrink MM, Hauptmann M, Lambalk CB, Burger CW, et al. Risk of cancer in children and young adults conceived by assisted reproductive technology. *Hum Reprod.* 2019;34(4):740–50.
40. Science Media Centre. Expert reaction to study looking at association between IVF and risk of childhood cancers 2019. Available from: www.sciencemediacentre.org/expert-reaction-to-study-looking-at-association-between-ivf-and-risk-of-childhood-cancers/.
41. Wang TT, Chen LZ, Yang TB, Wang LS, Zhao LJ, Zhang SM, et al. Cancer risk among children conceived by fertility treatment. *Int J Cancer.* 2019;144(12):3001–13.
42. Kramer S, Ward E, Meadows AT, Malone KE. Medical and drug risk factors associated with neuroblastoma: A case-control study. *J Natl Cancer Inst.* 1987;78(5):797–804.
43. Marees T, Dommering CJ, Imhof SM, Kors WA, Ringens PJ, van Leeuwen FE, et al. Incidence of retinoblastoma in Dutch children conceived by IVF: An expanded study. *Hum Reprod.* 2009;24(12):3220–4.

44. Hargreave M, Jensen A, Toender A, Andersen KK, Kjaer SK. Fertility treatment and childhood cancer risk: A systematic meta-analysis. *Fertil Steril*. 2013;100(1):150–61.
45. Kallen B, Finnstrom O, Nygren KG, Olausson PO. In vitro fertilization in Sweden: Child morbidity including cancer risk. *Fertil Steril*. 2005;84(3):605–10.
46. Williams CL, Bunch KJ, Sutcliffe AG. Cancer risk among children born after assisted conception. *N Engl J Med*. 2014;370(10):975–6.
47. Hargreave M, Jensen A, Hansen MK, Dehlendorff C, Winther JF, Schmiegelow K, et al. Association between fertility treatment and cancer risk in children. *JAMA: J Am Med Assoc*. 2019;322(22):2203–10.

14

Obstetric and perinatal outcomes using a gestational carrier

Marieke O. Verhoeven, Henrike E. Peters, and Cornelis B. Lambalk

Introduction

In vitro fertilization (IVF) in combination with the use of a gestational carrier is a treatment first reported in the United States in 1985 (1). Oocytes are usually retrieved from the intended mother after ovarian stimulation and fertilized in vitro with sperm cells of the intended father. The resulting embryo is transferred into the uterus of a gestational carrier. The gestational carrier is pregnant of a child not genetically related to her. This kind of treatment enables couples to have their own genetic offspring when there is no possibility to carry a pregnancy. In traditional surrogacy the oocyte of the surrogate is fertilized with sperm cells of the intended father by insemination. The surrogate is carrying a child genetically related to her. This chapter will discuss the procedure of IVF in combination with a gestational carrier.

The reasons for not being able to carry a pregnancy are various. The most clear indication is if the intended parents are a male with a female partner without a functional uterus. This could be the result of congenital absence of the uterus or the result of a hysterectomy because of medical reasons (for example, due to cancer or because of postpartum hemorrhage). Another reason for a woman not able to carry a pregnancy is a maternal illness not compatible with a pregnancy. Furthermore, gestational carriers are involved in cases of recurrent miscarriage, recurrent implantation failure, and for single fathers or for male couples. The gestational carrier procedure can be thus combined with oocyte donation but also with sperm donation.

Gestational carrier treatment is controversial. It is not allowed by law in a number of countries in Europe (2). Worldwide, in some of the states of the United States, Australia, Canada, and Israel it is practiced substantially (3–14). In Europe, in the United Kingdom, Belgium, the Netherlands, and Greece it is allowed under strict rules (15–18). Legislation differs between the various countries, going from commercially available gestational carrier agencies to only altruistic gestational carrier procedures.

Live birth rate

Reproductive outcomes of gestational carrier treatments have been reported from many countries (3–20). Whereas some authors particularly report the live birth rate for intended parents to show the success rate of their programs (6, 10, 11, 14, 16–18, 20), others have published about perinatal and obstetric outcomes as well (Table 14.1) (3–5, 7–9, 12, 13, 15, 19). Both features are important for the counseling of intended parents and gestational carriers (and their partners) to manage expectation of success of the treatment and give a realistic perception of the risks for the gestational carrier and child during the treatment. The live birth rates ranged from 15% in the earlier published studies up to around 60% in the current programs (3–7, 9–11, 13–18, 20). The live birth rates differed among the various

TABLE 14.1

Pregnancy Outcomes Using a Gestational Carrier

Pregnancy Outcomes	Reported Incidence in the Literature
Live birth rates	15%–60%
Miscarriage	3%–49%
Extrauterine pregnancy	Not reported
Hypertensive disorders and placental dysfunction	
Pregnancy-induced hypertension	4%–14%
Preeclampsia	1.9%–2.9%
Hemolysis, elevated liver enzymes, low platelets	2.9%
Low birth weight for gestational age	Associated with multiple pregnancies
Gestational diabetes	1.6%–18%
Placental disease	0.8%–4.9%
Cesarean section	8.8%–70%
Postpartum hemorrhage	2%–9%
Serious complications	3 cases
Postpartum depression	5%–11%
Premature delivery	10%
Birth defects	Not increased

indications for gestational carrier procedures, with the highest rates in the case of an absent uterus (59.3%–66.7%) (9, 15). Some authors reported similar live birth rates as with regular IVF programs (15, 16), whereas others report higher rates (3, 9), indicating that gestational carrier programs are as successful or even more successful for couples to fulfill their desire to have a child in case the intended parents are not able to carry a pregnancy.

Miscarriage

The percentage of miscarriage in the various programs vary greatly from 3% to 49% (3, 5, 7, 9, 11, 13, 15, 16, 18). Some programs found higher numbers of miscarriage compared to natural conception (7, 9, 13, 16, 18). This could indicate that the interaction of a genetically unrelated pregnancy with the carrier is different in comparison to women pregnant with a genetically related child. However, other programs do not report higher miscarriage percentages at all (3, 5, 11, 15).

The consequences of a miscarriage for the intended parents and the gestational carrier both should not be underestimated. Gestational carriers can feel rather guilty in case of a miscarriage. They usually had a history of previously uncomplicated pregnancies of their own children and want to help the intended parents but then have the feeling their body failed them when they lose the desired child of the intended parents. The intended parents grieve for not receiving a child and can have guilty feelings towards the gestational carrier for her going through the difficulties of a miscarriage.

Extrauterine pregnancies

No results are reported about extrauterine pregnancies. It seems there is no indication that this outcome would be different among gestational carriers than in regular couples undergoing IVF or in natural conception in multiparous women, since there are no reports of different incidences of extrauterine pregnancy in gestational carriers compared to regular pregnant women in the current literature.

Hypertensive disorders and placental dysfunction

Several complications of hypertensive disorders in pregnancy have been reported in gestational carriers. The incidence of pregnancy-induced hypertension ranges from 4.9% to 14.7%, being about the same or slightly higher compared to the general IVF population (3, 8, 15, 20, 21). Studies showed higher pregnancy-induced hypertension in gestational carriers compared to the previous pregnancies of the same women (3). Preeclampsia was present in 1.9%–2.9% of gestational carriers (3, 15). Hemolysis, elevated liver enzymes, and low platelets (HELLP syndrome) was reported in one program in 2.9% of the cases (15). The incidence of pregnancy-induced hypertension disorders seems to be higher than that in assisted reproductive technology pregnancies without the use of a gestational carrier or that of multiparous with natural conception (22). However, it should be realized that reported rates of hypertensive disorders in oocyte donation pregnancies are even higher (16%–40%) (23).

In the placenta of oocyte donor pregnancies, histological and immunohistochemical reactions are described, which could represent a host-versus-graft rejection–like phenomenon (24). For gestational carriers, it has been speculated that "a healthy carrier with a normal reproductive background might somehow compensate for atypical immunological reactions related to a foreign embryo" (25). Moreover, it has been reported that the incidence of a hypertensive disorder is higher if an oocyte donor is genetically completely unrelated to the recipient (20% versus 8%) (23).

Children born with low birth weight after a gestational carrier procedure were almost always associated with multiple pregnancies (4, 7, 8, 13). Some authors found a higher mean birth weight in singletons born after gestational carrier procedures compared to IVF programs without gestational carriers (5, 9, 12, 19), but others reported a higher incidence of low birth weight in singletons compared to the general population (13). Woo et al. compared the gestational pregnancies in the carrier with their own previous pregnancies and saw that the children after the gestational pregnancies had lower birth weight than after their own previous pregnancies of the same gestational carriers (3).

Gestational diabetes

Gestational diabetes was reported by various authors (3, 8, 13, 20). The incidence ranged from 1.6% to 18%, with the incidence of 18% in the smallest cohort (20). One study reports a significantly higher incidence of gestational diabetes in the gestational pregnancy compared with their previous natural pregnancies. So far the available data do not allow firm conclusions here.

Placental disease

Parkinson et al. reported placenta previa and abruption together with an incidence of 4.9% (8). None of the other studies reported an incidence of abruption. Dar et al. reported an incidence of placenta previa of 0.8% (13). Woo et al. reported an incidence of 4.9% of placenta previa in their gestational carriers (3). So far, the available data do not allow firm conclusions here about placental diseases in gestational carriers. Of the spontaneous conceived pregnancies, 0.56% are complicated by placenta previa and 0.4%–1 % are complicated by placental abruption (26).

Cesarean section

The incidence of cesarean section ranged from 8.8% to 70% (3, 8, 13, 15, 20). Parkinson et al. showed that the percentage reported in the gestational surrogacy program was the same as in the general population (8). Woo et al. reported an incidence of 8.7% of cesarean sections in the naturally conceived pregnancies compared to 19.8% in the pregnancies conceived in the gestational carrier program (3). Peters et al. show that the cesarean section rate was higher in gestational carriers compared to regular multiparous mothers (15). The different reported cesarean section rates in the gestational carriers is likely dependent on local clinical routines, patient preferences, and attitudes towards the cesarean section procedure.

Postpartum hemorrhage

The incidence of postpartum hemorrhage ranged from 2% to 9% (3, 15). These numbers were reported higher compared to the incidence in other multiparous women or to previous pregnancies of the gestational carriers (3, 15, 27). In general, oocyte donation pregnancies are reported to be associated with postpartum hemorrhage with an incidence between 0% and 17.3% (28).

Serious complications

A few serious complications are reported in the literature (15, 29). One hysterectomy was performed 16 days postpartum because of severe persistent postpartum hemorrhage after a cesarean section of a triplet pregnancy after a transfer of three embryos (29).

Another gestational carrier with three previous vaginal deliveries experienced a uterus rupture during induction of labor. She required a massive blood transfusion, a postpartum hysterectomy, and a left salpingo-oophorectomy (29).

In another reported series one patient with postpartum hemorrhage lost 4 liters of blood and also required a massive blood transfusion and an evacuation of the cavum of the uterus in the operating theater due to retention of placental tissue (15).

Premature delivery

Most premature deliveries in gestational carriers were associated with multiple pregnancies (4, 8). Some authors report a lower gestational age at birth for children born after gestational carrier procedures than after regular IVF programs (12). But Sunkara et al. showed a non-significantly lower preterm birth rate in gestational carriers compared to regular IVF pregnancies (19). Woo et al. compared the gestational pregnancies in the carrier with their own previous pregnancies and found a higher incidence of preterm delivery after a gestational pregnancy (3). No preterm births were reported in a gestational carrier program in the Netherlands (15).

Birth defects

From the studies reporting on birth defects, it seems that there is no increased risk compared to the general population (8, 13, 15, 17, 19, 29).

Postpartum depression

Two studies reported on postpartum blues or depression (8, 20). The first study reported 5 mild cases of postpartum blues or depression in a group of 95 gestational carriers. The second study reported 2 cases in a group of 17 gestational carriers. One of the cases needed antidepressant medication and psychotherapy (20). It should be realized that there is a need for special close care during the postpartum period for gestational carriers. During the pregnancy there is a lot of attention for the carrier by the intended parents and the social network. After delivery this attention shifts to the intended parents and their child. The gestational carrier experiences the difficulties of the postpartum period without caring for a newborn baby. This can give the gestational carrier a feeling of desolation.

Keeping the risks low

While a pregnancy is never without risks for any woman, the risks for gestational carriers seem to be increased in comparison to their own earlier pregnancies and in comparison to regular multiparous pregnancies, while their risk is not always increased when compared to pregnancies from normal IVF programs. Most programs select only women as gestational carriers with uncomplicated pregnancies and deliveries in their history. The selection of the gestational carrier probably influences the risks found in the different programs. However, there should be a discussion about what is an uncomplicated pregnancy or delivery. For example, the question is whether an uncomplicated planned cesarean section for a breech is an uncomplicated delivery. A cesarean section in a medical history increases the risk of a rupture during a next delivery. Is this risk high enough to refuse these women in a gestational carrier program? Or is it acceptable to include her after extensive counseling in a gestational program, as she is willing to take this risk? This is an ethical dilemma in which the values of the autonomy of the carrier versus "do no harm" of the doctor collide. In order to reduce the risk as much as possible, it is important to choose inclusion and exclusion criteria for the gestational carrier carefully. However, too strict criteria could make it impossible for intended parents to find a suitable gestational carrier.

Furthermore, many of the risks reported were increased in multiple pregnancies. Since multiple embryo transfer leads to more multiple pregnancies, it seems mandatory to use only single embryo transfers in gestational carrier programs.

It is very important that all parties involved in gestational carrier programs are counseled extensively over the possible outcomes for both the gestational carriers and the children born after the gestational carrier procedure in order to make an informed decision regarding such a procedure.

Conclusions

- Gestational carrier procedures imply psychological, legal, and medical risks.
- It is important to monitor the outcomes of gestational carrier programs for live birth rates but also for risks and complications of gestational carriers. These outcomes should be compared to the outcomes of the previous pregnancies of gestational carriers or other multiparous women, rather than those of a population undergoing IVF treatment. This will show the true additional risk for a woman entering in a gestational carrier program as a carrier.
- In such a program the inclusion criteria for being a possible gestational carrier should be carefully designed. Accepting anyone will increase the pregnancy and delivery risks, while applying too strict criteria could result in the impossibility for intended parents to find a suitable gestational carrier.
- Since multiple pregnancies will increase additional risks, these are to be avoided, and only single embryo transfers should be carried out in gestational carriers.
- Extensive counseling and regular contact with all parties before and during IVF treatment, pregnancy, and in the postpartum period are mandatory.

REFERENCES

1. Utian WH, Sheean L, Goldfarb JM, Kiwi R. Successful pregnancy after in vitro fertilization and embryo transfer from an infertile woman to a surrogate. *N Engl J Med*. 1985;313(21):1351–2.
2. Gianaroli L, Ferraretti AP, Magli MC, Sgargi S. Current regulatory arrangements for assisted conception treatment in European countries. *Eur J Obstet Gynecol Reprod Biol*. 2016;207:211–3.

3. Woo I, Hindoyan R, Landay M, Ho J, Ingles SA, McGinnis LK, et al. Perinatal outcomes after natural conception versus In Vitro Fertilization (IVF) in gestational surrogates: A model to evaluate IVF treatment versus maternal effects. *Fertil Steril.* 2017;108(6):993–8.
4. Wang AY, Dill SK, Bowman M, Sullivan EA. Gestational surrogacy in Australia 2004–2011: Treatment, pregnancy and birth outcomes. *Aust N Z J Obstet Gynaecol.* 2016;56(3):255–9.
5. Segal TR, Kim K, Mumford SL, Goldfarb JM, Weinerman RS. How much does the uterus matter? Perinatal outcomes are improved when donor oocyte embryos are transferred to gestational carriers compared to intended parent recipients. *Fertil Steril.* 2018;110(5):888–95.
6. Raziel A, Schachter M, Strassburger D, Komarovsky D, Ron-El R, Friedler S. Eight years' experience with an IVF surrogate gestational pregnancy programme. *Reprod Biomed Online.* 2005;11(2):254–8.
7. Perkins KM, Boulet SL, Jamieson DJ, Kissin DM, National Assisted Reproductive Technology Surveillance System G. Trends and outcomes of gestational surrogacy in the United States. *Fertil Steril.* 2016;106(2):435–42 e2.
8. Parkinson J, Tran C, Tan T, Nelson J, Batzofin J, Serafini P. Perinatal outcome after in-vitro fertilization-surrogacy. *Hum Reprod.* 1999;14(3):671–6.
9. Murugappan G, Farland LV, Missmer SA, Correia KF, Anchan RM, Ginsburg ES. Gestational carrier in assisted reproductive technology. *Fertil Steril.* 2018;109(3):420–8.
10. Grover SA, Shmorgun Z, Moskovtsev SI, Baratz A, Librach CL. Assisted reproduction in a cohort of same-sex male couples and single men. *Reprod Biomed Online.* 2013;27(2):217–21.
11. Goldfarb JM, Austin C, Peskin B, Lisbona H, Desai N, de Mola JR. Fifteen years experience with an in-vitro fertilization surrogate gestational pregnancy programme. *Hum Reprod.* 2000;15(5):1075–8.
12. Gibbons WE, Cedars M, Ness RB, Society for Assisted Reproductive Technologies Writing G. Toward understanding obstetrical outcome in advanced assisted reproduction: Varying sperm, oocyte, and uterine source and diagnosis. *Fertil Steril.* 2011;95(5):1645–9 e1.
13. Dar S, Lazer T, Swanson S, Silverman J, Wasser C, Moskovtsev SI, et al. Assisted reproduction involving gestational surrogacy: An analysis of the medical, psychosocial and legal issues: Experience from a large surrogacy program. *Hum Reprod.* 2015;30(2):345–52.
14. Corson SL, Kelly M, Braverman AM, English ME. Gestational carrier pregnancy. *Fertil Steril.* 1998;69(4):670–4.
15. Peters HE, Schats R, Verhoeven MO, Mijatovic V, de Groot CJM, Sandberg JL, et al. Gestational surrogacy: Results of 10 years of experience in the Netherlands. *Reprod Biomed Online.* 2018;37(6):725–31.
16. Meniru GI, Craft IL. Experience with gestational surrogacy as a treatment for sterility resulting from hysterectomy. *Hum Reprod.* 1997;12(1):51–4.
17. Dermout S, van de Wiel H, Heintz P, Jansen K, Ankum W. Non-commercial surrogacy: An account of patient management in the first Dutch Centre for IVF Surrogacy, from 1997 to 2004. *Hum Reprod.* 2010;25(2):443–9.
18. Brinsden PR, Appleton TC, Murray E, Hussein M, Akagbosu F, Marcus SF. Treatment by in vitro fertilisation with surrogacy: Experience of one British centre. *BMJ.* 2000;320(7239):924–8.
19. Sunkara SK, Antonisamy B, Selliah HY, Kamath MS. Perinatal outcomes after gestational surrogacy versus autologous IVF: Analysis of national data. *Reprod Biomed Online.* 2017;35(6):708–14.
20. Soderstrom-Anttila V, Blomqvist T, Foudila T, Hippelainen M, Kurunmaki H, Siegberg R, et al. Experience of in vitro fertilization surrogacy in Finland. *Acta Obstet Gynecol Scand.* 2002;81(8):747–52.
21. Reame NE, Parker PJ. Surrogate pregnancy: Clinical features of forty-four cases. *Am J Obstet Gynecol.* 1990;162(5):1220–5.
22. Masoudian P, Nasr A, de Nanassy J, Fung-Kee-Fung K, Bainbridge SA, El Demellawy D. Oocyte donation pregnancies and the risk of preeclampsia or gestational hypertension: A systematic review and metaanalysis. *Am J Obstet Gynecol.* 2016;214(3):328–39.
23. van der Hoorn ML, Lashley EE, Bianchi DW, Claas FH, Schonkeren CM, Scherjon SA. Clinical and immunologic aspects of egg donation pregnancies: A systematic review. *Hum Reprod Update.* 2010;16(6):704–12.
24. Gundogan F, Bianchi DW, Scherjon SA, Roberts DJ. Placental pathology in egg donor pregnancies. *Fertil Steril.* 2010;93(2):397–404.
25. Soderstrom-Anttila V, Wennerholm UB, Loft A, Pinborg A, Aittomaki K, Romundstad LB, et al. Surrogacy: Outcomes for surrogate mothers, children and the resulting families-a systematic review. *Hum Reprod Update.* 2016;22(2):260–76.

26. Jauniaux E, Gronbeck L, Bunce C, Langhoff-Roos J, Collins SL. Epidemiology of placenta previa accreta: A systematic review and meta-analysis. *BMJ Open.* 2019;9(11):e031193.
27. Bolten N, de Jonge A, Zwagerman E, Zwagerman P, Klomp T, Zwart JJ, et al. Effect of planned place of birth on obstetric interventions and maternal outcomes among low-risk women: A cohort study in the Netherlands. *BMC Pregnancy Childbirth.* 2016;16(1):329.
28. Storgaard M, Loft A, Bergh C, Wennerholm UB, Soderstrom-Anttila V, Romundstad LB, et al. Obstetric and neonatal complications in pregnancies conceived after oocyte donation: A systematic review and meta-analysis. *BJOG.* 2017;124(4):561–72.
29. Duffy DA, Nulsen JC, Maier DB, Engmann L, Schmidt D, Benadiva CA. Obstetrical complications in gestational carrier pregnancies. *Fertil Steril.* 2005;83(3):749–54.

15

Birth outcomes of children born after treatments still considered innovative

In vitro oocyte maturation

Julie Labrosse, Daniela Nogueira, and Christophe Sifer

Introduction

History

In vitro maturation (IVM) was first defined by Pincus and Enzmann (1935) (1), later by Edwards et al. (1965) (2), as the culture of immature cumulus-oocyte complexes retrieved from small antral follicles for 24–48 hours. The first live birth successfully obtained after IVM was described in 1991 in a patient suffering from premature ovarian insufficiency (3). Subsequently, Trounson et al. reported the first pregnancy obtained by IVM using oocytes retrieved after ultrasound-guided pick-up from a patient with polycystic ovary syndrome (PCOS) (4). Since then, IVM appears to be a promising technique with a potential for wider clinical applications to be used in everyday routine practice in medically assisted reproduction (MAR) centers (5, 6). Today, worldwide, up to 5,000 children were born using IVM (7).

Indications and protocols

IVM consists in retrieving immature cumulus-oocyte complexes at the GV (germinal vesicle) stage and maturing them in vitro until the metaphase II stage (5). Thus, the original IVM protocol does not include any ovarian hormonal stimulation or final in vivo maturation (8). Some assisted reproductive technique (ART) teams have attempted variations of the initial IVM protocol in order to enhance pregnancy and live birth rates after IVM, such as the use of low-dose ovarian priming with follicle-stimulating hormone (FSH) (9, 10) or ovulation triggering by human chorionic gonadotropin (hCG) or gonadotropin-releasing hormone (GnRH) agonists (11–13). However, so far, no advantage of such protocols has clearly been demonstrated (14).

In Europe, in 2015, a total of 265 treatments with IVM were reported, and 154 transfers of embryos obtained after IVM resulted in 45 pregnancies and 33 deliveries (15). Altogether, the number of IVM cycles performed in ART centers is still inferior to that of ovarian stimulation prior to in vitro fertilization (IVF) or intracytoplasmic sperm injection (ICSI). Although IVM was first developed for patients with PCOS, since it avoids the risk of ovarian hyperstimulation syndrome (16), indications of IVM have expanded. IVM has become a major option for fertility preservation, notably when ovarian stimulation is unfeasible or contraindicated (17, 18). One of the great advantages of IVM is that it can be performed at any stage of the menstrual cycle, which is particularly appropriate when urgent fertility preservation is required, for instance, prior to oncological treatments (19). Indeed, the retrospective analysis of 192 IVM cycles performed in 164 cancer patients showed no difference between IVM performed during the early follicular, late follicular, and luteal phases in terms of the number of oocytes collected, maturation rates, number of cryopreserved oocytes and embryos, and fertilization rates (20). Furthermore, the prospective analysis of 248 breast cancer patients who underwent fertility preservation prior to neoadjuvant chemotherapy showed that results were similar whether the oocyte retrieval was performed in the follicular or luteal phase of the cycle (21). Another indication of IVM are cases of resistant ovary syndrome. These patients suffer from gonadotropin resistance, showing elevated serum FSH and luteinizing hormone (LH) levels in spite of normal levels of anti-Müllerian hormone (AMH) and normal antral follicle counts (22, 23). Although resistant ovary syndrome might be genetic or immunologic, it often remains unexplained. In all, IVM appears to be the only alternative to egg donation for these patients whose ovaries do not respond to classical ovarian stimulation. Furthermore, poor responders to controlled ovarian stimulation in general can be candidates for IVM (24), as well as women without specific risks who are simply reluctant to undergo hormonal stimulation. IVM might also be an interesting option for endometriotic patients before surgery (25). Finally, IVM for the purpose of oocyte donation has also been described (26).

Nevertheless, ovarian stimulation for retrieval of mature oocytes remains the option to be privileged when possible, as significantly higher implantation rates, clinical pregnancy rates, number of available embryos, and live birth rates have been described in IVF compared to IVM (27). Altogether, the advantages of IVM include oocyte retrieval at any cycle phase, simplified and shortened treatment, increased patient convenience since less monitoring is required, reduction in cost since there is no medication for ovarian stimulation, and avoidance of side effects associated with ovarian stimulation by gonadotropins (28).

Health of children using ART with controlled ovarian stimulation

Children born after MAR following ovarian stimulation were reported to have adverse perinatal effects compared to children conceived naturally (29–34). A systematic review and meta-analysis described that in the same mother, a child conceived with MAR had a poorer outcome compared to a sibling conceived naturally, notably with a higher risk of preterm birth (29). Similarly, another systematic review and meta-analysis including 2,112 children conceived after IVF-ICSI procedures and 4,096 children conceived naturally demonstrated statistically higher blood pressures in the case of IVF-ICSI (30). MAR was also reported to be at higher risk of congenital abnormalities and birth complications such as low birth weight, very low birth weight, small for gestational age, preterm labor, congenital heart defects, central nervous system abnormalities, urogenital system abnormalities, and musculoskeletal disorders (31–33). Another study found that placental volume and other first-trimester parameters were modified by IVF with fresh embryo transfer or frozen embryo transfer (FET) compared to spontaneous conceptions, but with opposite trends, and that hormonal treatment per se may have a major effect on pregnancy outcomes through the modification of placental invasiveness (35). Data available concerning the risk of malignancies seem reassuring (36).

In all, the underlying mechanisms of these poorer obstetric and neonatal outcomes with MAR compared to natural conception are still poorly understood (37–42). A major challenge is the difficulty in distinguishing the effect of intrinsic maternal or paternal factors related to subfertility from the MAR treatment in itself. Children born after MAR may have altered epigenetic profiles, and these alterations may be one of the key areas to explore to improve our understanding of adverse child outcomes. Characteristics of the cellular process of fetal growth and epigenetic regulation during preimplantation are still in question (43). Intrauterine growth potential may be affected by epigenetic changes in the early embryonic stages during freezing and thawing (44). Culture conditions used in MAR may also play a role.

Compared to protocols of ovarian stimulation with high doses of gonadotropins, protocols involving lower doses of gonadotropins such as intrauterine inseminations are associated with lower perinatal risks. However, the fact that risks are still higher compared to natural conception even when relatively low doses of gonadotropins are involved suggests that both infertility and MAR influence perinatal outcomes.

Health of children using IVM

IVM of immature oocytes extends the in vitro culture to the early meiotic phase. Hence, the IVM technique raises the question of whether a prolonged in vitro culture and the maturation of oocytes under artificial conditions might have a negative impact on neonatal outcomes. High rates of chromosomal abnormalities in embryos fertilized following IVM have been reported. The longer the period of maturation in vitro, the higher the rate of abnormalities (45). This may in part explain the higher rate of miscarriage observed in IVM pregnancies. IVM might induce permanent changes in the expression of imprinted genes (epigenetic changes) (45). However, data from animal models were reassuring concerning imprinting establishment in cultured oocytes (46). Due to the potential impact of IVM on oocyte competence, on subsequent embryo development, and on placentation, IVM might affect pregnancy and neonatal outcomes and the long term development of children compared to ovarian stimulation or natural conception. Consequently, an increasing number of studies have addressed the maternal and neonatal outcomes and the health of children after conception by IVM.

Preterm births

Compared to ovarian stimulation, the risk of preterm birth does not seem to be increased with IVM (47–51). The highest rate of children born preterm reported in a study was 19% (48). However, the heterogeneity of data and populations on which studies are based make conclusions difficult to establish. The risk does not seem increased when considering only PCOS patients undergoing IVM compared to controls (49, 51). No difference was found when analyzing multiple pregnancies obtained with IVM compared to IVF (47, 48, 50, 51). Altogether, there is no sufficient evidence supporting that IVM increases the risk of preterm birth.

Birth weight

Birth weight of singletons born after IVM do not seem to differ compared to ovarian stimulation cycles (52). To date, only one study suggested that the birth weight of IVM children delivered at term was significantly higher compared to ICSI cycles, even after adjusting on maternal age, gestational age, and gender (47). No difference was found when considering IVM in PCOS patients only compared to IVF (49, 51). Furthermore, IVM with or without ovulation priming did not affect the birth weight of newborns (49, 51). Birth weight with IVM was not significantly increased compared to IVF for multiple pregnancies either (47, 48, 50, 51). These results confirm previous data showing that birth weight of children from IVM cycles are within the range of children in the general population (53).

Apgar scores and neonatal intensive care unit admissions

Apgar scores of children born with IVM are within normal range. Less than 3% of children were reported to have an Apgar score <7. Moreover, the rate of hospitalizations in an intensive care unit were not higher for IVM children (52).

Malformation rates

Children born with IVM do not display higher malformation rates compared to children born after IVF (52) or children conceived naturally (54). Analysis of IVM in PCOS patients only or IVM with or without ovulation priming by hCG did not affect results (49). Nevertheless, studies led so far on this subject lack a clear and homogenous definition of which malformations are considered minor and which are considered major. Furthermore, none of them has based its conclusions on the Classification of Diseases code for congenital anomalies (55). Hence, these results have to be confirmed on larger cohorts and homogenous studies, as the risk of malformations might be underestimated.

Short term development

Data on the short term development of children born after IVM are scarce. To date, only six studies addressed the health of IVM children up to 2 years (50, 53, 56–59). According to them, at the age of 2 years old, mean height and mean weight of children born after IVM were similar to children born after ovarian stimulation (50, 57) and to naturally conceived children (56). Interestingly, waist circumference at the age of 2 years old appears significantly higher in children born after IVM for mothers with PCOS compared to the general population. These observations might be imputable to the underlying maternal PCOS, favorizing metabolic syndrome and affecting the overall glucose and lipidic metabolisms (56).

Regarding mental abilities, IVM children show no delay in mental development compared to controlled ovarian stimulation at the age of 2 years old (50). However, when considering MAR techniques in general (IVM, IVF, and ICSI), the mental development of children as assessed by Bayley scales was significantly lower compared to children conceived naturally (52). Nevertheless, scores remain within normal range. Data are still too scarce to firmly conclude, although it seems that children develop normally.

Long term outcomes

So far, only one study reported the long term outcome of children born after IVM at a mean age of 7.5 ± 2.3 years, including seven children followed up until 19 years old (51). Mean height and mean weight with respect to age were similar between IVM and ovarian stimulation and were within the range of the general population. IVM was not associated with a higher rate of hospitalizations during childhood. At the age of 4 years old, three children born after IVM (two from a singleton pregnancy and one from a twin pregnancy) had a minor delay in development affecting speech and fine motor skills versus two children born after ovarian stimulation (corresponding to 1.7% of singletons and 1.4% of multiple pregnancies for IVM versus 0.4% of singletons and 0.7% of multiple pregnancies for controlled ovarian stimulation). No difference was observed between singletons and twins. This delay was resolutive at age 6 in two-thirds of the children.

Special case: IVM in cancer patients

Very few data exist on the obstetric and neonatal outcomes in cases of IVM performed in an oncologic context due to the small number of cases performed so far and lack of distance. Indeed, the first live births from aspirated immature oocytes for IVM in cancer patients was reported (60, 61). The oocytes were inseminated and subsequent embryos were vitrified and transferred a few years later when the patients were determined to be disease-free. The types of oncological conditions were not specified by the authors for each of the patients, but the children were deemed healthy. Recently, the first IVM live birth from *vitrified oocytes* has been reported (62). The patient had been diagnosed with invasive breast cancer at the age of 29 years old. Ovarian stimulation was contraindicated in this context due to positive nodal involvement. The patient had been addressed for fertility preservation prior to adjuvant chemotherapy treatment. Among the two possible options (IVM and/or ovarian tissue cryopreservation), the patient chose to undergo IVM only. IVM was performed promptly on cycle day 22 after previous assessment of ovarian parameters. Seven immature oocytes were retrieved after transvaginal ultrasound-guided pick-up. Oocyte-cumulus complexes were matured in vitro. After 48 hours of IVM, a total of six metaphase II oocytes were vitrified. Five years after IVM had been performed, and once oncology treatment had been completed, the patient used her IVM oocytes after endometrial preparation with hormonal replacement therapy and became pregnant after the transfer of one cleavage-stage embryo. She delivered a healthy boy at term.

Lately, a live birth 9 years after *zygotes* have been cryopreserved after IVM was reported in a breast cancer patient (62). A total of two out of four immature oocytes reached maturation. After microinjection, two zygotes were obtained and were cryopreserved. They were thawed 9 years later to be cultured until day 3 which resulted in a healthy baby at term. The patient was 42 years old on the day of transfer and had been attempting to conceive naturally without success for 5 years. Subsequently, a second pregnancy has been achieved of *vitrified oocytes* after IVM in a cancer patient (personal data).

This patient was diagnosed with breast cancer and IVM was performed prior her neoadjuvant oncological treatment at the age of 35 years old. Eight immature oocytes were retrieved, with five maturing 24 hours after IVM. Four years later when the patient was deemed disease-free, she returned with ovarian insufficiency and, following survival of four oocytes, one five-cell embryo was transferred in an artificial cycle. The patient delivered a healthy boy in November 2021 (personal data).

Altogether, cases of pregnancy after IVM in cancer patients are recent and data remain scarce. The reasons for the rare outcomes in the field of IVM using oocyte vitrification procedure are both relatively uncommon technology and low rate of patient return. Another additional reason for the scarce data is the existence of few specialized centers targeting this technology. So far, the few cases reported support the idea that fertility preservation by means of IVM is a relevant and safe option for cancer patients.

Conclusions

- IVM appears to be a safe and reliable technique in terms of neonatal outcomes.
- No significant adverse impact of IVM on children's health has been established so far, notably in terms of preterm birth, birth weight, malformations, and short term and long term development.
- While a considerable number of high-quality studies have been published investigating neonatal outcomes of children born after controlled ovarian stimulation, a similar analysis on IVM is still lacking.
- Most studies on IVM are limited in their size and design, and too few enable a clear comparison between children born with IVM, those born with other types of ART, and those conceived naturally.
- Controlled analyses of long term development are also required comparing IVM both to IVF and natural conception. Given these limitations, we must be cautious in drawing conclusions from the current literature.
- As IVM is gaining importance in the clinical realm, larger and more robust studies investigating both the short term and long term health of these children are warranted.

REFERENCES

1. Pincus G, Enzmann EV. The comparative behavior of mammalian eggs in vivo and in vitro : I. the activation of ovarian eggs. *J Exp Med*. 1935 Oct 31;62(5):665–75.
2. Edwards RG. Maturation in vitro of human ovarian oocyte. *The Lancet*. 1965 Nov 6;286(7419):926–9.
3. Cha KY, Koo JJ, Ko JJ, Choi DH, Han SY, Yoon TK. Pregnancy after in vitro fertilization of human follicular oocytes collected from nonstimulated cycles, their culture in vitro and their transfer in a donor oocyte program. *Fertil Steril*. 1991 Jan;55(1):109–13.
4. Trounson A, Wood C, Kausche A. In vitro maturation and the fertilization and developmental competence of oocytes recovered from untreated polycystic ovarian patients. *Fertil Steril*. 1994 Aug;62(2):353–62.
5. In vitro maturation: A committee opinion. *Fertil Steril*. 2021 Feb 1;115(2):298–304. Practice Committees of the American Society for Reproductive Medicine, the Society of Reproductive Biologists and Technologists, and the Society for Assisted Reproductive Technology.
6. Yang Z-Y, Chian R-C. Development of in vitro maturation techniques for clinical applications. *Fertil Steril*. 2017 Oct 1;108(4):577–84.
7. Sauerbrun-Cutler M-T, Vega M, Keltz M, McGovern PG. In vitro maturation and its role in clinical assisted reproductive technology. *Obstet Gynecol Surv*. 2015 Jan;70(1):45–57.
8. De Vos M, Smitz J, Thompson JG, Gilchrist RB. The definition of IVM is clear-variations need defining. *Hum Reprod Oxf Engl*. 2016 Nov;31(11):2411–15.
9. Suikkari AM, Tulppala M, Tuuri T, Hovatta O, Barnes F. Luteal phase start of low-dose FSH priming of follicles results in an efficient recovery, maturation and fertilization of immature human oocytes. *Hum Reprod Oxf Engl*. 2000 Apr;15(4):747–51.
10. Mikkelsen AL, Lindenberg S. Benefit of FSH priming of women with PCOS to the in vitro maturation procedure and the outcome: A randomized prospective study. *Reprod Camb Engl*. 2001 Oct;122(4):587–92.
11. Chian RC, Buckett WM, Tulandi T, Tan SL. Prospective randomized study of human chorionic gonadotrophin priming before immature oocyte retrieval from unstimulated women with polycystic ovarian syndrome. *Hum Reprod*. 2000 Jan 1;15(1):165–70.

12. Son W-Y, Chung J-T, Chian R-C, Herrero B, Demirtas E, Elizur S, et al. A 38 h interval between hCG priming and oocyte retrieval increases in vivo and in vitro oocyte maturation rate in programmed IVM cycles. *Hum Reprod Oxf Engl.* 2008 Sep;23(9):2010–6.
13. Sonigo C, Le Conte G, Boubaya M, Ohanyan H, Pressé M, El Hachem H, et al. Priming before in vitro maturation cycles in cancer patients undergoing urgent fertility preservation: A randomized controlled study. *Reprod Sci Thousand Oaks Calif.* 2020 Dec;27(12):2247–56.
14. Reavey J, Vincent K, Child T, Granne IE. Human chorionic gonadotrophin priming for fertility treatment with in vitro maturation. *Cochrane Database Syst Rev.* 2016 Nov 16;11:CD008720.
15. De Geyter C, Calhaz-Jorge C, Kupka MS, Wyns C, Mocanu E, Motrenko T, et al. ART in Europe, 2015: Results generated from European registries by ESHRE. *Hum Reprod Open.* 2020;2020(1):hoz038.
16. Siristatidis CS, Maheshwari A, Vaidakis D, Bhattacharya S. In vitro maturation in subfertile women with polycystic ovarian syndrome undergoing assisted reproduction. *Cochrane Database Syst Rev* [Internet]. 2018 Nov 15 [cited 2021 May 9];2018(11). Available from: www.ncbi.nlm.nih.gov/pmc/articles/PMC6517219/.
17. Donnez J, Dolmans M-M. Fertility preservation in women. *N Engl J Med.* 2018 Jan 25;378(4):400–1.
18. Grynberg M, Sonigo C, Santulli P. Fertility preservation in women. *N Engl J Med.* 2018 Jan 25;378(4):400.
19. De Vos M, Smitz J, Woodruff TK. Fertility preservation in women with cancer. *Lancet Lond Engl.* 2014 Oct 4;384(9950):1302–10.
20. Creux H, Monnier P, Son W-Y, Tulandi T, Buckett W. Immature oocyte retrieval and in vitro oocyte maturation at different phases of the menstrual cycle in women with cancer who require urgent gonadotoxic treatment. *Fertil Steril.* 2017 Jan;107(1):198–204.
21. Grynberg M, Poulain M, le Parco S, Sifer C, Fanchin R, Frydman N. Similar in vitro maturation rates of oocytes retrieved during the follicular or luteal phase offer flexible options for urgent fertility preservation in breast cancer patients. *Hum Reprod Oxf Engl.* 2016 Mar;31(3):623–9.
22. Galvão A, Segers I, Smitz J, Tournaye H, De Vos M. In Vitro Maturation (IVM) of oocytes in patients with resistant ovary syndrome and in patients with repeated deficient oocyte maturation. *J Assist Reprod Genet.* 2018 Dec;35(12):2161–71.
23. Grynberg M, Peltoketo H, Christin-Maître S, Poulain M, Bouchard P, Fanchin R. First birth achieved after in vitro maturation of oocytes from a woman endowed with multiple antral follicles unresponsive to follicle-stimulating hormone. *J Clin Endocrinol Metab.* 2013 Nov;98(11):4493–8.
24. Child TJ, Abdul-Jalil AK, Gulekli B, Tan SL. In vitro maturation and fertilization of oocytes from unstimulated normal ovaries, polycystic ovaries, and women with polycystic ovary syndrome. *Fertil Steril.* 2001 Nov;76(5):936–42.
25. Grynberg M, El Hachem H, de Bantel A, Benard J, le Parco S, Fanchin R. In vitro maturation of oocytes: Uncommon indications. *Fertil Steril.* 2013 Apr;99(5):1182–8.
26. Holzer H, Scharf E, Chian R-C, Demirtas E, Buckett W, Tan SL. In vitro maturation of oocytes collected from unstimulated ovaries for oocyte donation. *Fertil Steril.* 2007 Jul;88(1):62–7.
27. Gremeau A-S, Andreadis N, Fatum M, Craig J, Turner K, McVeigh E, et al. In vitro maturation or in vitro fertilization for women with polycystic ovaries? A case-control study of 194 treatment cycles. *Fertil Steril.* 2012 Aug;98(2):355–60.
28. Vuong LN, Le AH, Ho VNA, Pham TD, Sanchez F, Romero S, et al. Live births after oocyte in vitro maturation with a prematuration step in women with polycystic ovary syndrome. *J Assist Reprod Genet.* 2020 Feb;37(2):347–57.
29. Pinborg A, Wennerholm UB, Romundstad LB, Loft A, Aittomaki K, Söderström-Anttila V, et al. Why do singletons conceived after assisted reproduction technology have adverse perinatal outcome? Systematic review and meta-analysis. *Hum Reprod Update.* 2013 Apr;19(2):87–104.
30. Guo X-Y, Liu X-M, Jin L, Wang T-T, Ullah K, Sheng J-Z, et al. Cardiovascular and metabolic profiles of offspring conceived by assisted reproductive technologies: A systematic review and meta-analysis. *Fertil Steril.* 2017 Mar;107(3):622–631.e5.
31. Hoorsan H, Mirmiran P, Chaichian S, Moradi Y, Hoorsan R, Jesmi F. Congenital malformations in infants of mothers undergoing assisted reproductive technologies: A systematic review and meta-analysis study. *J Prev Med Pub Health.* 2017 Nov;50(6):347–60.
32. Qin J, Sheng X, Wu D, Gao S, You Y, Yang T, et al. Adverse obstetric outcomes associated with in vitro fertilization in singleton pregnancies. *Reprod Sci Thousand Oaks Calif.* 2017;24(4):595–608.

33. Giorgione V, Parazzini F, Fesslova V, Cipriani S, Candiani M, Inversetti A, et al. Congenital heart defects in IVF/ICSI pregnancy: Systematic review and meta-analysis. *Ultrasound Obstet Gynecol Off J Int Soc Ultrasound Obstet Gynecol*. 2018 Jan;51(1):33–42.
34. Maheshwari A, Pandey S, Amalraj Raja E, Shetty A, Hamilton M, Bhattacharya S. Is frozen embryo transfer better for mothers and babies? Can cumulative meta-analysis provide a definitive answer? *Hum Reprod Update*. 2018 Jan 1;24(1):35–58.
35. Choux C, Ginod P, Barberet J, Rousseau T, Bruno C, Sagot P, et al. Placental volume and other first-trimester outcomes: Are there differences between fresh embryo transfer, frozen-thawed embryo transfer and natural conception? *Reprod Biomed Online*. 2019 Apr;38(4):538–48.
36. Berntsen S, Söderström-Anttila V, Wennerholm U-B, Laivuori H, Loft A, Oldereid NB, et al. The health of children conceived by ART: "The chicken or the egg?" *Hum Reprod Update*. 2019 Mar 1; 25(2):137–58.
37. Pinborg A, Loft A, Aaris Henningsen A-K, Rasmussen S, Andersen AN. Infant outcome of 957 singletons born after frozen embryo replacement: The Danish National Cohort Study 1995–2006. *Fertil Steril*. 2010 Sep;94(4):1320–7.
38. Kondapalli LA, Perales-Puchalt A. Low birth weight: Is it related to assisted reproductive technology or underlying infertility? *Fertil Steril*. 2013 Feb;99(2):303–10.
39. Nakashima A, Araki R, Tani H, Ishihara O, Kuwahara A, Irahara M, et al. Implications of assisted reproductive technologies on term singleton birth weight: An analysis of 25,777 children in the national assisted reproduction registry of Japan. *Fertil Steril*. 2013 Feb 1;99(2):450–5.
40. Kalra SK, Ratcliffe SJ, Barnhart KT, Coutifaris C. Extended embryo culture and an increased risk of preterm delivery. *Obstet Gynecol*. 2012 Jul;120(1):69–75.
41. Cooper AR, O'Neill KE, Allsworth JE, Jungheim ES, Odibo AO, Gray DL, et al. Smaller fetal size in singletons after infertility therapies: The influence of technology and the underlying infertility. *Fertil Steril*. 2011 Nov;96(5):1100–6.
42. Litzky JF, Boulet SL, Esfandiari N, Zhang Y, Kissin DM, Theiler RN, et al. Effect of frozen/thawed embryo transfer on birthweight, macrosomia, and low birthweight rates in US singleton infants. *Am J Obstet Gynecol*. 2018 Apr 1;218(4):433.e1–e10.
43. Nelissen ECM, van Montfoort APA, Dumoulin JCM, Evers JLH. Epigenetics and the placenta. *Hum Reprod Update*. 2011 Jun;17(3):397–417.
44. Pinborg A, Wennerholm UB, Romundstad LB, Loft A, Aittomaki K, Söderström-Anttila V, et al. Why do singletons conceived after assisted reproduction technology have adverse perinatal outcome? Systematic review and meta-analysis. *Hum Reprod Update*. 2013 Apr;19(2):87–104.
45. Basatemur E, Sutcliffe A. Health of IVM children. *J Assist Reprod Genet*. 2011 Jun;28(6):489–93.
46. Anckaert E, De Rycke M, Smitz J. Culture of oocytes and risk of imprinting defects. *Hum Reprod Update*. 2013 Feb;19(1):52–66.
47. Fadini R, Mignini Renzini M, Guarnieri T, Dal Canto M, De Ponti E, Sutcliffe A, et al. Comparison of the obstetric and perinatal outcomes of children conceived from in vitro or in vivo matured oocytes in in vitro maturation treatments with births from conventional ICSI cycles. *Hum Reprod Oxf Engl*. 2012 Dec;27(12):3601–8.
48. Ho VNA, Braam SC, Pham TD, Mol BW, Vuong LN. The effectiveness and safety of in vitro maturation of oocytes versus in vitro fertilization in women with a high antral follicle count. *Hum Reprod Oxf Engl*. 2019 Jun 4;34(6):1055–64.
49. Mostinckx L, Segers I, Belva F, Buyl R, Santos-Ribeiro S, Blockeel C, et al. Obstetric and neonatal outcome of ART in patients with polycystic ovary syndrome: IVM of oocytes versus controlled ovarian stimulation. *Hum Reprod*. 2019 Aug 1;34(8):1595–607.
50. Roesner S, von Wolff M, Elsaesser M, Roesner K, Reuner G, Pietz J, et al. Two-year development of children conceived by IVM: A prospective controlled single-blinded study. *Hum Reprod Oxf Engl*. 2017 Jun 1;32(6):1341–50.
51. Yu EJ, Yoon TK, Lee WS, Park EA, Heo JY, Ko YK, et al. Obstetrical, neonatal, and long-term outcomes of children conceived from in vitro matured oocytes. *Fertil Steril*. 2019 Oct;112(4):691–9.
52. Strowitzki T, Bruckner T, Roesner S. Maternal and neonatal outcome and children's development after medically assisted reproduction with in-vitro matured oocytes-a systematic review and meta-analysis. *Hum Reprod Update*. 2021 Apr 21;27(3):460–73.

53. Söderström-Anttila V, Salokorpi T, Pihlaja M, Serenius-Sirve S, Suikkari A-M. Obstetric and perinatal outcome and preliminary results of development of children born after in vitro maturation of oocytes. *Hum Reprod.* 2006 Jun 1;21(6):1508–13.
54. Buckett WM, Chian R-C, Holzer H, Dean N, Usher R, Tan SL. Obstetric outcomes and congenital abnormalities after in vitro maturation, in vitro fertilization, and intracytoplasmic sperm injection. *Obstet Gynecol.* 2007 Oct;110(4):885–91.
55. 10cmguidelines-FY2020_final.pdf [Internet]. [cited 2021 May 28]. Available from: www.cdc.gov/nchs/data/icd/10cmguidelines-FY2020_final.pdf.
56. Belva F, Roelants M, Vermaning S, Desmyttere S, De Schepper J, Bonduelle M, et al. Growth and other health outcomes of 2-year-old singletons born after IVM versus controlled ovarian stimulation in mothers with polycystic ovary syndrome. *Hum Reprod Open.* 2020;2020(1):hoz043.
57. Foix-L'hélias L, Grynberg M, Ducot B, Frydman N, Kerbrat V, Bouyer J, et al. Growth development of French children born after in vitro maturation. *PloS One.* 2014 Feb 26;9:e89713.
58. Shu-Chi M, Jiann-Loung H, Yu-Hung L, Tseng-Chen S, Ming-I L, Tsu-Fuh Y. Growth and development of children conceived by in-vitro maturation of human oocytes. *Early Hum Dev.* 2006 Oct;82(10):677–82.
59. Yoshida H, Abe H, Arima T. Quality evaluation of IVM embryo and imprinting genes of IVM babies. *J Assist Reprod Genet.* 2013 Feb;30(2):221–5.
60. Creux H, Monnier P, Son W-Y, Buckett W. Thirteen years' experience in fertility preservation for cancer patients after in vitro fertilization and in vitro maturation treatments. *J Assist Reprod Genet.* 2018 Apr;35(4):583–92.
61. Kedem A. Outcome of immature oocytes collection of 119 cancer patients during ovarian tissue harvesting for fertility preservation. *J Assist Reprod Genet.* 2018;6.
62. Rodrigues P, Marques M, Pimentel S, Rato M, Carvalho P, Correia SC, et al. Oncofertility case report: Live birth 10 years after oocyte in vitro maturation and zygote cryopreservation. *J Assist Reprod Genet.* 2020 Dec;37(12):3089–94.

16

An overview on the clinical outcomes from ovarian tissue cryopreservation

Daniela Nogueira and Isabelle Demeestere

Introduction

Follicles, the basic functional components of the ovary, comprise two functional pools: resting and growing follicles. The resting follicle pool, localized at the ovarian cortical region, represents the "ovarian reserve" from which primordial follicles will be recruited for development throughout a woman's life. Ovarian tissue harvesting, either by an ovarian cortex biopsy or whole ovary, followed by ovarian tissue cryopreservation (OTC), is offered as an alternative to preserve fertility in young patients at risk of premature ovarian insufficiency (POI). POI may result because of genetic predispositions (Turner syndrome, galactosemia) that may affect the ovarian reserve or because of other benign conditions involving gonadotoxic treatments, such as alkylating agents for autoimmune disorders or as a conditioning regimen before hematopoietic stem cell transplantation (HSCT). However, more than 80% of the patients referred for OTC are patients scheduled to receive gonadotoxic therapy, i.e., chemotherapy or radiotherapy for cancers, including hematological (lymphoma or leukemia) and solid malignancies (breast cancer, sarcoma) (1). With the increase in life expectancy of patients diagnosed with most types of cancer due to advances in therapeutics and in early diagnosis, the possibility of fertility preservation has become crucial for patients' quality of life after treatment.

While OTC is offered as an alternative strategy alone or as a combined option with ovarian stimulation for oocyte cryopreservation in postpubertal women, it is currently the only reliable option for prepubertal girls. Alternatives to OTC for prepubertal girls, such as immature oocyte aspiration and ovarian stimulation for the collection of mature oocytes, have been sporadically reported (3, 4). These strategies raise ethical concerns since the quality of those retrieved prepubertal oocytes have not yet been sufficiently evaluated, and thus the risks of the procedure cannot be outweighed by the unknown benefits. Hence, it is of ultimate importance to gather information on the outcomes of OTC following ovarian tissue transplantation (OTT) (4) which, in prepubertal girls, is the medically rational conduct to follow. Cryopreserved ovarian tissue using the slow-freezing procedure and stored for more than 14 years has been transplanted with success (1), and long storage for up to 18 years did not affect follicular morphology and survival (5). OTC has also been suggested as an option for women requesting fertility preservation for age-related fertility loss or for delaying menopause (6), but this is of questionable recommendation and still controversial.

Selection criteria include patients younger than 35 years old with >50% of risk of POI, with a relatively good prognosis (7, 8). OTC has also been recommended in women aged up to 42 years or even 49 years (9–12). However, no pregnancies have been reported after 38 years (1) and rarely in women older than 35 years, with a better option being oocyte cryopreservation (13).

OTC is actually considered effective in restoring fertility in postpubertal patients (2, 18); however, data on efficacy and safety are still limited. Although the American Society for Reproductive Medicine (ASRM) suggested considering it as an established option for selected patients (15), European Society of Human Reproduction and Embryology (ESHRE) fertility preservation guideline commission categorizes it rather as an "innovative" technology since long term safety data for patients and their children have yet to be accomplished (16, 17).

Patient (maternal) risks and outcomes of ovarian tissue transplantation

The sole current option to restore fertility by using cryopreserved ovarian tissue remains OTT. After OTT, patients can attempt natural conception or standard ART procedures with the possibility of repetitive interventions for tissue replacement (1). Following the first restoration of ovarian function and embryo development subsequent to an heterotopic OTT (14, 15), as well as the first birth after orthotopic OTT (20), many other case reports of live births have subsequently followed. Nowadays this technology offers a 40% estimated success rate defined as at least one live birth per transplanted procedure (1). But overall, the usage rate of cryopreserved ovarian tissue remains low (13, 17). In general, in cancer patients, an interval of at least 1 year following chemotherapy completion should be considered before attempting a pregnancy to reduce the risk of pregnancy complications.

Apart from possible maternal risks associated with the disease itself and its treatment, there are other safety issues to be considered related to the OTT per se. Theoretically, two main safety aspects should be taken into consideration. A first consideration is related to the surgical procedure itself in view of its invasiveness and possible need for repeated reimplantation procedures. With the mean graft longevity of about 24 months but with large variation from 4 to 144 months, several patients seem to require two reimplantation procedures to achieve pregnancy (14), while a third OTT has been offered in less than 1% of patients (1). Complications related to OTT procedures are rarely reported irrespective of the technique of tissue replacement, whether orthotopically or heterotopically. In 770 cases of OTC, five minor complications and two severe complications were reported (10, 21). More than 60% of pregnancies occurred spontaneously after orthotopic auto-transplantation, but the pregnancies obtained after transplantation at the peritoneal site succeeded after in vitro fertilization (IVF) (1). Heterotopic transplantation subcutaneously in the forearm or to the abdominal wall is less invasive and efficient to restore endocrine function (22). However, only one live birth has been reported so far after transplantation to the anterior abdominal wall (23). For patients with specific ovarian risks, such as *BRCA* mutation carriers, the choice of the transplantation site should be made by taking into consideration the need to remove the grafted ovary after pregnancy (24).

An allograft between monozygotic twins of fresh or frozen tissue has also been reported with success when one of the sisters developed POI (25). However, in view of other well-established alternatives such as oocyte donation, this allograft strategy is generally not adopted in view of its rather unfavorable risk/benefit balance.

A second aspect to consider in OTT is the risk of disease transmission posttransplantation in cases of malignancies. This is due to the fact that ovarian metastases were found in more than 20% of female autopsies from non-gynecological malignancies, both hematological and solid tumors. Therefore, it is safer to recommend screening of the tissue before OTT (26), which may include immunohistology, molecular markers, and/or a xenograft model when available. However, in more than 300 cases of OTT, there have been no reports of relapse related to the original cancer in connection with OTT (1), except for a case of granulosa cell tumor that developed as a new cancer after grafting (23). For patients where the ovary was involved in the malignancy, experts do not recommend OTT since the putative risk of reintroducing cancer cells seems to outweigh the benefits of the OTT procedure (17). Alternatively, collection ex vivo of immature oocytes from the ovarian tissue for in vitro maturation (IVM) is an option to be considered, since five live births have been reported from this methodology without congenital malformations in the newborn (27–29). This option is also used for prepubertal ovaries since, at time of preparation for ovarian cryoconservation, it is possible to recover immature oocytes that would otherwise be discarded. These oocytes may serve as a surplus source of material for research and, in view of the investigations, its possible use in the future (30).

Neonatal outcomes

The key parameter to evaluate the effect that transplanted frozen-thawed ovarian tissues may have on the developmental capacity of its follicle-enclosed oocytes is the outcome of live births. The birth rate per ovarian tissue transplantation varies between 20% and 40%. In the latest series ever published with data produced worldwide, more than 400 patients underwent ovarian tissue replacement, resulting in more than 140 pregnancies and more than 100 children born (1, 14, 31–33). Over 90 live births were reported, but neonatal data have been evaluated for only about half of these births (1). The median gestational age was 38 weeks for singletons and 37 for twin pregnancies with median baby birth weights of 3,168 and 2,650 g. Sex ratio was 1:1 for boys and girls (34).

All these children were born healthy, except one who was affected by fetal arthrogryposis (35). In a recent French study on the fertility outcomes after OTT in 22 patients who received first-line chemotherapy before OTC, 13 pregnancies were reported in 7 patients, resulting in 8 healthy children (4).

Taken altogether, no evidence of additional risk of congenital abnormalities or genetic disorders after OTT has been reported (1, 32, 35, 36). The rate of congenital abnormalities in the children was estimated to be 1.2%, which is comparable to the rate of major malformation occurring in the general population (14).

A first live birth of an autografted ovarian tissue that was cryopreserved at the age of 14 years, before menarche, reassures the feasibility of the procedure when performed during childhood (37).

However, the number of live births from these procedures remains low and may be insufficient to make reliable conclusions. Large cohort studies with collection of long term follow-up data of the babies, including data on congenital and other possible abnormalities in the offspring, are still warranted.

Conclusions

- The most reliable application of OTC/OTT is in patients undergoing moderate-/high-risk gonadotoxic treatment.
- OTC/OTT is effective in restoring fertility with reasonable chances of achieving a live birth.
- OTC and OTT are considered safe procedures in adults and children if non-surgical contraindications exist.
- There is no evidence of risk of relapse related to the original cancer; nevertheless, tissue evaluation prior to reimplantation in cases of malignancies is strongly recommended.
- OTC is considered effective in restoring fertility in postpubertal patients; however, its efficacy to achieve live birth for patients over 36 years and/or with low ovarian reserve is uncertain.
- Orthotopic transplantation is mostly current and allows possible natural conception.
- There appears to be no increased risk of congenital abnormalities for children born, but OTC/OTT should still be categorized as "innovative" since long term follow-up data are still insufficient.

REFERENCES

1. Gellert SE, Pors SE, Kristensen SG, Bay-Bjørn AM, Ernst E, Yding Andersen C. Transplantation of frozen-thawed ovarian tissue: An update on worldwide activity published in peer-reviewed papers and on the Danish cohort. *J Assist Reprod Genet.* 2018 Apr;35(4):561–70.
2. Azem F, Brener A, Malinger G, Reches A, Many A, Yogev Y, et al. Bypassing physiological puberty, a novel procedure of oocyte cryopreservation at age 7: A case report and review of the literature. *Fertility and Sterility.* 2020 Aug 1;114(2):374–8.
3. Hanson BM, Franasiak JM. Ovarian tissue cryopreservation is standard of care in prepubertal patients, but does it have to be? *Fertility and Sterility.* 2020 Aug 1;114(2):277–8.
4. Poirot C, Fortin A, Lacorte JM, Akakpo JP, Genestie C, Vernant JP, et al. Impact of cancer chemotherapy before ovarian cortex cryopreservation on ovarian tissue transplantation. *Human Reproduction.* 2019 Jun 4;34(6):1083–94.
5. Fabbri R, Macciocca M, Vicenti R, Pasquinelli G, Caprara G, Valente S, et al. Long-term storage does not impact the quality of cryopreserved human ovarian tissue. *J Ovarian Res.* 2016 Aug 24;9(1):50.

6. Anderson RA, Baird DT. The development of ovarian tissue cryopreservation in Edinburgh: Translation from a rodent model through validation in a large mammal and then into clinical practice. *Acta Obstetricia et Gynecologica Scandinavica.* 2019;98(5):545–9.
7. Wallace WHB, Smith AG, Kelsey TW, Edgar AE, Anderson RA. Fertility preservation for girls and young women with cancer: Population-based validation of criteria for ovarian tissue cryopreservation. *Lancet Oncol.* 2014 Sep;15(10):1129–36.
8. Donnez J, Dolmans M-M. Fertility preservation in women [Internet]. http://dx.doi.org/10.1056/NEJMra1614676. Massachusetts Medical Society; 2017 [cited 2021 May 28]. Available from: www.nejm.org/doi/10.1056/NEJMra1614676.
9. Backhus LE, Kondapalli LA, Chang RJ, Coutifaris C, Kazer R, Woodruff TK. Oncofertility consortium consensus statement: Guidelines for Ovarian Tissue Cryopreservation. In: Woodruff TK, Snyder KA, editors. *Oncofertility fertility preservation for cancer survivors* [Internet]. Boston, MA: Springer US; 2007 [cited 2021 May 28]. pp. 235–9. (Cancer Treatment and Research). Available from: https://doi.org/10.1007/978-0-387-72293-1_17.
10. Jadoul P, Guilmain A, Squifflet J, Luyckx M, Votino R, Wyns C, et al. Efficacy of ovarian tissue cryopreservation for fertility preservation: Lessons learned from 545 cases. *Human Reproduction.* 2017 May;32(5):1046–54.
11. Karavani G, Schachter-Safrai N, Chill HH, Mordechai Daniel T, Bauman D, Revel A. Single-incision laparoscopic surgery for Ovarian Tissue Cryopreservation. *J Minim Invasive Gynecol.* 2018 Apr;25(3):474–9.
12. Lotz L, Maktabi A, Hoffmann I, Findeklee S, Beckmann MW, Dittrich R. Ovarian tissue cryopreservation and retransplantation – what do patients think about it? *Reproductive BioMedicine Online.* 2016 Apr 1;32(4):394–400.
13. Diaz-Garcia C, Domingo J, Garcia-Velasco JA, Herraiz S, Mirabet V, Iniesta I, et al. Oocyte vitrification versus ovarian cortex transplantation in fertility preservation for adult women undergoing gonadotoxic treatments: A prospective cohort study. *Fertil Steril.* 2018 Mar;109(3):478–85.e2.
14. Pacheco F, Oktay K. Current Success and efficiency of autologous ovarian transplantation: A meta-analysis. *Reprod Sci.* 2017 Aug;24(8):1111–20.
15. Fertility preservation in patients undergoing gonadotoxic therapy or gonadectomy: A committee opinion. *Fertility and Sterility.* 2019 Dec;112(6):1022–33.
16. Provoost V, Tilleman K, D'Angelo A, De Sutter P, de Wert G, Nelen W, et al. Beyond the dichotomy: A tool for distinguishing between experimental, innovative and established treatment. *Hum Reprod.* 2014 Mar;29(3):413–17.
17. ESHRE Guideline Group on Female Fertility Preservation, Anderson RA, Amant F, Braat D, D'Angelo A, Chuva de Sousa Lopes SM, et al. ESHRE guideline: Female fertility preservation. *Hum Reprod Open.* 2020;2020(4):hoaa052.
18. Oktay K, Buyuk E, Veeck L, Zaninovic N, Xu K, Takeuchi T, et al. Embryo development after heterotopic transplantation of cryopreserved ovarian tissue. *The Lancet.* 2004 Mar 13;363(9412):837–40.
19. Oktay K, Karlikaya G. Ovarian function after transplantation of frozen, banked autologous ovarian tissue. *New England Journal of Medicine.* 2000 Jun 22;342(25):1919.
20. Donnez J, Dolmans MM, Demylle D, Jadoul P, Pirard C, Squifflet J, et al. Livebirth after orthotopic transplantation of cryopreserved ovarian tissue. *The Lancet.* 2004 Oct 16;364(9443):1405–10.
21. Hoekman EJ, Louwe LA, Rooijers M, van der Westerlaken LAJ, Klijn NF, Pilgram GSK, et al. Ovarian tissue cryopreservation: Low usage rates and high live-birth rate after transplantation. *Acta Obstet Gynecol Scand.* 2020 Feb;99(2):213–21.
22. Bystrova O, Lapina E, Kalugina A, Lisyanskaya A, Tapilskaya N, Manikhas G. Heterotopic transplantation of cryopreserved ovarian tissue in cancer patients: A case series. *Gynecological Endocrinology.* 2019 Dec 2;35(12):1043–9.
23. Stern CJ, Gook D, Hale LG, Agresta F, Oldham J, Rozen G, et al. Delivery of twins following heterotopic grafting of frozen-thawed ovarian tissue. *Human Reproduction.* 2014 Aug 1;29(8):1828.
24. Lambertini M, Goldrat O, Ferreira AR, Dechene J, Azim Jr HA, Desir J, et al. Reproductive potential and performance of fertility preservation strategies in BRCA-mutated breast cancer patients. *Annals of Oncology.* 2018 Jan;29(1):237–43.
25. Silber S, Kagawa N, Kuwayama M, Gosden R. Duration of fertility after fresh and frozen ovary transplantation. *Fertility and Sterility.* 2010 Nov;94(6):2191–6.

26. Bastings L, Beerendonk CCM, Westphal JR, Massuger LFAG, Kaal SEJ, van Leeuwen FE, et al. Autotransplantation of cryopreserved ovarian tissue in cancer survivors and the risk of reintroducing malignancy: A systematic review. *Human Reproduction Update*. 2013 Sep 1;19(5):483–506.
27. Prasath EB, Chan MLH, Wong WHW, Lim CJW, Tharmalingam MD, Hendricks M, et al. First pregnancy and live birth resulting from cryopreserved embryos obtained from in vitro matured oocytes after oophorectomy in an ovarian cancer patient. 3.
28. Segers I, Bardhi E, Mateizel I, Van Moer E, Schots R, Verheyen G, et al. Live births following fertility preservation using in-vitro maturation of ovarian tissue oocytes. *Human Reproduction*. 2020 Sep 1;35(9):2026–36.
29. Uzelac PS, Nakajima ST. Live birth following in vitro maturation of oocytes retrieved from extracorporeal ovarian tissue aspiration and embryo cryopreservation for 5 years. 2015;104(5):3.
30. Segers I, Mateizel I, Van Moer E, Smitz J, Tournaye H, Verheyen G, et al. In Vitro Maturation (IVM) of oocytes recovered from ovariectomy specimens in the laboratory: A promising "ex vivo" method of oocyte cryopreservation resulting in the first report of an ongoing pregnancy in Europe. *J Assist Reprod Genet*. 2015 Aug;32(8):1221–31.
31. Silber SJ, DeRosa M, Goldsmith S, Fan Y, Castleman L, Melnick J. Cryopreservation and transplantation of ovarian tissue: Results from one center in the USA. *J Assist Reprod Genet*. 2018 Dec;35(12):2205–13.
32. Shapira M, Dolmans M-M, Silber S, Meirow D. Evaluation of ovarian tissue transplantation: Results from three clinical centers. *Fertility and Sterility*. 2020 Aug 1;114(2):388–97.
33. Dolmans M-M, von Wolff M, Poirot C, Diaz-Garcia C, Cacciottola L, Boissel N, et al. Transplantation of cryopreserved ovarian tissue in a series of 285 women: A review of five leading European centers. *Fertil Steril*. 2021 May;115(5):1102–15.
34. Jensen AK, Macklon KT, Fedder J, Ernst E, Humaidan P, Andersen CY. 86 successful births and 9 ongoing pregnancies worldwide in women transplanted with frozen-thawed ovarian tissue: Focus on birth and perinatal outcome in 40 of these children. *J Assist Reprod Genet*. 2017 Mar;34(3):325–36.
35. Meirow D, Ra'anani H, Shapira M, Brenghausen M, Derech Chaim S, Aviel-Ronen S, et al. Transplantations of frozen-thawed ovarian tissue demonstrate high reproductive performance and the need to revise restrictive criteria. *Fertility and Sterility*. 2016 Aug;106(2):467–74.
36. Imbert R, Moffa F, Tsepelidis S, Simon P, Delbaere A, Devreker F, et al. Safety and usefulness of cryopreservation of ovarian tissue to preserve fertility: A 12-year retrospective analysis. *Human Reproduction*. 2014 Sep 1;29(9):1931–40.
37. Demeestere I, Simon P, Dedeken L, Moffa F, Tsépélidis S, Brachet C, et al. Live birth after autograft of ovarian tissue cryopreserved during childhood. *Hum Reprod*. 2015 Sep;30(9):2107–9.

17

In vitro embryo development

Implications for epigenetic regulation

Giovanni Coticchio and Andrea Borini

Introduction

Genotype, environment, lifestyle, and diet regulate the health and disease of the adult. However, increasing evidence from both animal and human studies indicates that parental factors – such as metabolism, stress, and diet – can affect the health of the offspring. Such parental influence does not act by altering the DNA sequence and its transmission through generations; rather, it interferes with epigenetic mechanisms that during embryonic and fetal life reprogram the expression of genes involved in the formation and metabolism of the new individual (1).

This notion, referred to as "developmental origins of health and disease" (DoHaD), calls for an increased awareness of the parental role – not only during gestation in the case of the mother but also in the period around conception – in determining the health of the conceptus (2). Indirectly, it also casts a spotlight on the possible implications of assisted reproduction technologies (ARTs). Indeed, in vitro fertilization (IVF) per se implies that conception occurs while gametes and embryos are exposed to multiple non-physiologic factors – including hormone stimulation, culture conditions, and invasive manipulation – which might equally interfere with epigenetic mechanisms. Therefore, the concept of DoHaD may be relevant to the health of ART children (3). In this chapter, we will introduce the general question of the epigenetic implications of ART, focusing on the specific risk associated with culture media.

Essential developmental pathways in preimplantation development

Fertilization, cleavage, compaction, and blastocyst formation

In vitro, ideally in 110–120 hours, the human embryo develops into a blastocyst (4). This path starts with the long, complex process of fertilization, which ends with the first mitotic cleavage usually by 24 hours postinsemination. During the following 54–58 hours, the embryo undertakes repeated mitotic cycles at intervals of 12–15 hours, forming an aggregate – the morula – of apparently identical 12–16 spherical blastomeres. At approximately 80 hours postinsemination the first morphogenetic event of development, referred to as compaction, occurs (5). Losing their sphericity to acquire a flattened epithelial-like shape with ill-defined margins, blastomeres localize either internally or externally in the embryo. Such a dramatic change underpins the first developmental decision. Mouse studies have shown that blastomeres that become totally internalized within the morula will exclusively form the inner cell mass (ICM), while blastomeres that remain external and exposed to the surrounding environment will contribute mainly to the trophectoderm (TE). At compaction, other newly formed cell-to-cell interactions also seal the margins of the most external cells, forming a cellular barrier between the embryo's internal intercellular space and the outside environment (6). Afterwards, active generation of a high ion concentration in the intercellular space facilitates movement of water down a concentration gradient from the extraembryonic environment, leading to the formation of the fluid-filled cavity of the blastocoel (7). Enlargement of the

DOI: 10.1201/9781003052524-17

blastocoel proceeds in parallel with the formation of the polarized conglomerate of cells of the ICM and with the increase in diameter of the epithelial-like wall of the TE.

Embryonic genome activation

The early stages of embryo development are largely under the molecular control of maternally inherited messenger RNAs (mRNAs) and regulatory proteins stockpiled throughout oogenesis. This initial maternal control of development is gradually superseded as the embryo expresses its own genes. The first studies in the human reported that embryonic genome activation (EGA) began at a four- to eight-cell stage (8), but details of the overall dynamics of gene expression during preimplantation development remained unclear for several years. More recent studies have revealed a more detailed and complex picture of EGA, which has relevance for the morula stage. The first signs of transcription in the human embryonic genome are detectable at the two-cell stage, much earlier than previously thought. Notably, analysis of the whole preimplantation period showed that EGA occurs in a multiphasic fashion at designated stages: a pattern seen mirrored in a range of mammalian embryos (9). A major wave of transcription activation occurs at the four- to six-cell stage, involving mainly genes with a role in the translation machinery. This sets the stage for the two following and more extensive transcriptional bursts, which take place towards the end of day 3 of development (from the eight- to ten-cell stage interval), i.e., shortly before compaction of the morula (10).

Metabolic shift

In both model species and the human, metabolism undergoes important phase-dependent modifications in response to specific requirements of the embryo (11). During the early cleavage stages, the embryo is comparatively quiescent. Cell divisions occur at a moderate pace without increase in mass, and adenosine triphosphate (ATP) production is satisfied by low levels of oxidation of pyruvate and lactate (12). This picture changes in the second half of preimplantation development starting from the morula stage, when the rate of cell division and embryo mass increase and active transport moves ions from the surrounding environment to intercellular spaces (13). The energy demands for such activities trigger a marked increase in metabolism (14–16). Glucose consumption also raises via aerobic glycolysis (17, 18). Crucially from the morula stage, the genes whose products participate in this metabolic shift are regulated at the transcriptional level and expressed in a timely fashion.

Epigenetic regulation

Historically, epigenesis and preformism are embryological theories dating back as early as the times of Aristotle. They presumed that the embryo develops from a fertilized egg by progressive unfolding of a developmental plan or by enlargement of preorganized structures, respectively. The modern vision of epigenetics concerns lineage-specific, mitotically transmissible modifications of the chromatin or DNA bases that can influence gene expression (19). Notably, this modality of gene expression regulation differs from transient changes in gene transcription, whose duration is determined solely by the time of exposure to a specific regulator. Epigenetics is therefore a key strategy by which basic gene expression profiles in cell lineages are established and maintained during development. Two major waves of epigenetic changes occur during mammalian development: starting from fertilization during the first rounds of cleavage and during the constitution of primordial germ cells (PGCs). Both these phases presumably operate to erase previous epigenetic marks and re-establish baseline conditions from which novel mitotically transmissible epigenetic instructions can give rise to different cell lines (20).

Main epigenetic mechanisms

DNA base modification is a classic example of epigenetic change found in mammals. It involves the covalent addition of a methyl group (CH3) to the cytosine 5′-carbon operated by the enzyme (DNMT) (21). Cytosine methylation occurs more frequently in CpG dinucleotides. Notably, such dinucleotides are much more represented in regions of DNA (CpG islands) that operate as regulatory elements of transcribed sequences. This has suggested that cytosine methylation may affect DNA transcription in a heritable fashion. Consistent with this hypothesis, addition of a methyl group creates new topological characteristics of the DNA double helix major groove. The new conformation can generate alternative opportunities for binding between DNA and proteins, leading to changes in chromatin organization and/or activity of regulatory sequences that prevent the transcription of adjacent sequences (22). Cytosine methylation is believed to play an important role in the epigenetic regulation of alleles that are differentially expressed depending on their parental origin (23). In its turn, cytosine methylation is subject to regulation. TET proteins can target 5'-methycytosine producing various oxidized cytosine forms, including 5'-hydromethylcytosine (24). This modified cytosine base is poorly recognized by factors that have high affinity to methylcytosine; it is also preferentially found in euchromatic regions. Therefore, oxidation of 5'-methycytosine could represent a possible mechanism to revert a previously imposed chromatin condensation and repression of transcription.

Numerous posttranscriptional histone covalent modifications can influence chromatin condensation and ultimately gene expression (25). Acetylation and methylation of specific lysin (K) positions in histone 3 (H3) are typical in that respect. For example, acetylation and trimethylation of lysine 9 and 4 (H3K9ac and H3K4me3, respectively) characterize euchromatin regions and facilitate the access of transcription factors to sequences that positively regulate transcription. Instead, transcriptionally silent heterochromatic regions are enriched in H3 histones (tri)methylated in lysin 27 and 9 (H3K27me3 and H3K9me3, respectively) (26). Genes with a potential role in development may be organized in chromatin domains with different combinations of histone modification. For example, in pluripotent embryonic stem cells (ESCs), the chromatin of key genes is marked by both activating and repressing histone modifications (H3K4me3 and H3K27me3, respectively). This dual regulation does not allow direct expression, but it generates a stand-by status that predisposes such genes to prompt expression when needed. Conversely, genes whose chromatin is solely enriched in H3K27me3 remain permanently repressed.

Intense and sophisticated interaction between cytosine methylation and histone modification greatly expand the opportunities for epigenetic regulation. Typically, cytosine methylation can trigger a protein binding cascade that culminates with recruitment of heterochromatin proteins, methylation of histone 3, and further binding of DNMT. This creates a positive feedback loop that promotes cytosine methylation, chromatin condensation, and gene silencing (27–29). It can also generate spreading of a wave of epigenetic changes throughout a region starting from a "nucleation" site (30).

Finally, a third – less widespread – mechanism of epigenetic modification relies on histone variants. In growing oocytes, the H3.3 variant provides stability for nucleosome organization and is distributed throughout the genome in association with transcriptionally active regions. In early mouse embryos, its synthesis remains constant, but its association with chromatin is more prominent in H3K4me3-rich regions (transcriptionally active) and less abundant in H3K27me3-rich regions (transcriptionally repressed). Therefore, overall, cytosine methylation, histone acetylation/methylation, and histone variants are interacting parts of a larger, more complex mechanism of epigenetic regulation.

Genomic imprinting, imprinting disorders, ART, and infertility

In mammals, the alleles of a restricted number of genes, approximately 200 in humans, are expressed or repressed depending on whether they are inherited maternally or paternally. The insulin-like growth factor II gene is a typical case, in which solely paternal alleles are expressed. Conversely, only the maternal copy of the H19 is expressed. The mechanisms that control differential or selective expression of the maternal and/or paternal alleles of a gene are epigenetic and often, but not exclusively, based on cytosine methylation. Epigenetic marks are established in the germline and preserved during preimplantation development to achieve correct gene expression during fetal development and in some cases adult life (31). This system, referred to as genomic imprinting, has probably evolved also to balance during pregnancy fetal growth and the mother's ability to give adequate metabolic support. Disorders of imprinted genes are rare, but a few of them emerge as conditions possibly associated with ART. For example, meta-analysis data indicate that children conceived by ART are exposed to a fivefold increased risk to developing Beckwith-Wiedemann syndrome (BWS) compared with natural conceptions. However, absolute rates remain low (1:2700 vs. 1/13,700, respectively) (32). Silver-Russell syndrome (SRS) also shows an association with ART; nevertheless, the number of affected children was extremely low and epidemiologically irrelevant (32).

In addition to the presentation of specific diseases, changes in epigenetic marks of specific tissues and cells may suggest imprinting disorders. The umbilical cord blood of children conceived spontaneously (53 specimens), via standard IVF (34) or intracytoplasmic sperm injection (ICSI) (89) was analyzed to compare genome-wide methylation of CpG sites. Although marginal differences were observed in approximately 0.1 of target sites in ART children, overall the DNA methylation landscape of the three groups was very similar and with normal variation ranges (33). In another study comparing the cord blood and placenta of ART (51 samples, IVF and ICSI) and spontaneously conceived children, some differences in epigenetic signatures emerged; both changes in DNA methylation and transcription of transposable elements occurred in the placental tissue of ART births, while the expression of transposable elements was altered in the cord blood of IVF/ICSI children (34). A third study comparing 101 IVF, 81 ICSI, and 82 natural conceptions confirmed that assisted reproduction is positively associated with alterations in DNA methylation and expression of imprinted gene networks in the cord blood (35).

The implications of such modifications in DNA methylation and expression of transposable elements and imprinted genes in the placenta of ART children are difficult to interpret clinically. Notably, however, imprinted genes regulate placental growth and its role in metabolism regulation and nutrient exchange with the fetus. Therefore, imprinting alterations found in the placenta might underlie well-documented adverse effects of ART births. A number of meta-analyses have compared ART and naturally conceived children, adjusting for confounding factors and focusing on perinatal endpoints. (36–40). Some of these studies were extensive, collecting data from hundreds of thousands of IVF/ICSI births (40). Overall, these investigations converge towards comparable conclusions, indicating multiple growth and maturity alterations of ART children at birth, following transfer of fresh embryos: preterm birth (PTB), very preterm birth (VPTB), low birth weight (LBW), very low birth weight (VLBW), and small for gestational age (SGA).

Nevertheless, other studies indicate that some forms of infertility per se can cause altered growth parameters at birth in addition to ART (41). Evidence also exists of associations between male infertility, epigenetic modifications, and developmental outcomes. Altered methylation at specific GpG sites of imprinted genes occurs in spermatozoa of men suffering from oligozoospermia or azoospermic subjects presenting with maturation arrest (42). In spermatozoa of normozoospermic individuals with a history of unexplained infertility, altered DNA methylation patterns and microRNA profiles are positively associated with poor blastocyst development in oocyte donor cycles (43). Earlier studies also highlighted that lower global levels of 5′methylcytosine staining observed in spermatozoa do not correlate with fertilization but are negatively associated with pregnancy rates (44). Therefore, the question of possible epigenetic effects of fertility treatments remains open and difficult to appraise.

Epigenetic risk: Focus on embryo culture and culture media

The possible sources of epigenetic risk associated with ART are diverse, including controlled ovarian stimulation, gamete/embryo cryopreservation, and endometrial preparation for embryo transfer (45). Among them, gamete and embryo culture has raised particular attention. This interest is justified, as in ART the embryo undertakes the periconception development – central to the DoHaD hypothesis – in an artificial culture environment while crucial epigenetic processes unfold (1). Concerns emerged when studies in the sheep associated use of serum as a macromolecular supplement of culture media with the growth of abnormal fetuses and delivery of unusually large lambs after transfer of the blastocyst to recipient ewes (46) – a phenomenon referred to as large offspring syndrome (LOS). At the molecular level, we do not have a complete picture of how exposure to serum during preimplantation development can cause such massive growth effects, presumably due to epigenetic perturbations. But in the sheep, serum is associated with loss of methylation and decreased expression of M6P/IGF-IIR, a gene involved in organogenesis (47). Serum also affects the ultrastructure and metabolism of mitochondria, causing abnormal development of cristae, reduced oxidative activity, and abnormally high production of lactate (46). Following such observations, serum has been excluded from culture media for animal use in the biotechnology industry, a measure that has eradicated the occurrence of LOS. In ART, the use of serum as a macromolecular supplement of culture media was discontinued in the late 1990s.

Many other investigations of possible links between embryo culture and epigenetic alterations have been carried out in the mouse model. In this species, early studies showed that embryos cultured in the presence of serum display reduced expression of the Grb7 gene and the imprinted H19 and insulin-like growth factor 2 genes due to enhanced methylation of upstream control regions. On the contrary, the imprinted Grb10 gene results are overexpressed (48).

Mouse research has also focused on IVF media in general, in addition to serum. Preimplantation embryos grown in five commercially available media or in vivo were compared assessing DNA methylation in H19, Peg3, and Snrpn imprinted loci. Loss of imprinted methylation, especially in the H19 locus, occurred after development in all culture media compared with in vivo controls (49). Recent mouse studies carried out with more advanced technology indicated a link between IVF conditions and imprinting disorders. For example, a comprehensive analysis of genome-wide epigenetic-associated changes evidenced that IVF causes alterations in 3% of methylated regions; enhanced euchromatic characteristics in 293 chromatin domains; and extensive transcriptomic changes in DNA sequences involved in pathways of stress signaling, development, and cardiac function (50).

However, the mouse can hardly be considered a good or ideal model for the human. In fact, metabolism, body size, ovarian cycle, implantation mechanism, and gestation are very different in the two species (51), preventing direct extrapolation from animal data. Therefore, focus on embryo culture and epigenetics has progressively shifted towards studies harnessing human data. The first analysis reporting a specific effect of culture conditions on perinatal outcome involved the comparison of two commercially available culture media sets: Vitrolife and Cook (52). Embryo cohorts of each patient were randomly assigned to culture with either of the two media. In 110 single live births of the Vitrolife group birth weight (3453 ± 53 g), when adjusted for gender and gestational age, was higher compared with that of 78 single live births obtained with Cook media (3208 ± 61 g). Type of culture media remained significantly associated with difference in birth weight as well after multiple regression analysis, including other factors with a potential impact on birth weight. The authors concluded that the type of culture media used to grow the embryo for 2–3 days can affect birth weight and explain the low birth weight of ART children compared with naturally conceived births. Because of its questions and conclusions, the study has raised great interest in the scientific community and the general public. However, several factors limit its significance, including the very small number of births and the study design, which – although prospective – did not meet the criteria of a randomized controlled trial. A few years later, comparing the same culture media, the same authors published another study, reporting an increased rate of births with low birth weight and low birth weight for gestational age associated with Cook media (53). They also reported that the difference in growth observed in babies derived from embryo culture in Vitrolife and Cook media was already detectable from the second trimester of pregnancy (54). In children derived from embryos grown in Cook media, a lower weight during the first 2 years from birth (55) and at the age of 9 (56) was also reported. In the same year, in singleton births derived from fresh (n = 358) and cryopreserved embryos (n = 159), another study compared Sage and HTF media in relation to birth weight and mean birth weight adjusted for parity, gender, and gestational age (57). Outcomes were entirely comparable between the two groups, although a higher mean birth weight characterized births from cryopreserved embryos. A further study extended the range of tested culture media, comparing Vitrolife G5, Global, and Quinn's advantage. In 1,201 singletons and 445 sets of twins, weight and length at birth were similar in all observation groups, while multiple linear regression analysis indicated that several factors, but not type of culture medium, were significantly associated with birth weight (58). A Danish study highlighted similar birth weight in babies developed from embryos grown in Cook (n = 974) or Medicult media, the latter with (n = 204) or without (n = 147) supplementation with the granulocyte-macrophage colony stimulation factor hormone (GM-CSF) (59). The impact of the time of embryo culture, 3 or 5 days, was included in another investigation that comparatively assessed Vitrolife G5, Global, and Quinn's advantage media. Birth weight of children derived from blastocyst transfers of the three groups were similar. Collectively, birth weight of babies born from day 5 transfers (n = 2,833) was higher compared to that of children from day 3 transfer (n = 96), but the large difference in size of the two group questions the robustness of this observation (60).

Conclusions

- Epigenetics involve mitotically transmissible methylation of the DNA or modifications of the chromatin that can influence gene expression.
- During mammalian preimplantation development, epigenetic regulation reprograms the expression of genes involved in morphogenesis and metabolism.
- In vivo, parental factors can affect the health of the offspring by interfering with epigenetic mechanisms taking place in the periconception period – a phenomenon referred to as DoHaD.
- In vitro embryos are exposed to conditions that may affect epigenetic reprogramming.
- DoHaD may be relevant to the health of children born from ART treatments.
- Collective evidence indicates that multiple growth and maturity alterations are associated with ART children at birth. However, some forms of infertility per se can cause altered growth parameters at birth, too.
- Collectively, ART studies do not conclusively confirm that culture media can affect imprint mechanisms and produce epigenetic disturbances in fetal development.

REFERENCES

1. Fleming TP, Watkins AJ, Velazquez MA, Mathers JC, Prentice AM, Stephenson J, et al. Origins of lifetime health around the time of conception: Causes and consequences. *Lancet.* 2018;391:1842–52.
2. Sinclair KD, Watkins AJ. Parental diet, pregnancy outcomes and offspring health: Metabolic determinants in developing oocytes and embryos. *Reprod Fertil Dev.* 2013;26:99–114.
3. Velazquez MA, Fleming TP, Watkins AJ. Periconceptional environment and the developmental origins of disease. *J Endocrinol.* 2019;242:T33–T49.
4. Balaban B, Brison D, Calderon G, et al. The Istanbul consensus workshop on embryo assessment: Proceedings of an expert meeting. *Human Reproduction* [Internet]. 2011 Apr;26(6):1270–83.
5. Coticchio G, Lagalla C, Sturmey R, Pennetta F, Borini A. The enigmatic morula: Mechanisms of development, cell fate determination, self-correction and implications for ART. *Hum Reprod Update.* 2019;25:422–38.
6. Zenker J, White MD, Gasnier M, et al. Expanding actin rings zipper the mouse embryo for blastocyst formation. *Cell.* 2018;173:776–91.e17.
7. Watson AJ, Barcroft LC. Regulation of blastocyst formation. *Front Biosci.* 2001;6:D708–30.
8. Braude P, Bolton V, Moore S. Human gene expression first occurs between the four- and eight-cell stages of preimplantation development. *Nature.* 1988;332:459–61.
9. Svoboda P, Franke V, Schultz RM. Sculpting the transcriptome during the oocyte-to-embryo transition in mouse. *Curr Top Dev Biol.* 2015;113:305–49.
10. Vassena R, Boué S, González-Roca E, et al. Waves of early transcriptional activation and pluripotency program initiation during human preimplantation development. *Development.* 2011;138:3699–709.
11. Leese HJ. Metabolism of the preimplantation embryo: 40 years on. *Reproduction.* 2012;143:417–27.
12. Smith DG, Sturmey RG. Parallels between embryo and cancer cell metabolism. *Biochem Soc Trans.* 2013;41:664–9.
13. Martin KL, Leese HJ. Role of developmental factors in the switch from pyruvate to glucose as the major exogenous energy substrate in the preimplantation mouse embryo. *Reprod Fertil Dev.* 1999;11:425–33.
14. Houghton FD, Sheth B, Moran B, et al. Expression and activity of hexokinase in the early mouse embryo. *Mol Hum Reprod.* 1996;2:793–8.
15. Houghton FD, Humpherson PG, Hawkhead JA, Hall CJ, Leese HJ. Na+, K+, ATPase activity in the human and bovine preimplantation embryo. *Dev Biol.* 2003;263:360–6.

16. Sturmey RG, Leese HJ. Energy metabolism in pig oocytes and early embryos. *Reproduction*. 2003; 126:197–204.
17. Gardner DK, Lane M, Stevens J, Schoolcraft WB. Noninvasive assessment of human embryo nutrient consumption as a measure of developmental potential. *Fertil Steril*. 2001;76:1175–80.
18. Krisher RL, Prather RS. A role for the Warburg effect in preimplantation embryo development: Metabolic modification to support rapid cell proliferation. *Mol Reprod Dev*. 2012;79:311–20.
19. Stäubli A, Peters AH. Mechanisms of maternal intergenerational epigenetic inheritance. *Curr Opin Genet Dev*. 2021;67:151–62.
20. Xu R, Li C, Liu X, Gao S. Insights into epigenetic patterns in mammalian early embryos. *Protein Cell*. 2021;12:7–28.
21. Bird A. DNA methylation patterns and epigenetic memory. *Genes Dev*. 2002;16:6–21.
22. Bogdanović O, Veenstra GJ. DNA methylation and methyl-CpG binding proteins: Developmental requirements and function. *Chromosoma*. 2009;118:549–65.
23. Wilkins JF. Genomic imprinting and methylation: Epigenetic canalization and conflict. *Trends Genet*. 2005;21:356–65.
24. Véron N, Peters AH. Epigenetics: Tet proteins in the limelight. *Nature*. 2011;473:293–4.
25. Lunyak VV, Rosenfeld MG. Epigenetic regulation of stem cell fate. *Hum Mol Genet*. 2008;17:R28–36.
26. Ringrose L, Paro R. Epigenetic regulation of cellular memory by the Polycomb and Trithorax group proteins. *Annu Rev Genet*. 2004;38:413–43.
27. Fuks F, Hurd PJ, Deplus R, Kouzarides T. The DNA methyltransferases associate with HP1 and the SUV39H1 histone methyltransferase. *Nucleic Acids Res*. 2003;31:2305–12.
28. Stewart MD, Li J, Wong J. Relationship between histone H3 lysine 9 methylation, transcription repression, and heterochromatin protein 1 recruitment. *Mol Cell Biol*. 2005;25:2525–38.
29. Sarraf SA, Stancheva I. Methyl-CpG binding protein MBD1 couples histone H3 methylation at lysine 9 by SETDB1 to DNA replication and chromatin assembly. *Mol Cell*. 2004;15:595–605.
30. Rountree MR, Bachman KE, Herman JG, Baylin SB. DNA methylation, chromatin inheritance, and cancer. *Oncogene*. 2001;20:3156–65.
31. Xu R, Li C, Liu X, Gao S. Insights into epigenetic patterns in mammalian early embryos. *Protein & Cell* [Internet]. 2020 July;12(1):7–28. https://doi.org/10.1007%2Fs13238-020-00757-z.
32. Vermeiden JP, Bernardus RE. Are imprinting disorders more prevalent after human in vitro fertilisation or intracytoplasmic sperm injection? *Fertil Steril*. 2013;99:642–51.
33. El HN, Haertle L, Dittrich M, et al. DNA methylation signatures in cord blood of ICSI children. *Hum Reprod*. 2017;32:1761–9.
34. Choux C, Binquet C, Carmignac V, et al. The epigenetic control of transposable elements and imprinted genes in newborns is affected by the mode of conception: ART versus spontaneous conception without underlying infertility. *Hum Reprod*. 2018;33:331–40.
35. Vincent RN, Gooding LD, Louie K, et al. Altered DNA methylation and expression of PLAGL1 in cord blood from assisted reproductive technology pregnancies compared with natural conceptions. *Fertil Steril*. 2016;106:739–48 e3.
36. Helmerhorst FM, Perquin DA, Donker D, Keirse MJ. Perinatal outcome of singletons and twins after assisted conception: A systematic review of controlled studies. *BMJ*. 2004;328:261.
37. Jackson RA, Gibson KA, Wu YW, Croughan MS. Perinatal outcomes in singletons following in vitro fertilisation: A meta-analysis. *Obstet Gynecol*. 2004;103:551–63.
38. McGovern PG, Llorens AJ, Skurnick JH, et al. Increased risk of preterm birth in singleton pregnancies resulting from in vitro fertilisation-embryo transfer or gamete intrafallopian transfer: A meta-analysis. *Fertil Steril*. 2004;82:1514–20.
39. Marino JL, Moore VM, Willson KJ, et al. Perinatal outcomes by mode of assisted conception and subfertility in an Australian data linkage cohort. *PLoS One*. 2014;9:e80398.
40. Qin JB, Sheng XQ, Wu D et al. Worldwide prevalence of adverse pregnancy outcomes among singleton pregnancies after in vitro fertilisation/intracytoplasmic sperm injection: A systematic review and meta-analysis. *Arch Gynecol Obstet*. 2017;295:285–301.
41. Davies MJ, Moore VM, Willson KJ, et al. Reproductive technologies and the risk of birth defects. *N Engl J Med*. 2012;366:1803–13.
42. Marques PI, Fernandes S, Carvalho F, et al. DNA methylation imprinting errors in spermatogenic cells from maturation arrest azoospermic patients. *Andrology*. 2017;5:451–9.

43. Denomme MM, McCallie BR, Parks JC, et al. Alterations in the sperm histone-retained epigenome are associated with unexplained male factor infertility and poor blastocyst development in donor oocyte IVF cycles. *Hum Reprod.* 2017;32:2443–55.
44. Benchaib M, Braun V, Ressnikof D, et al. Influence of global sperm DNA methylation on IVF results. *Hum Reprod.* 2005;20:768–73.
45. Berntsen S, Söderström-Anttila V, Wennerholm UB, et al. The health of children conceived by ART: "The chicken or the egg?" *Hum Reprod Update.* 2019;25:137–58.
46. Thompson JG, Gardner DK, Pugh PA, et al. Lamb birth weight is affected by culture system utilized during in vitro pre-elongation development of ovine embryos. *Biol Reprod.* 1995;53:1385–91.
47. Young LE, Fernandes K, McEvoy TG, et al. Epigenetic change in IGF2R is associated with fetal overgrowth after sheep embryo culture. *Nat Genet.* 2001;27:153.
48. Khosla S, Dean W, Brown D, Reik W, Feil R. Culture of preimplantation mouse embryos affects fetal development and the expression of imprinted genes. *Biol Reprod.* 2001;64:918–26.
49. Market-Velker BA, Fernandes AD, Mann MR. Side-by-side comparison of five commercial media systems in a mouse model: Suboptimal in vitro culture interferes with imprint maintenance. *Biol Reprod.* 2010;83:938–50.
50. Ruggeri E, Lira-Albarrán S, Grow EJ, et al. Sex-specific epigenetic profile of inner cell mass of mice conceived in vivo or by IVF. *Mol Hum Reprod.* 2020;26:866–78.
51. Hanna CW, Demond H, Kelsey G. Epigenetic regulation in development: Is the mouse a good model for the human? *Hum Reprod Update.* 2018;24:556–76.
52. Dumoulin JC, Land JA, Van MAP, et al. Effect of in vitro culture of human embryos on birthweight of newborns. *Hum Reprod.* 2010;25:605–12.
53. Nelissen EC, Van MAP, Coonen E, et al. Further evidence that culture media affect perinatal outcome: Findings after transfer of fresh and cryopreserved embryos. *Hum Reprod.* 2012;27:1966–76.
54. Nelissen EC, Van MAP, Smits LJ, et al. IVF culture medium affects human intrauterine growth as early as the second trimester of pregnancy. *Hum Reprod.* 2013;28:2067–74.
55. Kleijkers SHM, van Montfoort APA, Smits LJM, et al. IVF culture medium affects post-natal weight in humans during the first 2 years of life. *Hum Reprod.* 2014;29:661–9.
56. Zandstra H, Brentjens LBPM, Spauwen B, Touwslager RNH, Bons JAP, Mulder AL, Smits LJM, van der Hoeven MAHBM, van Golde RJT, Evers JLH, et al. Association of culture medium with growth, weight and cardiovascular development of IVF children at the age of 9 years. *Hum Reprod.* 2018;33:1645–56.
57. Vergouw CG, Kostelijk EH, Doejaaren E, Hompes PG, Lambalk CB, Schats R. The influence of the type of embryo culture medium on neonatal birthweight after single embryo transfer in IVF. *Hum Reprod.* 2012;27:2619–26.
58. Lin S, Li M, Lian Y, Chen L, Liu P. No effect of embryo culture media on birthweight and length of newborns. *Hum Reprod.* 2013;28:1762–7.
59. Lemmen JG, Pinborg A, Rasmussen S, Ziebe S. Birthweight distribution in ART singletons resulting from embryo culture in two different culture media compared with the national population. *Hum Reprod.* 2014;29:2326–32.
60. Zhu J, Lin S, Li M, Chen L, Lian Y, Liu P, et al. Effect of in vitro culture period on birthweight of singleton newborns. *Hum Reprod.* 2014;29:448–54.

18
Psychosocial effects of undergoing assisted reproductive technologies

Sofia Gameiro and Bethan Rowbottom

Introduction

Patients undergoing assisted reproductive technologies (ARTs) experience a series of psychosocial effects that simultaneously result from and determine their treatment pathway. This chapter adopts the conceptual approach taken by the European Society for Human Reproduction and Embryology's (ESHRE) sponsored psychosocial care in infertility and ART guidelines in mapping such effects by treatment period and domain of experience (1). By adopting this holistic approach, we aim to provide a comprehensive portrait of the typical experiences the majority of patients undergo as they progress in their ART treatment pathway. ESHRE and the UK Human Fertilisation and Embryology Authority (HFEA) recommend that all fertility clinic staff (doctors, nurses, midwives, counselors, social workers, psychologists, embryologists, and administrative personnel) are aware of patients' treatment experiences and engage in offering adequate psychosocial care in combination with the medical care they provide during their routine practice (1, 2). By doing so, fertility staff can ensure that they will address the most common needs of 80% of their patients (1–3). To access evidence-based best-practice recommendations on how to do so, readers are signposted to the ESHRE guidelines (1).

We acknowledge that a small proportion of patients can experience more severe emotional problems that will require referral (self or by staff) to specialized psychosocial care, which is the sole responsibility of mental health professionals. We also acknowledge that some patients will experience specific needs that will not be covered in this chapter, for instance, needs related with the use of fertility preservation techniques, third-party donation, preimplantation genetic testing, etc. Such issues are so complex that it is impossible to pay them due attention within the scope of this chapter, but there are many specialized book chapters and papers available for consultation.

Similarly to the ESHRE guidelines, we will describe patients' experiences across three treatment periods. The pretreatment period refers to the period starting as patients first visit the fertility clinic and extends up to the last consultation preceding the start of a first treatment cycle. The during-treatment period refers to the period that each treatment cycle takes to unfold, be it first-line treatment such as intrauterine insemination (IUI) or ART cycles, as well as the period within consecutive cycles. The post-treatment period refers to the period after patients undergo their last treatment cycle and covers the experience of both patients who conceive (pregnancy and early postpartum) and do not conceive with treatment. Consistent with the World Health Organization (WHO) definition of health as physical, mental, and social well-being, we adopted the ESHRE conceptualization of the effects of treatment as being behavioral (e.g., lifestyle, nutrition, compliance), relational and social (partner relationship if there is one, family, friends, the larger community, and work), emotional (mental health, well-being, and quality of life), and cognitive (e.g., knowledge, concerns, motivation). Table 18.1 presents a summary of patients' experiences, which are organized by period (pre, during, and post-treatment) and domain of experience (behavioral, relational, social, and cognitive).

The pretreatment period: From patient's first visit to the clinic to the start of a first treatment cycle

By their first appointment at a fertility clinic, it is likely patients have already endured a long journey in pursuit of their parenthood goals. It is important to note that access to funded ART often requires a referral. This referral can come from several different clinicians (e.g., general practitioner, obstetrician/gynecologist, etc.) (4) and a period of unprotected regular intercourse, in the absence of a known fertility problem, is usually required. For instance, in the UK, funded in vitro fertilization (IVF) is only recommended after 2 years of regular unprotected intercourse for women of reproductive age with an unknown cause of infertility (3). Furthermore, beyond these recommended "watchful waiting" periods, patients may experience other barriers that delay their referral for treatment, such as health care professionals lacking sufficient knowledge or willingness to make a timely referral (4–6) or extended waiting lists for public- or private-funded treatment. Considering these potential hurdles in accessing care, it is hardly surprising that when patients attend the clinic for the first time, they may perceive this is a notable step forward and feel empowered with the sense of doing something tangible towards achieving their parenthood goals (7).

Around 6% of patients referred for treatment decide not to proceed before diagnostic investigation, and just over 3% withdraw during diagnostic workup (8). When they do complete diagnostic workup, receiving an infertility diagnosis may affect their psychological status. One cross-sectional study indicated that women who received a diagnosis of male factor infertility reported higher levels of anxiety than women with other diagnoses such as female factor, mixed, or unexplained (9). However, another study reported higher anxiety and distress levels in women before treatment in general, and more so when the diagnosis was female factor (10). Higher clinical distress and psychiatric morbidity in males have also been reported following diagnosis, and in particular for male factor or mixed factor diagnoses (11). Overall, the evidence indicates a negative psychological effect of receiving an infertility diagnosis, although the possible interactions between gender and cause of infertility on such an effect are inconclusive.

If patients are recommended fertility treatment, it is their decision whether to proceed or not. Around a third of patients decide not to uptake ART after diagnostic workup (8), citing reasons such as objections to treatment (e.g. ethical concerns), relational problems, the anticipated physical and psychological burden (8, 12), and female psychological vulnerability (13).

More than 80% of women who proceed to treatment engage in lifestyle behaviors that may be detrimental to their general and fertility health (14, 15). At this stage fertility staff usually make suggestions to address unhealthy lifestyles (16). For example, a reduction in body mass index (BMI) can improve the chances of successful treatment (17, 18). Patients often report being prepared to make these changes, but a cross-sectional study of 250 women showed that a majority did not. More specifically, 79.6% of women who regularly consumed alcohol did not reduce their consumption (15). Some patients find the lifestyle change suggestions they receive at their initial clinic appointments irrelevant, as they were already aware of these factors and feel that they had already taken sufficient steps to address them (19), which may explain why further changes are not implemented.

Couples beginning fertility treatment reportedly have similar levels of marital satisfaction to the general population (20, 21). However, there are interrelational influences on satisfaction, and if views on the importance of parenthood or the perceived social impact of infertility (e.g., infertility-related isolation) differ, this may result in lower marital satisfaction (22). Some patients may engage in avoidant behaviors, such as avoiding pregnant women, but this is associated with higher fertility-specific marital and social distress (23).

At the beginning of treatment, patients are no more likely to express depressive symptoms compared to the general population but may experience similar or worse anxiety levels than normative controls, though findings on anxiety levels are inconclusive (24). The varied results reported in the literature may result from patients choosing to provide socially desirable answers, fearing they may be denied treatment if they appear to be experiencing psychological difficulties (25, 26). Gender differences in psychological stress have also been found, with women more likely to experience infertility-related stress, anxiety, and depression before treatment and men more likely to experience depression (23, 25, 27). This may be related to the different challenges ART poses to men and women. For instance, women often undergo more invasive diagnosis and treatment procedures, and men may feel a sense of helplessness in face of their partner's experience. In this context, having a supportive and responsive spouse and using active coping strategies such as goal-oriented problem solving have been shown to be protective (28, 29). Conversely, psychological vulnerability (e.g., depressive symptoms in self or partner) and using passive coping strategies (e.g., rumination) contributes to heightened infertility-specific distress (27).

Women express three key concerns when accessing fertility treatment: missing work or finances, medical aspects of the treatment, and achieving a live birth (30, 31). Most patients seek information before starting treatment, and this is primarily found on the internet (e.g., social media, Google), magazines, and books. Fertility clinic websites are arguably the first place patients should look for information; however, some research indicates these may lack comprehensive and accurate information (32). The internet allows patients to access support and to find out about other patients' experiences, but credibility, accuracy, and navigation ease of the information available vary considerably (33). More distressed patients are more likely to search the internet for information, but also more likely to report they are unable to find useful information (34), suggesting that internet-based resources may not be suitable for everyone.

In summary, patients in the pretreatment period report similar levels of depression and marital satisfaction as the general population. However, the type of infertility diagnosis may be associated with higher anxiety levels in both women and men. Coping strategies play an important role at this stage, and as couples may be facing a shared stressor for the first time in their partnership, sharing values and being responsive to one another are protective factors. Access to information at this stage is key, and for those who are more distressed, accurate and comprehensive information from clinic staff may be more beneficial than the internet.

The during-treatment period: Undergoing fertility treatment cycles

Each treatment cycle is a period of high emotional reactivity for patients. Women and men tend to present similar emotional patterns across the cycle, although emotional reactions (anxiety, depression, stress, and other psychological comorbidities) are more common and slightly more accentuated in women (35–37). Women and their partners tend to cope with treatment in similar ways, and this may explain similarities in emotional responses (22, 38).

At the start of a cycle patients tend to be in an optimistic frame of mind even if slightly anxious. Indeed, the start of a cycle is an empowering moment for patients: their actions are in line with their desire for children, they have some control over what is happening, and they can proactively participate in the process (for instance, by self-injecting hormones) (7, 39). At this moment, patients tend to have overly optimistic expectations about the cycle outcome. When compared with IVF prognosis models, on average women and men overestimate their chances of success by 46% and 51%, respectively (40). Paradoxically, the main concern patients express is the possibility of failure, and this does not subside as they undergo repeated cycles (31).

As the cycle unfolds, patients report higher anxiety and distress waiting for outcomes, in particular concerning oocyte pickup, fertilization, and pregnancy test. The 2-week waiting period after embryo transfer is particularly challenging. Indeed, as time passes patients feel increasingly anxious and less optimistic about the outcome of the cycle, and these emotions can be very hard to manage (41). Given that patients have low control over the cycle outcome, the most useful coping strategies are those that focus on managing emotions instead of trying to change outcomes. Examples are emotional expressive coping, for instance, expressing feelings to oneself or significant others, or positive reappraisal coping, which consists of paying as much attention to the positive aspects of a situation as one pays to the negatives. Avoidance coping strategies, for instance, avoiding being with people with children, are associated with higher stress (42, 43).

Having to face these and other challenges seems to make partners come together. Indeed, patients in a partnership experience more intimacy with their partner during a treatment cycle than a regular menstrual cycle. However, they also perceive lower support from significant others (35). Men, in particular, can feel socially isolated, and these feelings are heightened at the start of ovarian stimulation, at oocyte retrieval, and after the pregnancy test (44). Consistently, patients express they want their fertility team to fully involve both partners in the treatment process (45).

At the end of the cycle emotional reactions will differ according to outcome. Those who do not achieve pregnancy experience intense depressive symptoms, which can last for 6 months (46). For one in four women and one in ten men, these depressive symptoms are in the realm of a depressive disorder (46). This period is also marked by low engagement with the treatment process: regardless of the cycle outcome, overall patients feel more depressed and less willing to continue treatment than they felt at the start of the cycle. Such reactions, however, are heightened in those patients who received a negative pregnancy result, which means that it is precisely those patients who most need to remain engaged with the treatment process to achieve parenthood that are most likely to discontinue (7).

The period immediately after a failed cycle is therefore an effortful period during which patients strive to rebuild their hopes of success. This implies as initial appraisal of whether they are able to continue treatment. If that is not the case, patients temporarily step away to reconnect with themselves and rebuild hope and personal resources to be able to try again. This process can involve rebuilding supportive networks, finding ways to have more control over the treatment process (e.g., reclaiming treatment decision making from their fertility team), and reframing failure in a more positive way, for instance, as a learning opportunity that will inform new attempts and may therefore increase chances of success (47, 48). However, discontinuation research suggests that many patients are not able to build themselves up for a new attempt and end up discontinuing (49).

Treatment factors play a role in how patients react. IVF/intracytoplasmic sperm injection (ICSI) cycles place a higher physical and emotional burden on patients than first-line (e.g., IUI) treatment cycles. A study showed that patients undergoing mild stimulation IVF/ICSI are more likely to experience negative emotions at oocyte retrieval but less likely to experience these during hormonal stimulation and after a treatment cycle failure or cancellation (50). While emotional reactions during a cycle do not differ across consecutive attempts (51), discontinuation research suggests that undergoing multiple cycles depletes patients' personal resources (49).

Patients vary in their individual profiles, and some individual characteristics are known to make treatment more emotionally difficult (52). Individuals who have a history of mental health vulnerability or with neurotic personality traits are more likely to experience depression, anxiety, or other psychiatric morbidity during treatment (52). Patients who are less able to cope with health care in general will also be more negatively affected by each treatment cycle, while patients who highly value parenthood or have low acceptance of a child-free lifestyle are more likely to experience anxiety and depression if treatment cycles are unsuccessful (53, 54). Finally, some studies suggest that infertile women tend to be self-critical and that these negative self-appraisals have a negative impact on their well-being (55).

Considering how challenging each treatment cycle is, it does not come as a surprise that many patients discontinue treatment before achieving pregnancy. More precisely, around 1 in 12 patients discontinue first-line treatment (56) with the main reasons for discontinuation being postponement (i.e., stopping treatment for at least 1 year, as referred to earlier), logistics and practical reasons (e.g., travel distance to clinic, change of residence), rejection of treatment, perception of poor prognosis, and psychological burden (49). Discontinuation is higher during ART, with one in five patients discontinuing before undergoing three consecutive cycles, despite having the financial means needed and a favorable prognosis (12). Compliance rates decrease as patients progress through their treatment cycles (from 82% after the first cycle to 75% after the second), but the reasons for it tend to be similar and include financial issues, the physical and psychological burden of treatment, postponement (for over a year), and relational problems. Patients who stop treatment due to dissatisfaction with care tend to do it immediately after their first attempt, either changing clinics or discontinuing (49).

Many women think that their emotional distress can cause treatment failure, which feeds stress and accentuates perceptions of failure and self-criticism. Systematic reviews of the literature have produced conflicting results. While Boivin et al. and Nicoloro-SantaBarbara et al. (57, 58) concluded there is no significant association between stress and treatment outcome, Matthiesen et al. and Purewal et al. detected a small significant association (59, 60). Several aspects may explain this inconsistency in results, including the number of treatment cycles and time of assessment of emotional reactions. Overall the data seem to suggest that how a person feels at the start of a treatment cycle does not predict the outcome of that cycle. Changes in emotional reactions during the cycle can predict its outcome, but this happens because patients are reacting to information about poor within-cycle outcomes (e.g., low number of oocytes collected, low embryo quality, etc.). The data also suggest that emotional distress can decrease chances of conceiving across multiple cycles (61). For instance, more distressed people are more likely to overeat, smoke, and drink. There is a vast evidence that obesity (62, 63), smoking (64), and alcohol consumption (65) reduce the chances of success with fertility treatment. Stress can also indirectly affect outcomes by causing patients to discontinue treatment despite a good prognosis (49, 61).

Overall, these data indicate that fertility treatment is stressful and psychosocially burdensome to patients, in particular when they are waiting to find out about important treatment-related outcomes. Patients who adjust better tend to be psychologically resilient, to have good support networks, to better accept a child-free lifestyle, and to use coping skills that allow them to sustain hope throughout multiple cycles. It is important to note that people who undergo fertility treatment tend to come from favorable backgrounds (e.g., education, income) and have good support networks, factors we know are protective in the face of stressful life events. Indeed, most patients are able to cope with the challenges of treatment, and only 10%–20% experience severe psychological impairment (1). Undergoing fertility treatment allows people to pursue their dream of parenthood, but even those who fail to conceive recognize the benefit of reaching peace of mind in relation to having tried, as opposed to regret for not giving it a go (66). Patients also acknowledge that their infertility and treatment experience has a positive impact on their relationship with their partner (when there is one) (67), and one study reported lower rates of marital dissolution among ART patients then the general population (68).

The post-treatment period: The aftermath of unsuccessful ART treatment and pregnancy after ART

The aftermath of unsuccessful ART

Recent HFEA data show a maximum of 57% of patients will achieve parenthood after three cycles of IVF (69). While some patients ultimately conceive spontaneously and others seek parenthood in other ways, such as adoption, 13%–30% remain childless (70, 71) or with fewer children than desired. Some research suggests the additional failure of unsuccessful adoption may result in poorer adjustment than those who remained childless and chose not to pursue adoption when both these groups were compared to patients that ultimately adopted or conceived spontaneously (72). Overall, most unsuccessful patients experience a loss of their biological parenthood goal, or more generally their parenthood goals, and this affects all domains of their experience.

In this period, patients may return to behaviors that they had reduced or stopped while going through treatment, such as smoking and alcohol consumption. For example, 5 years after treatment, women who did not achieve parenthood are more likely to use sleeping pills, smoke, and drink than those who became parents (73). However, this may just reflect that their lifestyles are not constrained by parenthood responsibilities. With time, most people let go of their unrealized wish for children and refocus their lives on other meaningful goals, such as caring for other people or pets, advocating for the rights of infertile people, or traveling (74, 75). However, one study showed that 6% of women had not disengaged from their parenthood goal up to 17 years after treatment (54). The pursuit of other meaningful goals requires active effort to confront a future without children (74, 76); however, qualitative research shows the ability to reframe one's goals leads to a sense of fulfilment and life satisfaction (74) and results in better psychosocial adjustment (77, 78).

Patients who remain involuntary childless may encounter social isolation from their networks as they are unable to share parenthood experiences with their peers (76), and that experience may repeat itself as their peers reach new parenthood-related milestones, for instance, grandparenthood (74). Women can also actively decide to isolate themselves from those who have children (79). Although potentially protective in the short term, in the longer term this form of avoidance coping is associated with poorer adjustment. As highlighted previously, the experience of undergoing ART treatment itself is unlikely to negatively affect the patients' partnerships, and those who were a couple during their treatment are generally satisfied with their relationship after completion (73, 80). However, treatment does have a toll on the sexual relationship, and its impact can last for a long time (74, 81), with patients expressing a desire to receive psychosocial support to address this issue.

Several studies have investigated the long term effects of unsuccessful treatment on emotional adjustment, but often these studies are cross-sectional. A recent meta-analysis of long term adjustment following unsuccessful treatment suggests that patients who do not conceive experience worse mental-health and well-being, and moderation analyses suggests that poorer adjustment is associated with the inability to reach one's parenthood goal, rather than parenthood status per se (54). Although overall not being able to conceive with treatment results in a period of emotional adjustment, research suggests that this does not necessarily translate into increased rates of psychiatric disorders when compared to those who become parents (82, 83).

Overall, the literature indicates that ending unsuccessful ART treatment triggers an intense and prolonged grief response to the loss of one's parenthood goals (46, 75, 84). Over time most patients adjust to remaining childless (24, 71, 78, 85, 86), but adjustment is a slow process: 2 years after treatment 50% of patients still hold on to their child wish, but 11–17 years after only 6% hold such wish and only 10% report psychological maladjustment (54). Research shows that many factors facilitate adjustment: being able to live with the uncomfortable emotions and thoughts related with the unfulfilled child wish, engaging and actively pursuing alternative but meaningful goals (81, 87), constructing positive meanings of one's experience, having a supportive partner (70) and network (81), and the passage of time (85, 86). Positive adjustment often translates into a restored sense of equilibrium with the world and hope towards the future. Conversely, being psychologically vulnerable (70, 81), lacking adequate support (86, 88, 89), and avoiding confronting one's situation (81) are known to hinder adjustment, translating into the refusal of childlessness and low mental health.

At the cognitive level, patients may experience a sense of loss and disruption to their views of the world as fair and logical. Engagement in cognitive efforts to try to make meaning of their situation may involve reviewing past efforts to conceive and/or the decisions and context that led to the end of treatment without a pregnancy. Patients find positively (re)framing their treatment experiences easier when they feel they were well counseled, involved in decision making, and had control over the decision to end treatment (54). Examples of positive meaning-making are reaching a sense they had done all they could (90) or that ending treatment meant someone else could pursue it. Consideration of their present situation often results in re-evaluation of their values and life priorities (75, 76) and their role in society. In this process, patients may question their society's representations of femininity (79) or masculinity or what it means to be a family (75), often leading to patients breaking away from more conservative views that do not account for their current status.

Overall, the literature shows that ending ART treatment without realizing one's parenthood goals triggers an intense loss that disrupts the core of one's identity and existential beliefs and demands a profound reconceptualization of what one's life and future can look like. Working through these challenges is a process that inevitably takes time, but is achievable for most patients, with only a minority being unable to overcome this major life event.

Pregnancy and early parenting after ART

Most research indicates that pregnancies after ART treatment are overall similar to pregnancies after spontaneous conception (91). First, patients do not experience worse mental health or quality of life, nor do they perceive themselves in a more negative way than people who conceive spontaneously (92). Second, they relate with their fetus in a similar way (92). Third, the quality of the partnership and perceived support are also similar (e.g., 93). Finally, lifestyle behaviors during pregnancy are overall healthy and similar across the two groups (94). The one difference that has been consistently found is that women who conceive with IVF tend to express more worries and anxieties about their pregnancies than women who conceive spontaneously (92). Risk factors for poorer mental health during pregnancy are psychological vulnerability (that would also have manifested in higher stress levels during treatment) and experiencing additional challenges during treatment and the pregnancy period, for instance, repeated cycle failure and multiple pregnancies (92, 95).

Psychosocial effects of undergoing ART 175

TABLE 18.1

Summary of the Psychosocial Effects of Undergoing ART: Organized by Domain of Experience (Vertical Axis) and Stage of Treatment (Horizontal Axis)

	Pre-Treatment	During Treatment	Pregnancy and Early Postpartum	Post-Treatment Unsuccessful Treatment
Behavioral	– 1 in 10 patients do not start ART. – Many patients report unhealthy lifestyle behaviors and do not change these before starting treatment. – More depressed patients are less likely to start treatment.	– Many patients report unhealthy lifestyles during treatment. – 1 in every 12 patients discontinues first-line treatment. – 1 in every 5 patients discontinues ART.	– Patients who achieve pregnancy with ART report similar lifestyle behaviors to people who get pregnant without treatment.	– Childless women may be more likely to engage in unhealthy lifestyle behaviors than women who achieve parenthood – With time around 90% of patients let go of their child wish.
Relational and Social	– Patients report similar marital and sexual relationships to the general population. – The way each member of the couple copes with infertility affects the other member. – Differences in personal values between a couple, e.g., importance of parenthood, may result in lower marital satisfaction.	– Satisfaction with relationship is similar at start and end of a treatment cycle. – Couples experience higher intimacy and social support during a treatment cycle than during a menstrual cycle. – Men feel more isolated than women during an ART cycle. – Undergoing treatment has benefits for the partnership.	– The partnership quality and partner support are similar in patients who achieve pregnancy with and without ART.	– Childless individuals experience social isolation from peers who have children and avoid social situations with children. – Childless individuals report being satisfied with their partnership.
Emotional	– Patients report similar levels of depression to the general population or matched control, but findings on anxiety are mixed. – Gender differences reported in depression, anxiety, and social and infertility-related stress. – Psychologically vulnerable patients and those using avoidance coping are at higher risk for emotional problems, while patients with a supportive spouse and using active coping strategies (e.g., problem solving) are at lower risk.	– Patients experience high emotional reactivity during a cycle. – Women are more likely to experience anxiety, depression, and other psychological comorbidity than men. – Anxiety and stress are higher when patients are waiting for results (oocyte pickup, fertilization, embryo transfer, pregnancy test). – Patients experience high emotional distress when given bad news, in particular of treatment failure. – Treatment stress can indirectly influence its outcome via unhealthy lifestyles and discontinuation.	– Achieving parenthood with ART is associated with higher life satisfaction and self-esteem. – Patients who achieve pregnancy with ART report more specific anxiety about the health of their pregnancies and fetus than patients who achieve it without ART.	– Patients are likely to experience intense and prolonged grief reactions. – Unsuccessful ART is associated with poor mental health and well-being but not with psychiatric disorders. – Patients who are willing to live with the pain of their unfulfilled child wish engage and actively pursue alternative life goals, construct positive meanings of their experience, have a supportive partner and network, and are likely to adjust. – Psychologically vulnerable patients who lack adequate support, avoid confronting their situation, and hold on to their child wish are likely to exhibit adjustment difficulties.
Cognitive	– Women express key concerns when accessing fertility treatment. – Most patients seek information prior to starting treatment.	– Patients have overoptimistic expectations about the chances of their cycle being successful. – Patients experience low engagement with treatment at the end of the cycle. – After a failed cycle, patients focus on rebuilding hope of success and personal resources to do more cycles.	– Patients who achieve pregnancy with ART are more likely to express pregnancy-related concerns than women who get pregnant without ART.	– Patients experience a sense of loss and engage in cognitive efforts to make meaning of their situation. – Patients question their cultural beliefs on the meanings of femininity, masculinity, family, etc. – Most patients are able to reframe their experience in a positive way.

For infertile patients, parenthood may seem like the long-promised dream that miraculously came true. Nonetheless. it is important to note that multiple research studies show that infertility resolution results in increased life satisfaction and self-esteem (e.g., 96), but it does not protect against the high risk for psychopathology usually observed during the early postpartum period.

Conclusions

- The psychosocial effects of ART are multidimensional and differ across the stages of treatment. Clinics need to tailor support to address such multidimensional impacts during and after treatment, be it successful or not.
- The ESHRE psychosocial care guidelines describe the minimum care standards clinics should strive to achieve and the required know-how to achieve it (1).
- Staff can use evidence-based psychosocial interventions and mobile and web-based apps to support patients during treatment (97, 98).
- There is a lack of research-informed support for patients who underwent unsuccessful treatment, with only one evaluated intervention (99) and the myjourney.pt web app (100) being available.

REFERENCES

1. Gameiro S, Boivin J, Dancet E, de Klerk C, Emery M, Lewis-Jones C, et al. ESHRE guideline: Routine psychosocial care in infertility and medically assisted reproduction-a guide for fertility staff. *Human Reproduction*. 2015;30(11):2476–85.
2. HFEA. *Code of practice*. 9th ed. London, UK: Human Fertilisation and Embryology Authority; 2018.
3. NICE. *Fertility: Assessment and treatment for people with fertility problems*. London, UK: National Collaborating Centre for Women's and Children's Health; 2013.
4. Klitzman R. Gatekeepers for infertility treatment? Views of ART providers concerning referrals by non-ART providers. *Reproductive Biomedicine & Society Online*. 2018;5:17–30.
5. Revelli A, Razzano A, Delle Piane L, Casano S, Benedetto C. Awareness of the effects of postponing motherhood among hospital gynecologists: Is their knowledge sufficient to offer appropriate help to patients? *J Assist Reprod Genet*. 2016;33(2):215–20.
6. Franklin S, Johnson MH. Are assisted reproduction health professionals still letting down their patients? *Reproductive Biomedicine Online*. 2013;27(5):451–2.
7. Gameiro S, Mesquita da Silva S, Gordon U, Baccino G, Boivin J, editors. In-depth analysis of what influences wether patients commit to achieve parenthood and undergo fertility treatment before and after a treatment cycle. 36th Annual Meeting of the European Society of Human Reproduction and Embryology, Virtual: Huma Reproduction; 2020.
8. Brandes M, Van Der Steen JOM, Bokdam SB, Hamilton C, De Bruin JP, Nelen W, et al. When and why do subfertile couples discontinue their fertility care? A longitudinal cohort study in a secondary care subfertility population. *Human Reproduction*. 2009;24(12):3127–35.
9. Lykeridou K, Gourounti K, Deltsidou A, Loutradis D, Vaslamatzis G. The impact of infertility diagnosis on psychological status of women undergoing fertility treatment. *Journal of Reproductive and Infant Psychology*. 2009;27(3):223–37.
10. Massarotti C, Gentile G, Ferreccio C, Scaruffi P, Remorgida V, Anserini P. Impact of infertility and infertility treatments on quality of life and levels of anxiety and depression in women undergoing in vitro fertilization. *Gynecological Endocrinology*. 2019;35(6):485–9.
11. Warchol-Biedermann K. The risk of psychiatric morbidity and course of distress in males undergoing infertility evaluation is affected by their factor of infertility. *American Journal of Men's Health*. 2019;13(1):1557988318823904.
12. Gameiro S, Verhaak CM, Kremer JAM, Boivin J. Why we should talk about compliance with Assisted Reproductive Technologies (ART): A systematic review and meta-analysis of ART compliance rates. *Human Reproduction Update*. 2013;19(2):124–35.

13. Crawford NM, Hoff HS, Mersereau JE. Infertile women who screen positive for depression are less likely to initiate fertility treatments. *Human Reproduction.* 2017;32(3):582–7.
14. Sharma R, Biedenharn KR, Fedor JM, Agarwal A. Lifestyle factors and reproductive health: Taking control of your fertility. *Reproductive Biology and Endocrinology.* 2013;11(1):66.
15. Gormack AA, Peek JC, Derraik JGB, Gluckman PD, Young NL, Cutfield WS. Many women undergoing fertility treatment make poor lifestyle choices that may affect treatment outcomes. *Human Reproduction.* 2015;30(7):1617–24.
16. Anderson K, Nisenblat V, Norman R. Lifestyle factors in people seeking infertility treatment: A review. *Australian and New Zealand Journal of Obstetrics and Gynaecology.* 2010;50(1):8–20.
17. Bellver J, Melo MAB, Bosch E, Serra V, Remohí J, Pellicer A. Obesity and poor reproductive outcome: The potential role of the endometrium. *Fertility and Sterility.* 2007;88(2):446–51.
18. Moran L, Tsagareli V, Norman R, Noakes M. Diet and IVF pilot study: Short-term weight loss improves pregnancy rates in overweight/obese women undertaking IVF. *Australian and New Zealand Journal of Obstetrics and Gynaecology.* 2011;51(5):455–9.
19. Porter M, Bhattacharya S. Helping themselves to get pregnant: A qualitative longitudinal study on the information-seeking behaviour of infertile couples. *Human Reproduction.* 2008;23(3):567–72.
20. Verhaak CM, Smeenk JMJ, Eugster A, Van Minnen A, Kremer JAM, Kraaimaat FW. Stress and marital satisfaction among women before and after their first cycle of in vitro fertilization and intracytoplasmic sperm injection. *Fertility and Sterility.* 2001;76(3):525–31.
21. Verhaak CM, Smeenk JMJ, Van Minnen A, Kremer JAM, Kraaimaat FW. A longitudinal, prospective study on emotional adjustment before, during and after consecutive fertility treatment cycles. *Human Reproduction.* 2005;20(8):2253–60.
22. Peterson BD, Newton CR, Rosen KH. Examining congruence between partners' perceived infertility-related stress and its relationship to marital adjustment and depression in infertile couples. *Family Process.* 2003;42:59–70.
23. Peterson BD, Pirritano M, Christensen U, Schmidt L. The impact of partner coping in couples experiencing infertility. *Human Reproduction.* 2008;23(5):1128–37.
24. Verhaak CM, Smeenk JM, Evers AWM, Kremer JAM, Kraaimaat FW, Braat DDM. Women's emotional adjustment to IVF: A systematic review of 25 years of research. *Human Reproduction Update.* 2006;13(1):27–36.
25. Demyttenaere K, Bonte L, Gheldof M, Vervaeke M, Meuleman C, Vanderschuerem D, et al. Coping style and depression level influence outcome in in vitro fertilization. *Fertility and Sterility.* 1998;69(6):1026–33.
26. Galst JP. The elusive connection between stress and infertility: A research review with clinical implications. *Journal of Psychotherapy Integration.* 2018;28(1):1.
27. Peterson BD, Sejbaek CS, Pirritano M, Schmidt L. Are severe depressive symptoms associated with infertility-related distress in individuals and their partners? *Human Reproduction.* 2014;29(1):76–82.
28. Van den Broeck U, Emery M, Wischmann T, Thorn P. Counselling in infertility: Individual, couple and group interventions. *Patient Education and Counseling.* 2010;81(3):422–8.
29. Donarelli Z, Lo Coco G, Gullo S, Marino A, Volpes A, Allegra A. Are attachment dimensions associated with infertility-related stress in couples undergoing their first IVF treatment? A study on the individual and cross-partner effect. *Human Reproduction.* 2012;27(11):3215–25.
30. Klonoff-Cohen H, Natarajan L. The Concerns during Assisted Reproductive Technologies (CART) scale and pregnancy outcomes. *Fertility and Sterility.* 2004;81(4):982–8.
31. Klonoff-Cohen H, Natarajan L, Klonoff E. Validation of a new scale for measuring concerns of women undergoing assisted reproductive technologies (CART). *Journal of Health Psychology.* 2007;12:352–6.
32. Hammarberg K, Prentice T, Purcell I, Johnson L. Quality of information about success rates provided on assisted reproductive technology clinic websites in Australia and New Zealand. *Australian and New Zealand Journal of Obstetrics and Gynaecology.* 2018;58(3):330–4.
33. Marriott JV, Stec P, El-Toukhy T, Khalaf Y, Braude P, Coomarasamy A. Infertility information on the World Wide Web: A cross-sectional survey of quality of infertility information on the internet in the UK. *Human Reproduction.* 2008;23(7):1520–5.
34. Brochu F, Robins S, Miner SA, Grunberg PH, Chan P, Lo K, et al. Searching the Internet for infertility information: A survey of patient needs and preferences. *Journal of Medical Internet Research.* 2019;21(12):e15132.

35. Boivin J, Andersson L, Skoog-Svanberg A, Hjelmstedt A, Collins A, Bergh T. Psychological reactions during in-vitro fertilization: Similar response pattern in husbands and wives. *Human Reproduction.* 1998;13:3262–7.
36. Montagnini HML, Blay SL, Novo NF, Freitas V, Cedenho AP. Estados emocionais de casais submetidos à fertilização in vitro [Emotional states of couples undergoing in vitro fertilization]. *Estudos de Psicologia.* 2009;26(4):475–81.
37. Chiaffarino F, Baldini M, Scarduelli C, Bommarito F, Ambrosio S, D'Orsi C, et al. Prevalence and incidence of depressive and anxious symptoms in couples undergoing assisted reproductive treatment in an Italian infertility department. *European Journal of Obstetrics, Gynecology, and Reproductive Biology.* 2011;158:235–41.
38. Knoll N, Schwarzer R, Pfuller B, Kienle R. Transmission of depressive symptoms: A study with couples undergoing assisted-reproduction treatment. *European Psychologist.* 2009;14(1):7–17.
39. Leiblum SR, Kemmann E, Lane MK. The psychological concomitants of in-vitro fertilization. *Journal of Psychosomatics, Obstetrics and Gynaecology.* 1987;6:165–78.
40. Peeraer K, Devroe J, D'Hooghe T, Boivin J, Vriens J, Dancet E. The realism of men and women's expected IVF live birth rates. 36th Annual Meeting of the European Society for Human Reproduction and Embryology: Human Reproduction; 2020. p. i81.
41. Boivin J, Lancastle D. Medical waiting periods: Imminence, emotions and coping. *Women's Health.* 2010;6:59–69.
42. Panagopoulou E, Vedhara K, Gaintarzti C, Tarlatzis B. Emotionally expressive coping reduces pregnancy rates in patients undergoing in vitro fertilization. *Fertility and Sterility.* 2006;86(3):672–7.
43. Ockhuijsen HDL, van den Hoogen A, Eijkemans M, Macklon N, Boivin J. Clarifying the benefits of the positive reappraisal coping intervention for the women waiting for the outcome of IVF. *Human Reproduction.* 2014;29(12):2712–8.
44. Agostini F, Monti F, De Pascalis L, Paterlini M, La Sala GB, Blickstein I. Psychosocial support for infertile couples during assisted reproductive technology treatment. *Fertility and Sterility.* 2011;95(2):707–10.
45. Dancet EAF, Nelen WLDM, Sermeus W, De Leeuw L, Kremer JAM, D'Hooghe TM. The patients' perspective on fertility care: A systematic review. *Human Reproduction Update.* 2010;16:467–87.
46. Verhaak CM, Smeenk JM, Evers AWM, Kremer JM, Kraaimaat FW, Braat DM. Women's emotional adjustment to IVF: A systematic review of 25 years of research. *Human Reproduction Update.* 2007;13(1):27–36.
47. Bailey A, Ellis-Caird H, Croft C. Living through unsuccessful conception attempts: A grounded theory of resilience among women undergoing fertility treatment. *Journal of Reproductive and Infant Psychology.* 2017;35(4):324–33.
48. Mesquita da Silva S, Place JM, Boivin J, Gameiro S. Failure after fertility treatment: Regulation strategies when facing a blocked parenthood goal. *Human Fertility.* 2020;23(3):179–85.
49. Gameiro S, Boivin J, Peronace LA, Verhaak CM. Why do patients discontinue fertility treatment? A systematic review of reasons and predictors of discontinuation in fertility treatment. *Human Reproduction Update.* 2012;18(6):652–69.
50. de Klerk C, Heijnen EMEW, Macklon NS, Duivenvoorden HJ, Fauser BCJM, Passchier J, et al. The psychological impact of mild ovarian stimulation combined with single embryo transfer compared with conventional IVF. *Human Reproduction.* 2006;21:721–7.
51. Turner K, Reynolds-May MF, Zitek EM, Tisdale RL, Carlisle AB, Westphal LM. Stress and anxiety scores in first and repeated IVF cycles: A pilot study. *Plos One.* 2013;8(5):e63743.
52. Rockliff HE, Lightman SL, Rhidian E, Buchanan H, Gordon U, Vedhara K. A systematic review of psychosocial factors associated with emotional adjustment in vitro fertilization patients. *Human Reproduction Update.* 2014;20(4):594–613.
53. Verhaak CM, Smeenk JM, van Minnen A, Kremer JM, Kraaimaat FW. Predicting emotional response to unsuccessful fertility treatment: A prospective study. *Journal of Behavior Medicine.* 2005;28(2):181–90.
54. Gameiro S, van den Belt-Dusebout AW, Smeenk J, Braat D, van Leeuwen FE, Verhaak CM. Women's adjustment trajectories during IVF and impact on mental health 11–17 years later. *Human Reproduction.* 2016;31(8):1788–98.

55. Galhardo A, Cunha M, Pinto-Gouveia J, Matos M. The mediator role of emotion regulation processes on infertility-related stress. *Journal of Clinical Psychology in Medical Settings*. 2013;20:497–507.
56. Brandes M, van der Steen JOM, Bokdam SB, Hamilton CJCM, de Bruin JP, Nelen WLDM, et al. When and why do subfertile couples discontinue their fertility care? A longitudinal cohort study in a secondary care subfertility population. *Human Reproduction*. 2009;24(12):3127–34.
57. Boivin J, Griffiths E, Venetis CA. Emotional distress in infertile women and failure of assisted reproductive technologies: Meta-analysis of prospective psychosocial studies. *British Medical Journal*. 2011;342(d223).
58. Nicoloro-SantaBarbara J, Busso C, Moyer A, Lobel M. Just relax and you'll get pregnant? Meta-analysis examing women's emotional distress and the outcome of assisted reproductive technology. *Social Science & Medicine*. 2018;213:54–62.
59. Matthiesen SM, Frederiksen Y, Ingerlev HJ, Zachariae R. Stress, distress and outcome of Assisted Reproductive Technology (ART): A meta-analysis. *Human Reproduction*. 2011;2011(26):2763–76.
60. Purewal S, Chapman SCE, van den Akker O. Depression and state anxiety scores during assisted reproductive treatment are associated with outcome: A meta-analysis. *Reproductive BioMedicine Online*. 2018;36(6):646–57.
61. Boivin J, Domar AD, Shapiro DB, Wischmann T, Fauser BC, Verhaak CM. Tackling burden in ART: An integrated approach for medical staff. *Human Reproduction*. 2012;27(4):941–50.
62. Pinborg A, Gaarslev C, Hougaard CO, Nyboe Anderson A, Kragh Anderson P, Boivin J, et al. The influence of female body weight on assisted reproductive technology (ART) procedures and live birth rates: A longitudinal multi-centre cohort study of 487 infertile couples. *Reproductive BioMedicine Online*. 2011;23(4):490–9.
63. Campbell JM, Lane MK, Owens JA, Bakos HW. Paternal obesity negatively affects male fertility and assisted reproduction outcomes: A systematic review and meta-analysis. *Reproductive BioMedicine Online*. 2015;31(5):593–604.
64. Waylen AL, Metwally M, Jones GL, Wilkinson AJ, Ledger WL. Effects of cigarette smoking upon clinical outcomes of assisted reproduction: A meta-analysis. *Human Reproduction Update*. 2009;15:31–44.
65. Nicolau P, Miralpeix E, Solà I, Carreras R, Checa MA. Alcohol consumption and in vitro fertilization: A review of the literature. *Gynecological Endocrinology*. 2014;30(11):759–63.
66. Mesquita da Silva S. *It's not over until it's over: Self and dyadic regulation and wellbeing when facing a blocked parenthood goal*. Cardiff: Cardiff University; 2016.
67. Schmidt L, Holstein B, Christensen U, Boivin J. Does infertility cause marital benefit? An epidemiological study of 2250 women and men in infertility treatment. *Patient Education and Counselling*. 2005;59:244–51.
68. Martins MV, Vassard D, Hougaard CO, Schimdt L. The impact of ART of union dissolution: A register-based study in Denmark 1994–2010. *Human Reproduction*. 2018;23:434–40.
69. McLernon DJ, Maheshwari A, Lee AJ, Bhattacharya S. Cumulative live birth rates after one or more complete cycles of IVF: A population-based study of linked cycle data from 178,898 women. *Human Reproduction*. 2016;31(3):572–81.
70. Fisher JRW, Baker GHW, Hammarberg K. Long-term health, well-being, life satisfaction, and attitudes toward parenthood in men diagnosed as infertile: Challenges to gender stereotypes and implications for practice. *Fertility and Sterility*. 2010;94(2):574–80.
71. Wischmann T, Korge K, Scherg H, Strowitzki T, Verres R. A 10-year follow-up study of psychosocial factors affecting couples after infertility treatment. *Human Reproduction*. 2012;27(11):3226–32.
72. Bryson CA, Sykes DH, Traub AI. In vitro fertilization: A long-term follow-up after treatment failure. *Human Fertility*. 2000;3(3):214–20.
73. Johansson M, Adolfsson A, Berg M, Francis J, Hogström L, Olof Janson P, et al. Quality of life for couples 4–5.5 years after unsuccessful IVF treatment. *Acta obstetricia et gynecologica Scandinavica*. 2009;88(3):291–300.
74. Wirtberg I, Möller A, Hogström L, Tronstad SE, Lalos A. Life 20 years after unsuccessful infertility treatment. *Human Reproduction*. 2007;22(2):598–604.
75. Daniluk JC. Reconstructing their lives: A longitudinal, qualitative analysis of the transition to biological childlessness for infertile couples. *Journal of Counseling & Development*. 2001;79(4):439–49.

76. McCarthy MP. Women's lived experience of infertility after unsuccessful medical intervention. *J Midwifery Women Health*. 2008;53(4):319–24.
77. Heckhausen J, Wrosch C, Fleeson W. Developmental regulation before and after a developmental deadline: The sample case of "biological clock" for childbearing. *Psychology and Aging*. 2001;16(3):400.
78. Martins MV, Basto-Pereira M, Pedro J, Peterson B, Almeida V, Schmidt L, et al. Male psychological adaptation to unsuccessful medically assisted reproduction treatments: A systematic review. *Human Reproduction Update*. 2016;22(4):466–78.
79. Johansson M, Berg M. Women's experiences of childlessness 2 years after the end of in vitro fertilization treatment. *Scand J Caring Sci*. 2005;19(1):58–63.
80. Sydsjö G, Ekholm K, Wadsby M, Kjellberg S, Sydsjö A. Relationships in couples after failed IVF treatment: A prospective follow-up study. *Human Reproduction*. 2005;20(7):1952–7.
81. Daniluk JC, Tench E. Long-term adjustment of infertile couples following unsuccessful medical intervention. *Journal of Counseling & Development*. 2007;85(1):89–100.
82. Yli-Kuha AN, Gissler M, Klemetti R, Luoto R, Koivisto E, Hemminki E. Psychiatric disorders leading to hospitalization before and after infertility treatments. *Human Reproduction*. 2010;25(8):2018–23.
83. Volgsten H, Schmidt L, Skoog Svanberg A, Ekselius L, Sundström Poromaa I. Psychiatric disorders in women and men up to five years after undergoing assisted reproductive technology treatment: A prospective cohort study. *Human Fertility*. 2019;22(4):277–82.
84. Volgsten H, Svanberg A, Olsson P. Unresolved grief in women and men in Sweden three years after undergoing unsuccessful in vitro fertilization treatment. *Acta Obstet Gynecol Scand*. 2010;89(10):1290–7.
85. Kuivasaari-Pirinen P, Koivumaa-Honkanen H, Hippeläinen M, Raatikainen K, Heinonen S. Outcome of Assisted Reproductive Technology (ART) and subsequent self-reported life satisfaction. *PloS One*. 2014;9(11):e112540.
86. Gameiro S, Van Den Belt-dusebout AW, Smeenk JMJ, Braat DDM, Van Leeuwen FE, Verhaak CM. Women's adjustment trajectories during IVF and impact on mental health 11–17 years later. *Human Reproduction*. 2016;31(8):1788–98.
87. Verhaak CM, Smeenk JMJ, Nahuis MJ, Kremer JAM, Braat DDM. Long-term psychological adjustment to IVF/ICSI treatment in women. *Human Reproduction*. 2007;22(1):305–8.
88. Sydsjö G, Vikström J, Bladh M, Jablonowska B, Svanberg AS. Men report good mental health 20 to 23 years after in vitro fertilisation treatment. *BMC Public Health*. 2015;15(1):1175.
89. Vikström J, Josefsson A, Bladh M, Sydsjö G. Mental health in women 20–23 years after IVF treatment: A Swedish cross-sectional study. *BMJ Open*. 2015;5(10).
90. Throsby K. "No-one will ever call me mummy": Making sense of the end of IVF treatment. London School of Economics, Gender Institute; 2001.
91. Hammarberg K, Fisher JR, Wynter KH. Psychological and social aspects of pregnancy, childbirth and early parenting after assisted conception: A systematic review. *Human Reproduction Update*. 2008;14:395–414.
92. Hammarberg K, Astbury J, Baker HWG. Women's experience of IVF: A follow-up study. *Human Reproduction*. 2001;16(2):374–83.
93. Cebert M, Silva S, Stevenson EL. Are there differences in marital-role quality between women and their male partners who conceived via IVF and those who did not? *Journal of Best Practices in Health Professions Diversity: Research, Education and Policy*. 2019;11(2):135–49.
94. Fisher J, Wynter KH, Hammarberg K, McBain J, Gibson F, Boivin J, et al. Age, model of conception, health service use and pregnancy health: A prospective cohort study of Australian women. *BMC Pregnancy and Childbirth*. 2013;13:88.
95. García-Blanco A, Diago V, Hervás D, Ghosn F, Vento M, Chaáfer-Pericás C. Anxiety and depressive symptoms, and stress biomarkers in pregnant women after in vitro fertilization. *Human Reproduction*. 2018;33(7):1237–46.
96. Shreffler KM, Greil AL, Tiemeyer S, McQuillan J. In infertility resolution associated with a change in women's well-being? *Human Reproduction*. 2020;35(3):605–16.
97. Frederiksen Y, Farver-Vestergaard I, Skovgård NG, Ingerslev HJ, Zachariae R. Efficacy of psychosocial interventions for psychological and pregnancy outcomes in infertile women and men: A systematic review and meta-analysis. *BMJ Open*. 2015;5:e006592.

98. Meyers AJ, Domar AD. Research-supported mobile applications and internet-based technologies to mediate the psychological effects of infertility: A review. *Reproductive BioMedicine Online*. 2020;42(3):679–85.
99. Kraaij V, Garnefski N, Fles H, Brands A, van Tricht S. Effects of a self-help program on depressed mood for women with an unfulfilled child wish. *Journal of Loss and Trauma*. 2016;21(4):275–85.
100. Rowbottom B, Gameiro S, editors. Prospective acceptability study of a psychological online self-help intervention for individuals with an unmet parenthood goal. 36th Annual Meeting of the European Society for Human Reproduction and Embryology, European Society for Human Reproduction and Embryology; 2020.

19

Psychosocial adjustment in offspring conceived through assisted reproductive technologies

Childhood, adolescence, and young adulthood

Catherine McMahon and Caitlin Macmillan

In 1969, publication of the first scientific paper about in vitro fertilization (IVF) in humans provoked *Life* magazine (1) to devote a special issue asking their readers to speculate about the impact on sex and family relationships: Would parents be able to love a child conceived in this way? While readers were open to the new opportunities offered by this reproductive revolution, there were also concerns about negative consequences for children and the institution of the family. Twenty years later, theologian Anthony Fisher warned "It would be surprising, in fact, if there were not psychological ill-effects from the IVF program" (2) (p. 73). Pioneering physiologist Robert Edwards took a different view: "If there is no undue risk of deformity additional to those in natural conception, and publicity is avoided, the children should grow up and develop normally and be no more misfits than other children born today after some form of medical help" (p. 12) (3). Now, more than 40 years since Louise Brown, the first baby conceived through IVF, was born in 1979, there are more than 8 million children worldwide who have been conceived through assisted reproductive technologies (ARTs) (4). This chapter reviews three decades of empirical evidence to see if concerns about the psychological well-being of children conceived through ART are justified.

We begin with a brief overview of developmental theory and research regarding predictors of psychological health and resilience in children and young adults. Erik Erikson (5) outlined key developmental tasks that needed to be mastered as children progress through the lifespan: the young infant needs to develop a sense of trust; the toddler grapples with emerging autonomy; the school-aged child needs to master learning and peer relationships. Erikson is perhaps most famous for his seminal work on the identity struggles of adolescence, particularly pertinent in the context of the complex family structures enabled through ART.

Parents scaffold psychological development, and their task is to provide developmentally graded support as children negotiate these developmental challenges. Secure attachment to parents provides the child with a sense of self-worth and trust in others that is protective against psychopathology across the lifespan. (6) Responsive, sensitive parenting is fundamental; parents need to comfort and support their child when distressed, providing a safe haven. They also need to encourage exploration, learning, and autonomy, providing a secure base for the child's wider engagement with the world. Parents need to balance respect for the child's perspective and preferences with a capacity to take charge, regulate, and monitor risk in developmentally appropriate ways (7). Children develop poorly regulated behavior when the balance is skewed towards parental control, with too little warmth and perspective taking (authoritarian parenting). A failure to regulate and provide developmentally appropriate structure can also contribute to dependency and immaturity (8). The worst-case scenario is the parent who is physically or psychologically absent; child outcomes are worst when there is low parental warmth as well as low control (9).

What are the determinants of parenting, and how might conception through ART influence parenting quality? Belsky (10) provides a simple model: parenting quality is determined by characteristics of the parents, the child, and the context. With respect to parent characteristics, extensive research confirms that how an adult was cared for in early childhood is a key predictor of later capacity for warm, emotionally available parenting (11). Depression and anxiety can compromise parenting capacity (12), while older age, higher levels of education, and psychological maturity predict more optimal parenting (13). Parent-child relationships are transactional and reciprocal; some children are poorly regulated from birth with temperamental styles or special needs that make caring for them more challenging (14). The social context is crucial: social disadvantage, substandard housing, and unstable family structures make parenting difficult and compromise child well-being, while support from an extended family and a well-resourced community are protective (15).

There are a number of psychosocial protective factors in the ART context, notably older parental age, higher education, and financial security, which may be a prerequisite for accessing the technology. On the other hand, the process is stressful, leading to emotional distress, and the new family structures made possible by ART may lead to problematic relations with extended family, complex relationships with donors, and stigma from the wider community which can compromise both parent and child well-being (16, 17).

Early life deficits in socioemotional processes and atypical social development are antecedents of later behavioral and psychological problems (18). We examine research evidence on parenting, the parent-child relationship, and child psychological well-being and behavioral adjustment in the ART context. In the first section, we consider the transition to parenthood and the parent-child relationship in the early years after birth. As the child develops, attention and emotion regulation are key foundations for learning and mental health. Positive self-esteem and a coherent identity are crucial to psychological well-being during middle childhood and adolescence (5). The second part of the chapter focuses on adolescence and emerging evidence about adjustment in young adult offspring conceived through ART, particularly scenarios involving donor gametes and more complex family forms.

Risks for early child development associated with ART

Unique aspects of the ART context can influence parent adjustment during pregnancy with implications for the evolving parent-child relationship. These include the emotional toll of infertility and treatment, high levels of emotional investment in the pregnancy which might lead to unrealistic expectations of the child and parenthood, and defensive strategies to manage anxiety about the pregnancy outcome in the context of these expectations. Families formed using donated gametes (sperm, eggs, embryos) encounter additional challenges when forming parent-child relationships. They need to reconcile the absence of a genetic link with one or both parents and establish a family that does not conform to the traditional nuclear family model.

Emotionally depleted parents?

The physical, emotional, and financial demands of infertility and treatment can have a negative effect on expectant parents and on the couple's relationship. Some couples struggle with unresolved grief regarding infertility and previous reproductive losses (19). Relationship dynamics may be complicated when one partner carries the infertility diagnosis and the other is genetically related to the child. Parental psychological well-being provides the context for parent-child interactions and the parent-child relationship. There is a large body of evidence confirming that prenatal depression and anxiety are associated with less optimal parenting and child development (20). The ART treatment process is highly stressful (see Chapter 18). While vulnerability to pregnancy-focused anxiety is well established (21, 22), a study of a large sample of women (n = 592) conceiving through ART showed no evidence of elevated depression during pregnancy (22), nor at 4 (23) and 18 months (24) after birth. There has been very little research on adjustment to pregnancy after conception using donated eggs or embryos. The process of conception is more complex and costly, with greater health risks (25, 26).

Overvalued pregnancies and unrealistic expectations?

Pregnancies characterized by heightened emotional (and financial) investment juxtaposed with heightened risk (real or imagined) have been described as overvalued (27). There is a lot at stake, the couple may be older, and the pregnancy may be their only chance to have a child. A perception of risk can change the subjective experience of pregnancy, leading to anxiety about the outcome (discussed earlier) and a defensive "emotional cushioning" as parents struggle to contain their expectations and hold back from reverie about the child (28). This may be compounded by unrealistically high expectations of the long-awaited child (the term "messianic" was used in the early days of IVF) (2) and parenthood (19), leading to inevitable disappointment when the fantasy has to be reconciled with reality. There is evidence that parents conceiving through ART tend to view their infant as "special" and "vulnerable" (29) which could lead to overprotective parenting. These feelings may be intensified for women conceiving with donated eggs (30).

Physiological pathways affecting child regulation

There is a large and growing body of evidence that maternal stress in pregnancy can have a negative impact on the developing fetal hypothalamic-pituitary-adrenal (HPA) axis and central nervous system, leading to problems with emotion and behavior regulation in infancy and childhood (31). Consistent evidence of elevated pregnancy-related anxiety and recent evidence that women pregnant through ART have elevated stress biomarkers (21) suggests offspring conceived through ART might be particularly at risk of these fetal programming effects.

Perinatal risks: Twins and triplets

Multiple births are more common after ART (when there is multiple embryo transfer) and are associated with increased likelihood of preterm birth and low birth weight. Low birth weight is also more common for singleton births (32). These perinatal risk factors are associated with difficult temperament and poorly regulated behavior in infancy. Preterm birth is a well-documented predictor of socioemotional problems and an independent risk factor for psychiatric disorder in childhood (18). Caring for twins involves additional parenting demands and likelihood of less one-on-one interaction (16); however, the risks associated with multiple birth after ART can be avoided by single embryo transfer.

Research evidence: Parent and child well-being in the early years

Three methodological approaches have been employed: self-report questionnaire measures (completed by parents and, in some studies, older children as well), narrative interviews which are more robust to socially desirable reporting (parents, older children), and observed parent-child interactions which can be coded blind to mode of conception. Some studies have also included projective tests of child representations of attachment and family relationships. Narrative interviews and observations provide the most convincing evidence, but they are labor intensive and difficult to administer and code in large samples.

Parenting and parent-child relationships after ART

Pregnancy and infancy

Parents undergoing fertility treatment develop an adaptive tolerance for contradictory and intense feelings during the treatment phase (33), and this may serve them well during the transition to parenthood, which is also a time of emotional ups and downs. Research findings regarding fetal attachment after ART support this interpretation. While it might be expected that elevated anxiety during pregnancy would compromise attachment to the fetus, mothers conceiving through ART generally report more intense and positive fetal attachment compared to naturally conceiving mothers (34). There is very little evidence regarding fetal attachment after egg and embryo donation. Two qualitative studies indicate that the process of forming an attachment is complex and individualized. The absence of a genetic connection is keenly felt; however, women conceiving through egg donation emphasize the importance of the gestational connection, nourishing the baby through their umbilical cord (30, 35). Nonetheless, some report struggling with feeling like an imposter and not a "real" mother (36).

How do these intense and often contradictory feelings play out after birth? Research findings reveal few differences in parental psychological well-being in the first 2 years after birth comparing parents conceiving through ART and naturally conceiving parents with respect to postnatal depression (23, 24) and parenting stress (24, 37), including when the mother has conceived using donor eggs (30). Observational measures of parent-infant interaction provide the most convincing evidence, and studies have showed no differences in parent sensitivity in Australian (38) and Belgian samples (39) when mothers are genetically related to offspring. Indeed, detailed microanalyses in a small Greek sample (40) showed that parents conceiving through ART were more attentive to their infant's distress and engaged in more soothing behaviors. Gibson and colleagues (38) found no differences in observed attachment security and emotional availability comparing a group of mothers whose toddlers had been conceived through ART (genetically related) and a demographically matched comparison group conceived without medical intervention. These studies involve parents of singletons. Studies have revealed higher anxiety and depression when parents of twins and triplets are compared to parents of singletons conceived through ART (41, 42), but few studies have compared twins conceived through ART with naturally conceived twins. In sum, evidence indicates positive psychological adjustment in pregnancy and early parenthood; however, most studies have examined only parents who are genetically related to their singleton infants.

Childhood and adolescence

Susan Golombok's research team has conducted a comprehensive program of research in the UK and Europe that reports cross-sectional and longitudinal comparisons between naturally conceiving parents; parents conceiving through IVF who are genetically related to the child; and more complex family scenarios involving donor sperm, eggs, embryos, and surrogacy. Several studies also include adoptive parents. Golombok (16, 17) synthesizes findings from this body of research and concludes that parents conceiving through ART (irrespective of the involvement of donor gametes and family form) show more similarities than differences when compared with spontaneously conceiving (SC) parents in psychological well-being (mood, parenting stress), parenting, and the parent-child relationship across middle childhood and into adolescence. In fact, parenting has frequently been found to be warmer and more emotionally involved in the ART families, including those using either sperm or egg donation to conceive, from middle childhood through to adolescence (16, 43).

Research examining parent-child relationships in lesbian families using ART to conceive with donor sperm has found the quality of parent-child relationships similar to heterosexual donor conception families (44). In some studies, lesbian mothers have been reported to show more parenting awareness skills (45). There is evidence that mothers who are not genetically or gestationally related to the child (nonbiological mothers) in lesbian families are more involved with their children than nonbiological fathers in donor-conceived families (46, 47) and show more parental concern than biological (genetically related) fathers in SC families (48). While solo mothers using ART to conceive (sperm donation) reported interacting less frequently with their young infants compared with mothers in heterosexual couple families (49), a subsequent follow-up of the sample showed that these differences were limited to infancy. As the child developed through toddlerhood, the solo mothers reported more joy, more pleasure, and less anger during interactions with their child (50).

Research is still limited with respect to parenting and child outcomes after conception through egg and embryo donation (numbers are small; children still young); however, emerging evidence suggests few differences early in the child's life. More sensitive parent responding (parent reported) has been found in egg donation compared with sperm donation families at different developmental periods (51, 52). Findings to date indicate no differences in mother-child relationship quality in families conceiving through embryo donation when compared to ART families where the mother is genetically related to the child (53, 54).

"Two-father" families are the most recent family form enabled by ART; typically one father is genetically related to the child and there is an egg donor and a gestational surrogate who carries the baby and gives birth. Gay men becoming fathers are defying social and traditional gender norms in pursuing fatherhood, which may evoke discrimination and negative attitudes (17). There is limited research. A recent review of child psychosocial outcomes for children of gay fathers (with a variety of pathways to parenthood, including adoption) concludes that gay fathers are no different from lesbian and heterosexual parents in their capacity for warmth, sensitivity, and fostering of secure attachments in their children and that their children are well adjusted (55). Research findings in the first in-depth study comparing 40 gay father surrogacy families with 55 lesbian mother families showed that compared with the lesbian mothers, gay fathers had comparably positive relationships with their children and their children showed lower levels of emotional problems, a finding corroborated by teacher ratings. Children in both groups were subject to stigma from peers, however, and greater stigmatization was associated with more behavior problems (56).

In-depth interviews, including with children conceived through ART, corroborate parent reports. Children from donor-conceiving and SC families generally report comparably warm and affectionate parenting (57). Parents conceiving through ART describe a high investment in parenthood, awareness of the importance of attentive parenting, and a lasting appreciation of the opportunity to parent that is enabled by ART – they tend to savor each moment and don't take anything for granted (17). While the bulk of the studies report no differences or more positive adjustment in ART families, in some studies donor-conceiving parents report persistent perceptions of their child as vulnerable and requiring protection (50, 58) (perhaps from negative effects of stigma), a relational dynamic that has the potential to lead to overinvolved parenting including infantilization and enmeshment (59), which may impede the development of autonomy and self-regulation (8, 60).

Child psychological well-being: Behavior regulation

There are two main risk pathways to problematic behavior. With regard to the first, poor parenting and problematic parent-child relationships, evidence discussed earlier suggests this is not a risk in the ART context. The second relates to the perinatal risks associated with ART conception.

Temperament and behavior in infancy and childhood

Given persistent evidence of pregnancy-focused anxiety in women conceiving through ART, it is surprising that, to our knowledge, there is no evidence of adverse impacts on offspring. Findings regarding infant temperament (the child's reactivity and capacity to self-regulate) have been inconsistent. While early follow-up studies found parents reported more difficult temperament in infancy and toddlerhood (38), these were not corroborated by *observed* differences in child behavior in interactive stress contexts at either age, suggesting it was parental concern rather than temperament difficulties that distinguished the two groups (38). More recent findings regarding child temperament from a larger sample indicated that while high maternal trait anxiety in pregnancy predicted difficult infant temperament for both ART and SC-conceived infants, there were no associations between pregnancy-focused anxiety (significantly higher in the women conceiving through ART) and difficult infant temperament. In fact, compared with SC mothers, the mothers conceiving through ART reported an *easier* temperament in their infants, controlling for gestational age and birth weight (61).

Could there be sleeper effects? Research in community samples suggests effects of exposure to pregnancy anxiety can persist throughout childhood (31). Recent evidence suggests behavior regulation and psychological adjustment during childhood and early adolescence in children conceived through ART is comparable with SC children (62–65), including self-reports from the children themselves (66). Findings from the UK Millennial Cohort Study suggest that overall children conceived through ART are not more at risk of psychosocial or behavioral problems (62). This study, like the studies on infant temperament reported earlier, notes some minor behavioral difficulties (with small effect sizes) from the parent perspective in early childhood, but these are no longer apparent by early adolescence. More research is needed, and interpretation of study findings is complex given the influence of protective factors (relative parental affluence, high education), on the one hand, and perinatal risk variables, on the other. Most research involves singletons, and neurodevelopmental and behavioral outcomes are likely to be more complicated with twins. See Chapter 5 for a more comprehensive overview of pediatric and neurodevelopmental outcomes.

Summary comments: Parent and child well-being

The findings noted indicate that the fundamental underpinnings of healthy child emotional development (warm, involved parenting and positive parent-child relationships) are present for children conceived through ART irrespective of genetic relatedness and that, overall, the "kids are alright" (67). This is likely to be due in part to the fact that parenting was planned and children very much wanted (17), as well as to the protective socioeconomic profile of older parental age, education, and financial security.

There are limitations to the research, however, including the use of volunteer and purposive samples and low response rates for families using gamete donation to conceive. Low disclosure rates about biological origin mean that our understanding of the psychological impact of disclosure on the ART-conceived person's mental health and well-being is still limited. The proliferation of unregulated donor arrangements that may make access to donor identity problematic into the future poses a challenge for families conceiving through ART and for researchers. Studies regarding disclosure have generally relied on parent reports. As older donor-conceived offspring who have had time to reflect on the consequences of their conception have begun to engage in research, some discrepancies between parent perceptions and donor-conceived people's personal experiences have presented. We explore these issues in the next section.

Psychological well-being of adolescent and young adult offspring conceived through ART

Adolescent development: Autonomy and identity

Adolescence is a time of psychological vulnerability, irrespective of mode of conception, and many parents struggle to cope with the transition to more autonomous behavior that is typical and normative in adolescent offspring. The young person experiences hormonal fluctuations related to puberty, erratic mood swings, and struggles with impulse control and emotion regulation. Significant neural reconfiguration supports new capacities for metacognition and complex thinking, which enable acute attunement to honest communication, authenticity, and hypocrisy. The adolescent needs to consolidate an integrated, coherent sense of self; an autonomous identity independent of parents that incorporates gender identity and sexuality (5). All adolescents and young adults engage in this process, but it may be more complex and more salient for donor-conceived offspring. There is an innate motivation to connect past, present, and future, which can be particularly challenging if available information cannot be integrated and components of identity are unknown, disorganized, or confused (68, 69).

Identity and genetic relatedness

Like adoptees, donor-conceived people find themselves in a precarious position in a society where kinship and genetic relatedness are fundamental to socially defined identity (68, 69). Those conceived by single donated gametes may seek to find their missing genetic parent, while those conceived through double donation and embryo donation are in a similar position to adoptees. There is considerable variability in the importance a young person places on being donor-conceived and finding genetic parents. Like adoptees, some will reflect deeply on their genetic non-relatedness and its meaning, while others will not (69–71). Some will experience acute grief and loss about the absence of a genetic connection (72). A willingness on the part of parents to provide accurate and complete information about genetic ties and the circumstances of their child's conception can assist them in resolving any grief and consolidating their genetic identity. This information may not be available to donor-conceived young people for a range of reasons. These include the donor being anonymous or a donor for whom there is limited information available (for example, if the donor lives in another country with different practices around record keeping and beliefs about offspring rights to information), having parents who are unwilling or unable to share information (e.g., deceased, can't remember), lost or destroyed records, or having learned conception history independent of parents, leading to an unwillingness to approach them about the matter.

Following decades of research confirming the importance of identity tracing for psychological well-being in adoptees (74) and advocacy from cohorts of donor offspring who could not access information about their donors, the rights of offspring to identifying information are now enshrined in legislation in many, but not all, developed Western countries and jurisdictions. Access to this information is generally not available until the child is 18 years old, towards the end of the critical developmental phase of adolescence (75).

Disclosure and secrecy

Disclosure of the child's genetic origins is the most vexed and challenging issue for parents conceiving using donated gametes. Favorable shifts in social attitudes and increased awareness of the importance of disclosure appear to be driving the growth in disclosure among families with young donor-conceived children; so, too, the increased use of ART among same-sex couples and solo parents who are unable to conceal the use of donor conception (16, 76). Among heterosexual couples whose donor-conceived children are now older, disclosure remains the exception rather than the rule (52, 77), although it is difficult to draw conclusions, as non-disclosing families and families with older children are less likely to engage in research (77, 78). Most research is based on parent reports (78–82), and when literature has included offspring they are recruited through their parents (e.g., 43, 57), favoring disclosing families.

There has been heated debate about the impact of disclosure or failure to disclose on donor-conceived people. Some have argued that evidence does not support the assumption that disclosure of donor conception to donor-conceived offspring is psychologically beneficial (80, 82). The view that nondisclosure is of no psychological concern does not acknowledge the increasing prevalence of donor-conceived people discovering their donor conception status independently of their parents, the impact this can have on family relationships and trust, and the fact that some report not communicating with their parents about it (71). Although true prevalence of this phenomenon is unknown, it is assumed to be increasing as non-disclosing parents frequently disclose to family and friends (83–85). Further, there is growing community interest in and understanding of genetics, increasing use of direct-to-consumer DNA testing (86, 87), and evolving legislation providing legal pathways for donors to contact offspring independent of their parents and irrespective of any prior anonymity agreements (88). The impact of unplanned or unintentional disclosure is not currently understood and to do so requires studies that include donor-conceived offspring recruited independently of their parents.

When disclosure has been late or accidental, donor-conceived people report that the feeling of being lied to negatively affects their relationships with their parents (70, 76, 89–91). However donor-conceived people who have learned of their donor conception status later in life also commonly report positive impacts on parent-child relationships, including the ability to recontextualize and review their relations with parents (92), which may be beneficial even in cases of previously tumultuous parent-child relationships (71).

Young children who have learned their donor conception status do not appear to differ emotionally or behaviorally from children who have not (58). However, within a multinational sample, disclosing families experienced less severe and less frequent disputes and children perceived their mothers as less strict (58). Further, when compared to SC families, parent-child relationships in non-disclosing families have been found to be less favorable (93). This challenges the beliefs of non-disclosing parents who report that protecting family relationships is the motivation for their secrecy (83, 94). When considering the age of disclosure, it appears that, as in the case of adoption, open communication from an early age is best (43, 76), reducing the likelihood of accidental disclosure and perceived deceit. Early disclosure also allows donor-conceived people to integrate their donor-conceived status as they develop their sense of identity.

Donor-conceived adult perspectives

Few studies to date have directly recruited donor-conceived *adults*, who have achieved adequate autonomy, maturity, and metacognitive capacities to reflect on their mode of conception and how it has affected them. Recruitment strategies largely work through online social networks, support groups, and registries due to the difficulty of identifying donor-conceived adults. This has potentially led to biased research samples composed of individuals struggling to reconcile their mode of conception or motivated by a sense of pain and injustice (82), and their perspectives are therefore often dismissed when they are at odds with mainstream narratives (95). Nonetheless, recruitment in this way is currently the most ethical and inclusive option while secrecy and nondisclosure remain so prevalent. It provides an opportunity to understand how those who may be most profoundly affected are impacted by their ART conception and the related policies and practices.

Donor-conceived adult reports encapsulate positive, neutral, and negative experiences (70, 89–92), which appear transient (72, 96). Curiosity is common (72, 76, 90, 97). Negative experiences include worry about not having a complete medical history and the unique situation of having multiple half-siblings, raising the risk for consanguineous relationships (73). Many jurisdictions have attempted to mitigate these concerns by limiting the number of families who can use a particular donor and giving parents the option of an identity-release donation or abolishing anonymous donation completely. Other concerns expressed by some donor-conceived people relate to incompatible parent-child relationships, feeling "different," and a sense of disrupted identity (70, 72, 89, 90, 97).

For some, identity formation is disrupted due to complex identity reappraisal and negotiation (70, 92, 98), which can be distressing (73). This is a well-documented experience of adoptees who have reported an intense, all-consuming curiosity and preoccupation with obtaining information in an attempt to ameliorate the confusion and uncertainty of missing genetic information (99). There is some anecdotal evidence that this experience may be particularly salient for those who discover they are donor conceived later in life (100). It may be that the disclosure experience fractures identity and disrupts a sense of continuity due to the required reassessment of identity and earlier assumptions about kinship. Symptoms of confusion, disruption, and uncertainty appear to be exacerbated for donor-conceived people when their attempts to obtain information are unsuccessful.

Many donor-conceived people, particularly those who have learned their conception history later in life, have attempted to seek contact with their donors, even if they are inaccessible due to anonymity (71, 92, 97). Family relationships can be challenged when a donor-conceived person reaches out to a donor or a donor's family (89). Some donor-conceived offspring choose not to share their donor contact-seeking with their parents (92), possibly to protect these relationships. Another possible reason is learned secrecy; non-disclosing families may be less emotionally available and disinclined to open communication more generally. It may also be an attempt to protect the parent's sense of identity, parenthood, and family; however, these explanations need to be confirmed empirically.

Conclusions

- Overall, there is consistent evidence in infancy and childhood of comparable psychological and behavioral adjustment in offspring conceived through ART compared with SC offspring from similar backgrounds.
- ART involving donated gametes is more complex, and the complexity hinges around parent struggles with disclosure, despite greater recognition of offspring rights to information about their biological (genetic) identity.
- ART-conceived offspring who learn their conception history later in life may encounter difficulties coming to terms with secrecy, feelings of being deceived, and the development of a coherent sense of self.
- Extant evidence is largely based on adjustment in early and middle childhood from volunteer samples; the voices of older offspring and offspring from families who do not participate in research are missing.
- Emerging research with adolescent and young adult ART offspring reveals a range of complex psychological processes evolving across the lifespan. Researchers and professionals need to prepare for the possibility that these narratives and experiences may not fully conform to mainstream perceptions of nonproblematic adjustment, in which case practices and the policy and social environment in which they operate may need adjustment.

REFERENCES

1. *Time Life Magazine.* 1969 Feb.
2. Fisher A. *IVF: The critical issues.* Victoria: Collins Dove; 1989.
3. Edwards RG, Glass B. Fertilization of human eggs in vitro: Morals, ethics and the law. *Quarterly Review of Biology.* 1976 Jan 1;51:367–91.
4. European IVF-monitoring Consortium (EIM)‡ for the European Society of Human Reproduction and Embryology (ESHRE), Wyns C, Bergh C, Calhaz-Jorge C, De Geyter C, Kupka MS, Motrenko T, Rugescu I, Smeenk J, Tandler-Schneider A, Vidakovic S, Goossens V. ART in Europe, 2016: Results generated from European registries by ESHRE. *Hum Reprod Open.* 2020 Jul 31;2020(3):hoaa032. doi: 10.1093/hropen/hoaa032. PMID: 32760812; PMCID: PMC7394132.
5. Erikson E. *Childhood and society.* New York: Norton; 1963.
6. Bowlby J. *Attachment and loss (Vol. I: Attachment).* London: Pimlico; 1969/1997.
7. Powell B, Cooper G, Hoffman K, Marvin B. *The circle of security intervention: Enhancing attachment in early parent-child relationships.* New York: Guilford Publications; 2013 Sep 26.
8. Baumrind D. Child care practices anteceding three patterns of preschool behavior. *Genetic Psychology Monographs.* 1967;75(1):43–88.
9. Maccoby EE. The role of parents in the socialization of children: An historical overview. *Dev Psych.* 1992;28:1006–17.
10. Belsky J. The determinants of parenting: A process model. *Child Dev.* 1984 Feb 1:83–96.
11. Verhage ML, Schuengel C, Madigan S, Fearon R, Oosterman M, Cassibba R, et al. Narrowing the transmission gap: A synthesis of three decades of research on intergenerational transmission of attachment. *Psych Bull.* 2016;142(4):337–66.
12. Murray L, Cooper P, Fearon P. Parenting difficulties and postnatal depression: Implications for primary healthcare assessment and intervention. *Community Practitioner.* 2014;87(11):34–8.
13. Bornstein MH, Putnick DL, Suwalsky JT, Gini M. Maternal chronological age, prenatal and perinatal history, social support, and parenting of infants. *Child Dev.* 2006 Jul;77(4):875–92.
14. Putnam SV, Sanson AV, Rothbart MK. Child temperament and parenting. In: Bornstein MH, editor. *Handbook of parenting.* 2nd ed. Vol. 1. Children and Parenting. New Jersey: Lawrence Erlbaum; 2002. pp. 255–77.
15. Easterbrooks A, Katz RC, Menon, M. Adolescent parenting. In: Bornstein MH, editor. *Handbook of parenting.* 3rd ed. Vol. 3. Being and Becoming a Parent. New York: Routledge; 2019. pp. 199–231.
16. Golombok S. *Modern families: Parents and children in new family forms.* Cambridge: Cambridge University Press; 2015.
17. Golombok S. Parenting and contemporary reproductive technologies. In: Bornstein MH, editor. *Handbook of parenting.* 3rd ed. Vol. 3. Being and Becoming a Parent. New York: Routledge; 2019. pp. 482–512.
18. Montagna A, Nosarti C. Social-emotional development following very pre-term birth: Pathways to psychopathology. *Front Psychol.* 2016;7:1–23.
19. Burns LH. Psychiatric aspects of infertility and infertility treatments. *Psychiat Clin N Am.* 2007;30: 689–716.
20. Madigan S, Oatley H, Racine N, Fearon RP, Schumacher L, Akbari E, Cooke JE, Tarabulsy GM. A meta-analysis of maternal prenatal depression and anxiety on child socioemotional development. *J Am Acad Child Psy.* 2018 Sep 1;57(9):645–57.
21. García-Blanco A, Diago V, Hervás D, Ghosn F, Vento M, Cháfer-Pericás C. Anxiety and depressive symptoms, and stress biomarkers in pregnant women after in vitro fertilization: A prospective cohort study. *Hum Reprod.* 2018 July 1;33(7):1237–46.
22. McMahon CA, Boivin J, Gibson FL, Hammarberg K, Wynter K, Saunders D, Fisher J. Age at first birth, mode of conception and psychological wellbeing in pregnancy: Findings from the Parental Age and Transition to Parenthood Australia (PATPA) study. *Hum Reprod.* 2011 June 1;26(6):1389–98.
23. McMahon CA, Boivin J, Gibson FL, Fisher JR, Hammarberg K, Wynter K, Saunders DM. Older first-time mothers and early postpartum depression: A prospective cohort study of women conceiving spontaneously or with assisted reproductive technologies. *Fertil Steril.* 2011 Nov 1;96(5):1218–24.
24. McMahon CA, Boivin J, Gibson FL, Hammarberg K, Wynter K, Fisher JR. Older maternal age and major depressive episodes in the first two years after birth: Findings from the Parental Age and Transition to Parenthood Australia (PATPA) study. *J Affect Disorders.* 2015 Apr 1;175:454–62.

25. Jeve YB, Potdar N, Opoku A, Khare M. Donor oocyte conception and pregnancy complications: A systematic review and meta-analysis. *BJOG: Int J Obstet Gynecol.* 2016 Aug;123(9):1471–80.
26. Moreno-Sepulveda J, Checa MA. Risk of adverse perinatal outcomes after oocyte donation: A systematic review and meta-analysis. *J Assist Reprod Gen.* 2019 Oct 1;36(10):2017–37.
27. Raphael-Leff J. *Psychological process of childbearing*. 4th ed. London: Routledge; 2009.
28. Markin RD, Zilcha-Mano S. Cultural processes in psychotherapy for perinatal loss: Breaking the cultural taboo against perinatal grief. *Psychother.* 2018 Mar;55(1):20.
29. Gibson FL, Ungerer JA, Tennant CC, Saunders DM. Parental adjustment and attitudes to parenting after in vitro fertilization. *Fertil Steril.* 2000 Mar 1;73(3):565–74.
30. Imrie S, Jadva V, Fishel S, Golombok S. Families created by egg donation: Parent – child relationship quality in infancy. *Child Dev.* 2019 Jul;90(4):1333–49.
31. Glover V, Ahmed-Salim Y, Capron L. Maternal anxiety, depression, and stress during pregnancy: Effects on the fetus and the child, and underlying mechanisms. *Fetal Dev.* 2016:213–227.
32. Wennerholm UB, Bergh C. Perinatal outcome in children born after assisted reproductive technologies. *Upsala J Med Sci.* 2020 Apr 2;125(2):158–66.
33. Bolvin J, Lancastle D. Medical waiting periods: Imminence, emotions and coping. *Women's Health.* 2010 Jan;6(1):59–69.
34. Hammarberg K, Fisher JR, Wynter KH. Psychological and social aspects of pregnancy, childbirth and early parenting after assisted conception: A systematic review. *Hum Reprod Update.* 2008 Sep 1;14(5):395–414.
35. Kirkman M. Being a "real"mum: Motherhood through donated eggs and embryos. *Women's Studies International Forum.* 2008 Jul 1;31(4):241–8. Pergamon.
36. Imrie S, Jadva V, Golombok S. "Making the child mine": Mothers' thoughts and feelings about the mother – infant relationship in egg donation families. *J Fam Psychol.* 2020 Jun;34(4):469–79.
37. Golombok S, Lycett E, MacCallum F, Jadva V, Murray C, Rust J, Abdalla H, Jenkins J, Margara R. Parenting infants conceived by gamete donation. *J Fam Psychol.* 2004 Sep;18(3):443.
38. Gibson FL, Ungerer JA, McMahon CA, Leslie GI, Saunders DM. The mother-child relationship following In Vitro Fertilisation (IVF): Infant attachment, responsivity, and maternal sensitivity. *J Child Psychol and Psyc.* 2000 Nov;41(8):1015–23.
39. Colpin H, Demyttenaere K, Vandemeulebroecke L. New reproductive technology and the family: The parent-child relationship following in vitro fertilization. *J Child Psychol Psychiatry.* 1995 Nov;36(8):1429–41.
40. Papaligoura Z, Trevarthen C. Mother – infant communication can be enhanced after conception by in-vitro fertilization. *Infant Mental Health Journal: Official Publication of the World Association for Infant Mental Health.* 2001 Nov;22(6):591–610.
41. Cook R, Bradley S, Golombok S. A preliminary study of parental stress and child behaviour in families with twins conceived by in-vitro fertilization. *Hum Reprod.* 1998 Nov 1;13(11):3244–6.
42. Olivennes F, Golombok S, Ramogida C, Rust J, Team FU. Behavioral and cognitive development as well as family functioning of twins conceived by assisted reproduction: Findings from a large population study. *Fertil Steril.* 2005 Sep 1;84(3):725–33.
43. Golombok S, Ilioi E, Blake L, Roman G, Jadva V. A longitudinal study of families formed through reproductive donation: Parent-adolescent relationships and adolescent adjustment at age 14. *Dev Psychol.* 2017 Oct;53(10):1966.
44. Hunfeld JA, Fauser BC, de Beaufort ID, Passchier J. Child development and quality of parenting in lesbian families: No psychosocial indications for a-priori withholding of infertility treatment. A systematic review. *Hum Reprod Update.* 2002 Nov 1;8(6):579–90.
45. Flaks DK, Ficher I, Masterpasqua F, Joseph G. Lesbians choosing motherhood: A comparative study of lesbian and heterosexual parents and their children. *Dev Psychol.* 1995 Jan;31(1):105.
46. Tasker F, Golombok S. The role of co-mothers in planned lesbian-led families. *J Lesbian Stud.* 1998 Sep 11;2(4):49–68.
47. Brewaeys A, Ponjaert I, Van Hall EV, Golombok S. Donor insemination: Child development and family functioning in lesbian mother families. *Hum Reprod.* 1997 Jun 1;12(6):1349–59.
48. Bos HM, Van Balen F, Van den Boom DC. Child adjustment and parenting in planned lesbian-parent families. *Am J Orthopsychiatry.* 2007 Jan;77(1):38–48.
49. Murray C, Golombok S. Going it alone: Solo mothers and their infants conceived by donor insemination. *Am J Orthopsychiatry.* 2005 Apr;75(2):242–53.

50. Murray C, Golombok S. Solo mothers and their donor insemination infants: Follow-up at age 2 years. *Hum Reprod.* 2005 Jun 1;20(6):1655–60.
51. Golombok S, Murray C, Brinsden P, Abdalla H. Social versus biological parenting: Family functioning and the socioemotional development of children conceived by egg or sperm donation. *J Child Psychol Psychiatry.* 1999 May;40(4):519–27.
52. Murray C, MacCallum F, Golombok S. Egg donation parents and their children: Follow-up at age 12 years. *Fertil Steril.* 2006 Mar 1;85(3):610–8.
53. MacCallum F, Golombok S, Brinsden P. Parenting and child development in families with a child conceived through embryo donation. *J Fam Psychol.* 2007 Jun;21(2):278.
54. MacCallum F, Keeley S. Embryo donation families: A follow-up in middle childhood. *J Fam Psychol.* 2008 Dec;22(6):799.
55. Carneiro FA, Tasker F, Salinas-Quiroz F, Leal I, Costa PA. Are the fathers alright? A systematic and critical review of studies on gay and bisexual fatherhood. *Front Psychol.* 2017 Sep 21;8:1636.
56. Golombok S, Blake L, Slutsky J, Raffanello E, Roman GD, Ehrhardt A. Parenting and the adjustment of children born to gay fathers through surrogacy. *Child Dev.* 2018 Jul;89(4):1223–33.
57. Blake L, Casey P, Jadva V, Golombok S. "I was quite amazed": Donor conception and parent – child relationships from the child's perspective. *Child Soc.* 2014 Nov;28(6):425–37.
58. Golombok S, Brewaeys A, Giavazzi MT, Guerra D, MacCallum F, Rust J. The European study of assisted reproduction families: The transition to adolescence. *Hum Reprod.* 2002 Mar 1;17(3): 830–40.
59. Garber BD. Parental alienation and the dynamics of the enmeshed parent – child dyad: Adultification, parentification, and infantilization. *Fam Court Rev.* 2011 Apr;49(2):322–35.
60. Zeinali A, Sharifi H, Enayati M, Asgari P, Pasha G. The mediational pathway among parenting styles, attachment styles and self-regulation with addiction susceptibility of adolescents. *J Res Med Sci.* 2011 Sep;16(9):1105.
61. McMahon CA, Boivin J, Gibson FL, Hammarberg K, Wynter K, Saunders D, Fisher J. Pregnancy-specific anxiety, ART conception and infant temperament at 4 months post-partum. *Hum Reprod.* 2013 Apr 1;28(4):997–1005.
62. Barbuscia A, Myrskylä M, Goisis A. The psychosocial health of children born after medically assisted reproduction: Evidence from the UK Millennium Cohort Study. *SSM-Population Health.* 2019 Apr 1;7:100355.
63. Hart R, Norman RJ. The longer-term health outcomes for children born as a result of IVF treatment: Part II-mental health and development outcomes. *Hum Reprod Update.* 2013;19:244–50.
64. Punamaki R-L, Tiitinen A, Lindblom J, Unkila-Kallio L, Flykt M, Vanska M, et al. Mental health and developmental outcomes for children born after ART: A comparative prospective study on child gender and treatment type. *Hum Reprod.* 2016;31(1):1–107.
65. Waganaar K, van Weissenbruch MM, Knol DI, Delemarre-Van de Waal HA, Huisman J. Behavior and socioemotional functioning in 9–18-year-old children born after in vitro fertilization. *Fertil Steril.* 2009;92(6):1907–14.
66. Waganaar K, van Weissenbruch MM, van Leeuwen FF, Cohen-Kettenis PT, Delemarre-Van de Waal HA, Schats R et al. Self-reported behavior and socioemotional functioning of 11–18-year-old adolescents conceived by in vitro fertilization. *Fertil Steril.* 2011;95(2):611–16.
67. Cholodenko L, Bening A, Moore J, Ruffalo M, Wasikowska M, Blumberg S. The kids are all right. Universal Studios; 2011.
68. Grotevant HD, Dunbar N, Kohler JK, Esau AM. Adoptive identity: How contexts within and beyond the family shape developmental pathways. *Fam Rela.* 2000 Oct;49(4):379–87.
69. Leon IG. Adoption losses: Naturally occurring or socially constructed? *Child Dev.* 2002 Mar;73(2):652–63.
70. Turner AJ, Coyle A. What does it mean to be a donor offspring? The identity experiences of adults conceived by donor insemination and the implications for counselling and therapy. *Hum Reprod.* 2000 Sep 1;15(9):2041–51.
71. Mogseth ME. Donor conception and unknown kin: Reconsidering identity and family through anonymous and deanonymized relations [Master's thesis]. Oslo, Norway: University of Oslo; 2019.
72. Hewitt G. Missing links: Identity issues of donor conceived people. *J Fertil Couns.* 2002; 9:14–19.
73. Marquardt E, Glenn ND, Clark K. My daddy's name is donor: A new study of young adults conceived through sperm donation. Institute for American Values; 2010.

74. Palacios J, Brodzinsky D. Adoption research: Trends, topics, outcomes. *Int J Behav Dev.* 2010;34(3): 270–84.
75. Erikson EH. *Identity: Youth and crisis* (No. 7). New York: WW Norton & Company; 1968.
76. Jadva V, Freeman T, Kramer W, Golombok S. The experiences of adolescents and adults conceived by sperm donation: Comparisons by age of disclosure and family type. *Hum Reprod.* 2009 Aug 1;24(8): 1909–19.
77. Gottlieb C, Lalos O, Lindblad F. Disclosure of donor insemination to the child: The impact of Swedish legislation on couples' attitudes. *Hum Reprod.* 2000 Sep 1;15(9):2052–6.
78. Nachtigall RD, Tschann JM, Quiroga SS, Pitcher L, Becker G. Stigma, disclosure, and family functioning among parents of children conceived through donor insemination. *Fertil Steril.* 1997 Jul 1;68(1):83–9.
79. Owen L, Golombok S. Families created by assisted reproduction: Parent–child relationships in late adolescence. *J Adol.* 2009 Aug 1;32(4):835–48.
80. Kovacs GT, Wise S, Finch S. Keeping a child's donor sperm conception secret is not linked to family and child functioning during middle childhood: An Australian comparative study. *Aust N Z J Obstet Gynaecol.* 2015 Aug;55(4):390–6.
81. Amor DJ, Lewis S, Kennedy J, Habgood E, McBain J, McLachlan RI, Rombauts LJ, Williams K, Halliday J. Health outcomes of school-aged children conceived using donor sperm. *Reprod Biomed Online.* 2017 Oct 1;35(4):445–52.
82. Pennings G. Disclosure of donor conception, age of disclosure and the well-being of donor offspring. *Hum Reprod.* 2017 May 1;32(5):969–73.
83. Cook R, Golombok S, Bish A, Murray C. Disclosure of donor insemination: Parental attitudes. *Am J Orthopsychiatry.* 1995 Oct;65(4):549–59.
84. Braverman AM, Boxer AS, Corson SL, Coutifaris C, Hendrix A. Characteristics and attitudes of parents of children born with the use of assisted reproductive technology. *Fertil Steril.* 1998 Nov 1;70(5):860–5.
85. Leiblum SR, Aviv AL. Disclosure issues and decisions of couples who conceived via donor insemination. *J Psychosom Obst Gyn.* 1997 Jan 1;18(4):292–300.
86. Harper JC, Kennett D, Reisel D. The end of donor anonymity: How genetic testing is likely to drive anonymous gamete donation out of business. *Hum Reprod.* 2016 Jun 1;31(6):1135–40.
87. Phillips AM. Only a click away – DTC genetics for ancestry, health, love . . . and more: A view of the business and regulatory landscape. *Appl Tansl Genomics.* 2016 Mar 1;8:16–22.
88. Graham S, Mohr S, Bourne K. Regulating the'good'donor: The expectations and experiences of sperm donors in Denmark and Victoria, Australia. In: *Regulating reproductive donation*. Cambridge: University Press; 2016. pp. 207–31.
89. Blyth E, Crawshaw M, Frith L, Jones C. Donor-conceived people's views and experiences of their genetic origins: A critical analysis of the research evidence. In: *Assistierte Reproduktion mit Hilfe Dritter*. Berlin: Springer; 2020. pp. 361–88.
90. Mahlstedt PP, LaBounty K, Kennedy WT. The views of adult offspring of sperm donation: Essential feedback for the development of ethical guidelines within the practice of assisted reproductive technology in the United States. *Fertil Steril.* 2010 May 1;93(7):2236–46.
91. Zweifel JE. Donor conception from the viewpoint of the child: Positives, negatives, and promoting the welfare of the child. *Fertil Steril.* 2015 Sep 1;104(3):513–19.
92. Daniels K. The perspective of adult donor conceived persons. In *Assistierte Reproduktion mit Hilfe Dritter*. Berlin: Springer; 2020. pp. 443–59.
93. Golombok S, Readings J, Blake L, Casey P, Mellish L, Marks A, Jadva V. Children conceived by gamete donation: Psychological adjustment and mother-child relationships at age 7. *J Fam Psychol.* 2011 Apr;25(2):230–9.
94. Laruelle C, Place I, Demeestere I, Englert Y, Delbaere A. Anonymity and secrecy options of recipient couples and donors, and ethnic origin influence in three types of oocyte donation. *Hum Reprod.* 2011 Feb 1;26(2):382–90.
95. Somerville M. Donor conception and children's rights: "First, do no harm". *CMAJ.* 2011 Feb 8;183(2):280.
96. Beeson DR, Jennings PK, Kramer W. Offspring searching for their sperm donors: How family type shapes the process. *Hum Reprod.* 2011 Sep 1;26(9):2415–24.
97. Macmillan CM, Allan S, Johnstone M, Stokes MA. Donor conception: How demographics and disclosure experiences impact donor-conceived adults' motivations for seeking information about, and contact with, sperm donors. *Reprod Biomed Online.* 2021 April 10. https://doi.org/10.1016/j.rbmo.2021.04.005

98. Cushing AL. "I just want more information about who I am": The search experience of sperm-donor offspring, searching for information about their donors and genetic heritage. *Inform Res*. 2010 Jun 1;15(2).
99. Sants HJ. Genealogical bewilderment in children with substitute parents. *Brit J Med Psychol*. 1964 Jun;37(2):133–42.
100. Allan S. Donor conception, secrecy, and the search for information. *J Law Med*. 2012 Jun 8;19(4).

20

The long term safety of assisted reproductive technologies

Ethical aspects

Lucy Frith, Heidi Mertes, and Nicola Jane Williams

Introduction

While the central place of safety in assisted reproductive technologies (ARTs) is self-evident, there are divergent opinions on which kinds of risks are admissible for whom and when and who gets to decide on the permissibility of risks. Key areas are how the welfare of the future child is to be balanced against the reproductive autonomy of prospective parents, how we can ensure that safety is not overtaken by other interests, and how to strike the right balance between ensuring safety and ensuring access to medical treatment, in addition to other areas. In this chapter, we will touch on several of these topics, giving an insight into some of the ethical principles and debates underlying certain policies, guidelines, and common practices in ART related to long term safety.

From bench to bedside

Responsible innovation in ART ideally proceeds through the following steps: preclinical research (in cells, animals, and/or embryos), clinical trials, and (long term) follow-up studies (1, 2). While the ethics of preclinical research on animals and of clinical trials on patients are well-rehearsed, issues that are particularly challenging in reproductive medicine are those related to research on human embryos and to long term follow-up of the resulting children (long term follow-up will be discussed in Section 4.3). Embryo research is controversial due to the potential instrumentalization of human creatures who are accorded varying degrees of moral status based either on their inherent value as members of the human species, or their potential to become a person, and/or based on their symbolic value (3). While many countries allow research on embryos that were created through in vitro fertilization (IVF) treatment but will not be transferred to the patient for various reasons, few allow the creation of a human embryo specifically for research purposes (4). Regulatory limitations on research should, however, not be seen as an excuse for introducing new treatments without proper risk assessments.

The technological imperative

Requiring 0% risk for the introduction of new reproductive technologies is unattainable, and attempting to approximate this zero-risk level would lead to the inaccessibility of many beneficial treatments, which is, given the high burden of disease, morally problematic (1). This means that difficult weighing efforts are needed to determine when a new treatment is ready for the clinic. One factor that is known to confound sound decision making in this regard is a phenomenon described as the *technological imperative*. Relying on the typology of the technological imperative in the context of health care put forward by Björn Hofmann (5), we can point to several potential ways in which the technological imperative might plead for a premature introduction of new reproductive technologies. First, the *imperative of possibility and action* appeals to the moral intuition that if we can help patients by means of a novel technology, we should (despite safety concerns), rather than abandoning them (e.g., grant access to uterus transplantation through clinical trials despite considerable risks). Second, the *imperative of demand* refers to the pressure that patients may put on clinicians to receive a certain treatment (e.g., a Turner syndrome patient demanding that she receives treatment just as other patients do). As long as we include the considerations noted earlier as elements in the weighing of pros and cons, there is no problem. However, once they become *imperatives* and can no longer be put in the balance alongside other considerations, such as safety concerns, an ethical problem arises.

Who decides which risks are acceptable?

In natural reproduction, the reproductive liberty of individuals is only restricted in very exceptional circumstances, for example, when people have a severe mental disability or during incarceration. This means that people are free to reproduce, even if they know that by doing so, they risk conceiving a child that will suffer from suboptimal life circumstances due to physical impairments or contextual factors. Some would argue that reproductive liberty also pleads against any kind of interference in assisted reproduction, both on a governance level and on the level of the hospital or health care workers whose assistance is sought. However, reproductive liberty is generally considered to be a liberty right, not a claim right, meaning that although I am free to reproduce as I wish, I cannot make a claim on others in terms of practical or financial assistance to support me in this pursuit. As physicians have sworn an oath not to harm their patients and are arguably co-responsible for the welfare of the children they help conceive, they can therefore legitimately refuse to perform certain procedures on certain patients when – according to their assessment – the risks for the parents and/or child are unacceptable (see 'Recipient welfare in ART' and 'The welfare and interests of children produced through ART'). Note that informed consent or a waiver of liability signed by a patient in no way removes the moral responsibility a health care professional has for the adverse effects of treatments on their patients and the resulting children. However, reasonable disagreement can exist between different parties involved concerning which risk is – or is not – acceptable.

Excessive risk reduction?

While most of the ethical concerns in the realm of risks in reproductive medicine are aimed at insufficient risk reduction, too *much* risk reduction may also prove problematic. For example, in the context of preimplantation genetic testing for aneuploidy screening (PGT-A), claims have been made that it would be irresponsible to transfer aneuploid embryos and that therefore all embryos need to be screened. Similarly, some patients only receive treatment after agreeing to take risk-reducing measures, e.g., preconception genetic screening, PGT-M, or weight loss, while single, same-sex, or "older" patients are completely denied treatment on the alleged basis of concerns over the well-being of the future children. What we notice here, is that the – in principle – morally laudable goal of risk reduction might be window dressing for other motives, either commercial (in the case of widespread PGT-A or preconception screening) or ideological (in the case of refusal of treatment for people with certain – mostly non-heteronormative – characteristics). In the context of genetic screening in particular, concerns are voiced regarding the message that such screening and selection requirements send to people with disabilities regarding the differential value of their lives (6). Thus, while risk reduction is needed to avoid serious risks, it is wise to keep in mind that we take numerous calculated risks on a daily basis in order to obtain the things we value in life. Reproduction, despite all the risk reduction measures we might take, remains an intrinsically risky endeavor.

Recipient welfare in ART

This edited collection has outlined a range of scenarios and possible risks to both those receiving ARTs (which for the purposes of this chapter we will call recipients) and those born from those procedures.

In this section we focus on the recipients of treatments and the ethical issues raised when decisions have to be made about who ought to receive fertility treatments and in what circumstances. When deciding who to treat, fertility clinicians have a number of factors to consider. Of overriding concern is the need to consider the welfare of potential recipients in ART and the welfare of any future child (which will be explored in Section 4). In determining the welfare of potential recipients, it is argued that in the absence of adequate reasons to the contrary, clinicians should promote the reproductive rights and respect the autonomy of their patients. In what follows we therefore outline these principles, explore their importance for individual welfare, and consider how these might be balanced against other considerations.

The right to reproduce

Questions of access to ART have been a contentious issue since the development of IVF in the late 1970s. One of the main arguments for not restricting access to ART is that the infertile have the same right to reproduce as the fertile. This is an area of debate that has been changed radically by the scientific development of ART, giving infertile people many more options to explore in terms of having a child. The right to reproduce free from interference is generally viewed as an important basic human right enshrined in both Article 16 of the United Nations Declaration on Human Rights and Article 12 of the European Convention on Human Rights as the right to marry and found a family. As mentioned earlier, these articles are usually understood as stipulating what can be called a liberty right or negative right, that is a right not to have one's reproductive capacities interfered with against one's will. An interest in reproduction is generally held to be of significant import, with one of IVF's pioneers Robert Edwards noting: "It is impossible to put a price on the benefits to society of producing wanted children raised in a caring environment."

The development and practice of ART can therefore provide those who experience infertility with the means to achieve their own reproductive aspirations and exercise their reproductive liberty. John Robertson (7) has put forward a rights-based argument to support the extended use of ART. He begins by arguing that the concept of procreative liberty should be given primacy when making policy decisions in this area. Procreative liberty is the freedom to decide whether, when, how, how often, and with whom to reproduce. At first sight, this appears to be a negative right, not to have one's reproductive capacities interfered with. However, Robertson endorses subsidiary enabling rights to procreation, that is, someone has the right to something if it can be regarded as a prerequisite for procreation. This effectively turns a negative right (not to be interfered with) into a positive right (to have something made available to one). Thus, individuals have a right to access ART in Robertson's account, since they enable those who experience infertility to exercise their reproductive rights in the same way as their fertile counterparts.

Robertson's claim could clearly be problematic. The feminist philosopher Laura Purdy (8) argues that Robertson adopts a position that blurs the distinction between negative and positive rights. He seems to infer that the strong right not to have one's reproductive capabilities interfered with implies an equally strong right to reproduce. Embedded in this discussion of reproductive rights is the assumption, made by Robertson, that the issues raised by natural reproduction are akin to those raised by assisted reproduction. Christine Overall (9), a feminist critic of ART, argues that the issues raised by the two forms of reproduction are fundamentally different, and correspondingly, the right to use ART needs a different burden of proof from the right to be free from reproductive interference.

As a result, it is by no means clear that good arguments can be provided to support the claims by scholars like Robertson that there is a positive right to reproduce (and accordingly that the infertile should have the means made available for them to reproduce or what the practical implications of such a right would be in terms of funding, etc.). It is not generally recognized that just because the means are available to achieve some end, people have a right to those means. In terms of providing the basis for access to ART, these arguments based on a conception of the positive right to reproduce have not had the significant practical effects that their proponents might have hoped. Most health care systems have limits on whether, when, and for whom ART will be funded as part of socialized or insurance-based medical care.

Reproductive choice and liberty

Another key principle to consider when discussing the risks that recipients of ART ought to be permitted to shoulder is that of reproductive choice. ART is often considered to broaden the range of *meaningful* reproductive options that are available to prospective parents. Any extension of choice is frequently portrayed as desirable, and this is often also claimed of reproductive choices. Appeals to the importance of reproductive choice have underpinned many arguments provided in favor of innovation in ART. Advocates of reproductive autonomy, for example, Savulescu (10) and Harris (11) endorse the pre-eminence of parental choice in most circumstances. The central tenet of this view is that personal reproductive decisions should be free from interference unless they will cause *serious harm to others* (12). As will be discussed in 'The welfare and interests of children produced through ART', it is unclear how concerns regarding the welfare of *future* persons should be weighed against reproductive liberty.

This view has significant philosophical pedigree, with many philosophers and jurists holding that individual freedom is the appropriate baseline assumption when discussing the permissibility of the acts and choices of moral agents. Mill, for example, held that "in practical matters, the burden of proof is supposed to be with those who are against liberty" (13). Locke held similarly that man is naturally in "a State of perfect Freedom to order their actions . . . as they see fit . . . without asking leave or depending upon the Will of any other Man" (14) and that this should place limits on the liberty-limiting abilities of the state, whose goal should be seen to preserve and protect natural liberties and property. More recent expression is also found in the work of Stanley Benn who suggests that "the burden of justification falls on the interferer, not on the person interfered with" (15), and Rawls who argues that in a just society "there is a general presumption against imposing legal and other restrictions on conduct without a sufficient reason" (16).

This argument is sometimes reinforced by claims that reproductive choices are "integral to a person's sense of being" (17), and any restrictions therefore require even more robust justification than less important choices (7). There is a belief that the more important the choice, the stronger the case for restricting it has to be. Hence, as reproductive choice is very important – the desire for a child is perceived by many as a fundamental need – allowing people to exercise it is a good in itself, and this good *outweighs the production of a certain level of harm* such as in cases where treatment is provided to women who have serious background medical conditions.

Balancing principles and rights

While respecting individuals' free choices to reproduce may, at first blush (prima facie), seem a good rule of thumb, attention to competing considerations may lead to different conclusions.

Balancing harms and benefits of treatments need to be considered at a number of levels, and it is important to think about what types of harm are relevant here. While clinicians may be concerned about harms experienced by the patients in front of them, there could be wider societal harms caused by the use and provision of ART. For example, while some feminists have argued that ART and techniques extend women's procreative choices by offering additional choices, others argue that desires to avail oneself of ART and techniques are, in some sense, inauthentic, as the harms of infertility are the result of problematic societal pressures and norms. Thus, the very existence of ART can constrain and influence choices, and their provision can reinforce and validate such pressures and norms, causing expressive harm. Here, what are presented as new options can quickly become seen as the standard of care that women have to actively refuse. Thus, some have claimed that the availability of such technologies has imposed upon potential reproducers a *forced choice* to either pursue or refuse to pursue new technological options (18), with childlessness no longer seen as an acceptable option unless women have tried to conceive by using ART.

It is argued that women are particularly susceptible to essentialist and pronatalist social pressures and norms surrounding reproduction and womanhood. Pronatalism is an attitude or policy that encourages reproduction and promotes the role of parenthood. Pronatalism particularly affects women, who are encouraged to become mothers. In a patriarchal society true femininity is often equated with childbearing, and motherhood is thereby regarded as a necessary aspect of womanhood, with women considered essentially or naturally parents. The way in which society pressures women to have children and the focus on genetic relationships can be said to be socially determined ways of constructing our reproductive relationships. It could be argued that we do not have to respond to such pressure to reproduce, and it is important to give women the freedom to choose to remain child free and have that choice be equally valued and respected (19). The wider social implications of the use of ART and its potential to forward or set back attempts to drive social change thus needs to be considered when weighing up their associated harms and benefits.

That our choices are both constrained and constructed by our social, economic, and political situations, however, is increasingly acknowledged and accepted in new theories of autonomy such as relational autonomy questioning the Western interpretation of autonomy as excessively individualistic (20) and depending on "an asocial, abstract conception of individuals" (21). These kinds of theories of autonomy consider the person in their wider context, and they might be more useful in deciding how decisions should be made and determining who should make them. Dove et al. define relational autonomy as "a conception of autonomy that places the individual in a socially embedded network of others" (22). It is often argued that people usually make important decisions by discussing them with people they are close to. Therefore, the notion of the individual as ideally atomistic and self-sufficient may be a misnomer in medical practice in general and particularly unhelpful in considering ART. ART has, as its focus, the creation of families and is therefore never solely about the risks to one person.

Professional responsibility

Health care professionals have a responsibility to act in the interests of the individuals who are presenting for treatment as well as any future offspring. Reasons for overriding the reproductive autonomy of a potential recipient might be that to treat them may result in undue harm to them, i.e., a women with cardiac problems for whom pregnancy would put an undue strain on them; or what is asked for is not legally allowed in the country where treatment is being offered, i.e., sex selection for social reasons is currently forbidden in the UK (Human Fertilisation and Embryology Act 1990: Schedule 2, 1ZB[1]); or payment or reimbursement systems will not pay for the treatment, i.e., in the UK limits are placed on the number of IVF cycles people can receive on the National Health Service (23). Therefore, it is often not in the fertility clinician's power to be able to give the recipient exactly what they want for reasons that may be regulatory or financial in nature or related to the particular patient. While physicians may be constrained by the context in which they practice, as medical professionals, they also have to weight their own duties to do no harm and promote beneficence for their patients. Therefore, in certain situations, it is not ethically desirable to accede to whatever the patient requests, but to act to further the patient's best interests and in line with professional codes that recognize such responsibilities. Often through discussion and counseling, recipients can see how certain actions, such as continuing IVF cycles when there is little chance of success, are not in their interests, and they can be supported to make the best decision in the circumstances for themselves and one that the medical team can also work with.

In order for physicians to adequately discharge these duties in this complex area, recipients need to be provided with the relevant information on all aspects of their treatment. Counseling is recommended to enable recipients to understand both the medical implications of the treatment and the psychosocial aspects of forming a family in this way. ART is much more than a form of medical treatment and is most appropriately seen as an exercise in family formation, and this should be born in mind when appraising recipients of the risks and benefits of ART and ensuring that recipients receive the necessary support to make sufficiently informed decisions for themselves and their future family and, if relevant, the implications of using donated reproductive material (i.e., gametes/embryos) (24). Even then, if conception does not take place, the feeling of failure and the stress, strain, and costly medical treatment can all take their toll (25).

In sum, while it is often argued that fertility clinicians should aim to respect their patient's autonomy, often this is not possible – societal harms have to be weighed against individual benefit, potential harms to the individual have be weighed, and sometimes patients need to be counseled and supported to act in their own best interests.

The welfare and interests of children produced through ART

Unlike many other arenas in medicine where safety concerns have as their primary focus the welfare of those who receive treatment, reproductive medicine differs in that its primary function is *the creation of an additional party*: a child. Thus, discussion of safety concerns in ART are complicated by the need to consider not only the safety of a procedure or intervention for the individuals and/or couples who seek them and how this should be balanced against a desire to respect the autonomy of prospective parents but also the welfare of the children that may be produced through ART who do not and cannot consent to the risks involved in treatment. Indeed, in cases where interventions affect the germline (such as mitochondrial replacement therapy and gene editing), safety concerns extend to children who may be born *many generations* into the future, leading to an even more pressing need to carefully consider the risks and burdens such treatments may impose on parties other than the intended parents over both the short and long term.

As noted by Robertson (26), with respect to child welfare, ART therefore has the following ethical structure:

> The use of [ART] may enable an infertile person or one who carries genes for serious disease to reproduce, but in doing so they risk having a child with diminished welfare. The degree, certainty, and kind of risk vary, as does the motivation for seeking reproductive assistance and the person's other options for reproducing. But they all pose a risk that the child will experience physical, psychological, or social limitations that ordinarily do not occur without the use of [ART].
>
> (p. 8)

Yet how risky is *too risky*? How should we calculate and weigh such risks in the face of uncertainty? And to what lengths ought practitioners and policymakers go in service of the aim of protecting the welfare of children born through ART? In this section we explore questions of *child welfare arising from safety concerns in ART*, such as the risks to the physical welfare of offspring posed by modifying, selecting, and manipulating gametes and embryos and from interventions such as IVF and ICSI.

Welfare standards and non-identity problems

As explained by Pennings et al. (27) there are different positions on determining acceptable risks to offspring, which can be identified as falling somewhere on a spectrum from accounts providing very minimal welfare requirements sitting at one end and accounts providing extremely strong welfare requirements sitting at the other. In this section we will explore standards from both ends of the spectrum (the so-called "maximal" and "minimal" welfare standards) and a more moderate position known as the "reasonable welfare standard".

According to the maximal welfare standard, medically assisted reproduction should not be provided "when it is indicated that the life conditions of the future child will not be optimal" (27). In this view, no risks of harm to children produced through ART should be considered acceptable, which would, given that no fertility treatment is risk free, preclude provision in all cases. Setting such a high bar when it comes to ART, however, is problematic, as those able to reproduce without assistance are not generally considered to be blameworthy when they (inevitably) bring children into the world in suboptimal conditions. Thus, it is often considered unfair or unreasonable to set the bar for responsible reproduction so high in one reproductive context but not others. At the other end of the scale is the "wrongful life" or "minimal welfare" standard. This view suggests that ART should be permitted so long as it does not result in the births of children whose lives have been variously described in the ethics literature surrounding assisted reproduction as "less than worth living" (28), "intractably miserable" (29), "dominated by pain and suffering" (30), and "worse than no life at all" (31). Given that the majority of individuals with even the most painful and life-limiting diseases and disabilities consider their own lives to be worth living, requirements regarding safety and risk to children produced through ART would, in this view, be incredibly permissive, with little requirement to even attempt to reduce any risks.

Given concerns regarding excessiveness and unfairness on the maximal standard, some have suggested that rather than maximizing child welfare or failing to account for it in all but the most significant cases, we should instead aim for sufficiency, accepting some risks in ART, but requiring that they are both reduced in so far as possible and fall below an acceptable or "reasonable" threshold for harm. Yet how should we determine what risks are acceptable or reasonable? Some suggest that natural conception should be used as the benchmark for acceptable levels of risk such that treatments and techniques which impose risks on offspring that are *greater* than those imposed by natural reproduction ought to be forbidden. Yet this threshold seems arbitrary and seems to make an unjustified leap from a descriptive statement about the world to a claim about how things ought to be. Others therefore suggest a more principled limit, suggesting that responsible reproductive policies (and reproducers) should make decisions regarding acceptable and unacceptable levels of risk to offspring on the basis of whether the children produced are likely to have "at least a *normal opportunity* for the good life" (8) or "the abilities and opportunities to realise those dimensions and goals that in general make a life valuable" (27).

However, while it seems self-evident that the welfare of children produced by ART should be of paramount importance to physicians, researchers, and prospective parents, many nations worldwide have incorporated child welfare requirements into legislation and policy governing assisted reproduction (26),[1] and so, too, do many professional bodies[2] – philosophically the matter is a little more complex. This is the result of a paradox known in philosophy as "the non-identity problem" (32) which arises in situations where the only means we have of protecting some individual (or group of individuals) from some particular (and negative) event or occurrence is to prevent their existence. Where this is the case, unless that individual's life is so bad that it fails to meet the "wrongful life" or "minimal welfare" standard discussed previously, they cannot be considered harmed. For even if their existence is marked by suffering, this is a condition of their very existence: it is unavoidable. They could not exist in any other state, and their existence is, on balance, a benefit to them. In the context of ART, many decisions to provide or not to provide treatments alter the timing and manner of conception and thus fall prey to the non-identity problem such as the use of fertility drugs, preimplantation genetic diagnosis followed by embryo selection, gamete donor selection decisions, and potentially, mitochondrial replacement therapy. Such cases force us to reconsider the ultimate "goals" of child welfare requirements in ART. Candidates include impersonal considerations such as a commitment to reducing levels of suffering and limited opportunity in the world regardless of who experiences it (33, 32) and public health goals to reduce the overall burden of disease and disability within a given society (34).

Weighing risks to offspring

In cases of ART that do not fall prey to the non-identity problem or where child welfare goals are motivated by impersonal and public health goals, attention should also be directed to questions of whether and when certain risks associated with ART should be considered to fall within the remit of safety considerations and how such risks should be weighted.

With respect to the former question, ought, for example, the social harms that may befall children conceived through gamete donation, mitochondrial replacement, surrogacy arrangements, and gene editing be counted as safety risks alongside the physical risks of such technologies? Such concerns, after all, may be considered to arise primarily as a result of discrimination and/or prevailing norms and attitudes regarding the importance of genetic and gestational ties for parenthood, which may be reduced through altering the social context rather than restricting the use of ART. A clear example where social solutions to the suffering of ART-conceived children may be deemed more appropriate can be found in cases where children born outside of heteronormative family structures experience discrimination as a result of the manner of their conception. A slightly more complicated case is that of the interests of donor-conceived children, who may claim that they are "harmed" when they are unable to access identifying information regarding their donors or by the very knowledge that they are donor conceived (35, 36). For while in some cases, risks and welfare concerns resulting from donor anonymity may clearly be related to considerations regarding safety such as a lack of knowledge regarding propensity to genetic disease, in others these decrements could be argued to be *primarily* caused by social norms and attitudes that privilege genetic ties between families and lead donor-conceived offspring to place significant value on finding out information and potentially cultivating relationships with their donors and donor siblings. Indeed, given increasing acceptance of the social nature of many of the harms associated with disability, it may also be found that the physical risks associated with the use of ART to children may be significantly reduced in their intensity through attending to the social context in which disability arises (37), and this, too, may affect calculations regarding risk.

Once we have determined which risks count within the remit of safety considerations, questions then move to focus on how we should weigh such risks given difficulties in both forecasting the long term risks of ART and their incidence, the catastrophic nature of some of those risks which may affect the germline, and in obtaining data through the long term follow-up studies of children born through ART. Ought we, as in other contexts, calculate the acceptability of risks by straightforwardly using expected value analysis, combining data we have regarding the probability of their occurrence with their disvalue? Ought we only to take into account *known* harms and risks, using a narrow evidence-based methodology (38)? Or, given the inevitability of uncertainty in this context and attendant difficulties in establishing causal connections between our activities and outcomes, ought we to take a more risk-averse approach by implementing a precautionary approach that assigns greater disvalue to small and/or uncertain risks of significant harm/damage than standard approaches to risk management (39)? One thing is certain: however we choose to weigh risks, proper attention to safety concerns in ART, as in all areas of medicine, requires robust preclinical research prior to application in humans and long term and wide-ranging follow-up of children born through ART in order to track both foreseen and unforeseen outcomes and improve technologies and techniques.

Long term follow-up of ART-conceived children

While proper attention to the long term safety risks of ART for children born requires research exploring outcomes for such children, difficulties in obtaining data over the long term are significant, and careful attention should be paid, as in all research contexts involving children, to principles relating to the best interests of the children involved, necessity, harm minimization, and informed consent. For patients and children, regular attendance at clinical appointments, for example, can impose significant physical, psychological, and financial costs. As a result, it is generally considered that attention should be directed to the question of compensation for research involvement; follow-up studies should involve only minimal risks to children; should be performed only when the results of research are considered to be in the best interests of the child or children generally, such as where the information collected over time is liable to affect the direction of treatment in the future; and where parties to the research are made aware of its purpose and appropriate consent/assent is provided by the parents and child and/or the child once they have reached majority (40).

Importantly, the crucial party to follow-up, the resulting child, cannot be asked for a long term commitment at the onset of treatment (2). Moreover, long term follow-up, and especially cross-generational follow-up, is also challenging, as it requires studies that continue over several years and decades, which are difficult to fund. These limitations lead to a situation in which it is oftentimes incorrect to label a treatment as "established", although it has surpassed the early experimental phase. For this reason, it was suggested that a third, intermediate label should be introduced, "innovative treatment", to better clarify to the patient that there is a continuum from experimental to established treatment and that uncertainties oftentimes remain even when treatments no longer have the "experimental" label (41). In order to gather sufficient data to be able to recategorize innovative treatments as established treatments, those collecting, collating, and analyzing such data must ensure long term sources of funding are available to support follow-up studies and establish long term risks.

Conclusions

- When judging whether long term risks in ART are justified, different aspects need to be balanced against one another.

- Discussions regarding the right to reproduce and liberty grant individuals significant autonomy with respect to reproductive decision making.
- The physician's responsibility to reduce harm to both recipients and offspring cast doubt on the paramount nature of individual autonomy in the context of reproduction, as do worries regarding problematic social pressures and norms.
- Worries regarding child welfare are also particularly difficult to weigh in this context, given both the implications of the non-identity problem and difficulties in long term follow-up of ART-conceived children.
- Our reproductive choices do not occur in a vacuum; as such, the wider social implications of ART must also be considered and principles of responsible innovation be adhered to, both in the clinic and in research contexts.

NOTES

1. In the UK, for example, it is held that in matters affecting the interests of children, their welfare is to be considered of paramount importance and that in the context of assisted reproduction, practices and procedures which pose *significant risks of physical and/or psychological harm* to children will be prohibited (Human Fertilisation and Embryology Act, 1990, s. 13[5]).
2. For example, European Society of Human Reproduction and Embryology's (ESHRE's) Ethics and Law Taskforce claims that "technology and research must always be subordinate to the welfare of the future offspring . . . the interests of future offspring must prevail on the development and progress of science" (Pennings et al., 2007, p. 2587).

REFERENCES

1. Dondorp W, de Wert G. Innovative reproductive technologies: Risks and responsibilities. *Human Reproduction*. 2011;26(7):1604–8.
2. Jans V, Dondorp W, Mastenbroek S, Mertes H, Pennings G, Smeets H, de Wert G. Between innovation and precaution: How did offspring safety considerations play a role in strategies of introducing new reproductive techniques? *Human Reproduction Open*. 2020;2:1–9.
3. ESHRE Task Force on Ethics and Law. The moral status of the pre-implantation embryo. *Human Reproduction*. 2011;16(5):1046–8. https://doi.org/10.1093/humrep/16.5.1046.
4. Mertes H. Understanding the ethical concerns that have shaped European regulation of human embryonic stem cell research. *Proceeding of the Belgian Royal Academies of Medicine*. 2012;1:127–39.
5. Hofmann B. Is there a technological imperative in health care? *International Journal of Technology Assessment in Health Care*. 2002;18(3):675–89.
6. Parens E, Asch, A. Disability rights critique of prenatal genetic testing: Reflections and recommendations. *Mental Retardation and Developmental Disabilities Research Reviews*. 2003;9(1):40–7.
7. Robertson JA. *Children of choice: Freedom and the new reproductive technologies*. Princeton: Princeton University Press; 1994.
8. Purdy LM. Genetic diseases: Can having children be immoral? In: Arras J and Rhoden NK, editors. *Ethical issues in modern medicine*. 3rd ed. California: Mayfield Publishing Company; 1989. pp. 311–17.
9. Overall C. *Human reproduction: Principles, practices, policies*. Toronto: Oxford University Press; 1993.
10. Savulescu J. Sex selection: The case for. *Medical Journal of Australia*. 1999;171:373–5.
11. Harris J. *On cloning: Thinking in action*. London, Routledge; 2004.
12. Feinberg J. *Social philosophy*. Engelwood Cliffs, NJ: Prentice Hall; 1973.
13. Mill JS. *The subjection of women*. London: Longmans, Green, Reader and Dyer; 1869.
14. Locke J. The second treatise of government. In: Laslett P, editor. *Two treatises of government*. Cambridge: Cambridge University Press; 1960/1689.
15. Benn SI. *A theory of freedom*. Cambridge: Cambridge University Press; 1988.

16. Rawls J. *Justice as fairness: A restatement.* Cambridge, MA: Belknap Press; 2001.
17. Jackson E. Rethinking the pre-conception welfare principle. In: Horsey K, Biggs H, editors. *Human fertilisation and embryology: Reproducing regulation.* London: Routledge-Cavendish; 2007.
18. Franklin S. Making miracles: Scientific progress and the facts of life. In: Franklin S, Ragone H, editors. *Reproducing reproduction.* Philadelphia: University of Pennsylvania Press; 1998. pp. 102–17.
19. Mertes H. The role of anticipated decision regret and the patient's best interest in sterilisation and medically assisted reproduction. *Journal of Medical Ethics.* 2017;43(5):314–18.
20. Mackenzie C, Stoljar N, editors. *Relational autonomy: Feminist perspectives on autonomy, agency, and the social self.* Oxford: Oxford University Press; 2000.
21. Donchin A. Understanding autonomy relationally: Toward a reconfiguration of bioethical principles. *J Med Philos.* 2001;26:365–86.
22. Dove E, et al. Beyond individualism: Is there a place for relational autonomy in clinical practice and research? *Clinical Ethics.* 2017;12(3):150–65.
23. National Health Service. Availability: IVF. 2021 [cited 2021 July 13]. Available from: www.nhs.uk/conditions/ivf/availability/.
24. Crawshaw M, et al. on behalf of the British Infertility Counselling Association. Counselling challenges associated with donor conception and surrogacy treatments – time for debate. *Human Fertility.* 2021. doi: 10.1080/14647273.2021.1950850.
25. Daniluk J. "If we had it to do over again . . .": Couples' reflections on their experiences of infertility treatments. *The Family Journal: Counseling and Therapy for Couples and Families.* 2001 Apr;2002;9(2):122–33.
26. Robertson JA. Procreative liberty and harm to offspring in assisted conception. *American Journal of Law and Medicine.* 2004;30:7–40.
27. Pennings G, de Wert G, Shenfield F, Cohen J, Tarlatzis B, Devroey P. ESHRE task force on ethics and law 13: The welfare of the child in medically assisted reproduction. *Human Reproduction.* 2007;22(10):2585–8.
28. Steinbock B. Wrongful life and procreative decisions. In: Roberts MA, Wasserman DT, editors. *Harming future persons: Ethics, genetics and the non-identity problem.* London: Springer; 2009. pp. 155–78.
29. Rakowski E. Who should pay for bad genes? *California Law Review.* 2002;90(5):1345–414.
30. Bennett R. The fallacy of the principle of procreative beneficence. *Bioethics.* 2009;23(5):265–73.
31. Brock DW. The non-identity problem and genetic harms: The case of wrongful handicaps. *Bioethics.* 1995;9:269–75.
32. Parfit D. *Reasons and persons.* Oxford: Clarendon Press; 1984.
33. Buchanan A, Brock DW, Daniels N, Wikler D. *From chance to choice: Genetics and justice.* New York: Cambridge University Press; 2000.
34. Williams NJ. Harms to "others" and the selection against disability view. *Journal of Medicine and Philosophy.* 2017;42(2):154–83.
35. Cohen IG. Prohibiting anonymous sperm donation and the child welfare error. *Hastings Centre Report.* 2011;41(5):13–14.
36. Wilkinson S. Gamete donor motives, payment, and child welfare. In: Golombok S, Scott R, Appleby JB, Richards M, Wilkinson S, editors. *Regulating reproductive donation.* Cambridge: Cambridge University Press; 2016. pp. 232–58.
37. Beaudry JS. Beyond (models of) disability? *Journal of Medicine and Philosophy.* 2016;41(2):210–28.
38. Read R, O'Riordan T. The precautionary principle under fire. *Environment: Science and Policy for Sustainable Development.* 2017;59(5):4–15.
39. Manson NA. Formulating the precautionary principle. *Environmental Ethics.* 2002;24(3):263–74.
40. Medical Research Council. MRC ethics guide: Medical research involving children. 2004 [cited 2021 July 4]. Available from: https://mrc.ukri.org/documents/pdf/medical-research-involving-children/.
41. Provoost V, Tilleman K, D'Angelo A, De Sutter P, de Wert G, Nelen W, Pennings G, Shenfield F, Dondorp W. Beyond the dichotomy: A tool for distinguishing between experimental, innovative and established treatment. *Human Reproduction.* 2014;29(3):413–17.

Index

Note: Page numbers in *italics* indicate a figure and page numbers in **bold** indicate a table on the corresponding page.

abortion: spontaneous 22, 89
acceptable risks 196, 200
acetylation 163
adenosine triphosphate (ATP) 162
adjusted odds ratio (aOR) 20, **23**, **32**, 42, **44**, 49, **51–2**, **55**, **75**, 76, 78–80, **113**
adoption 5, 62, 65, 99, 173, 186, 188
advanced maternal age (AMA) 20, 55, 79, 86–92, *87*, **88**, 98, 103, 105
alcohol consumption 173
alkylating agents 118, 122, 156
amenorrhea 117–18, 120, 122–3
American Reproductive Medicine Society 73
American Society for Reproductive Medicine (ASRM) 2, 68, 120, 156
amniocentesis 69
anemia 69; gestational 102
aneuploidies 86, 98; chromosomal 98
aneuploidy 89, 99, 196; autosomal trisomies 89
anovulatory women 8, 54
antepartum hemorrhage 45, 53, 111, **126**
anthracyclines 122
antimullerian hormone (AMH) 2–3, 5, 63, 120–2, 149
antral follicle count (AFC) 2–3, 5, **52**, **55**, 122
anxiety 170–2, **175**, 183–6
aorta: aorta root dilation 65; bicuspid aortic valve 62, 65; coarctation of 62, 65
aortic dissection 61–2
Apgar score 53, **55**, 91, 102, **126**, 150
Aristotle 162
aromatase inhibitors 48, 54, 119
array comparative genomic hybridization (array-CGH) 98, 102
ART-conceived children 31, 34, 37, 132–8, **134**, **135**, 189, 201–3
ascites 1, **2**, 5
assisted reproduction 98, *104*, 164, 197, 200–1, 203n1; safety of 61–65; *see also* assisted reproductive technologies
assisted reproductive technologies (ARTs) 76, 108, 161, 169, 182, 195–6; after cancer treatment 117–28; ethical aspects 195–203; long term outcomes of children conceived through 28–37, **36**; long term safety of 8–16, 61, 195–203; and maternal cancer risk 8–16; and maternal health 76, 195; maternal psychosocial effects of 169–76; psychosocial adjustment in offspring conceived through 182–9; and risks of childhood cancer 132–8; and Turner syndrome 62–5; *see also names of specific technologies/procedures*
asthma 32–3, **32**, 92

attention deficit hyperactivity disorder (ADHD) 21, **30**, 31
Australia **11**, **13**, **14**, **16**, **30**, 48, 109, *110*, 134, **134**, 137, 141, 185
autism 22, **30**, 35, **36**, 79, 91; *see also* autism spectrum disease; autism spectrum disorder
autism spectrum disease 21
autism spectrum disorder (ASD) **30**, 31, 87, 91
autoimmune diseases/disorders 61, 73, 156
autonomy 145, 182, 186–8, 197, 199–200, 203; reproductive 195, 198–9
azoospermia 21–2, 164

Bayley scales 151
Beckwith-Wiedemann syndrome (BWS) 21, 132, 164
Belgium **32**, **36**, 109, 141, 185
biopsy *see* blastocyst-stage biopsy; blastomere biopsy; polar body biopsy; trophectoderm biopsy
birth: live 1, 3, 20, 22, 43, 45, 48, 62–3, 70, 73, 86–8, **88**, 92, 98, 108–10, 120, 123–5, **127**, 141–2, **142**, 145, 148–9, 151, 157–8, 165, 171; *see also* birth defects; birth weight; cesarean deliveries/sections; preterm birth
birth defects 21–2, 24, 102, **142**, 144
birth weight (BW) 20–1, 34, 42, 44–5, **46**, 48–9, 53–4, 69–70, 81, 88, 92, **100**, 102–3, 134–5, 143, 150, 152, 158, 165–6, 186; *see also* low birth weight; very low birth weight
blastocysts 45, 48, 55, 98, 102–5, 109, 114, 161, 164–5; transfer of 45, 102–5, 114, 165
blastocyst-stage biopsy 104
blastocyst-stage biopsy and frozen embryo transfer (BB-FET) 99, **101**, 102–3
blastomere biopsy 98–9, **100–1**, 102–3, 105
blastomeres 98, 103, 161; *see also* blastomere biopsy
body mass index (BMI) **10**, **12**, **15**, 34, 42, **52**, **55**, 89, 92, 99, 103, 170
breast cancer 9, **10**, **11**, 16, **64**, 70, 90, 117–19, 122, 148, 151, 156
breastfeeding 9, 92
Brown, Louise 182

cabergoline 4–5
Canada 62, 141
cancer 9, 90, 92, 123, 125, **128**, 134–8, **134**, **135**, 156; central nervous system 136; childhood 92, 132–8, **134**, **135**; diagnosis 117–18, **126**; hematological 123; hormone-sensitive 8; and recall bias 8; recurrence 118, 120; risk of 8–9, **10**, **11**, **12**, **13**, 14–15, **15**, **16**, 35, 90, 120, 134–8, **135**; survivors 117, 122–5, **126**, **128**; treatment and obstetric outcomes 117–128;

205

see also breast cancer; carcinoma; cervical cancer; chemotherapy; endometrial cancer; leukemia; ovarian cancer; radiotherapy; retinoblastoma; tumors; uterine cancer
capillary permeability 3
carcinoma 123
cardiac defects 89
cardiovascular disorders/disease 31–2, **32**, 34, 37, 88, 90
Centers for Disease Control and Prevention (CDC) 108
cerebral palsy (CP) **30**, 31, 87, 91
cervical cancer 125
cesarean deliveries/sections 20, 22, **23**, **46**, 49, **51**, 54, 73–4, **75**, **77**, 78, 87, 89, 92, 99, **100**, 102, 111, **113**, 122, **128**, **142**, 143–5
chemotherapy 70, 73, 117–23, 125, **128**, 149, 151, 156–8
childbearing 198
childbirth 8, 62, 90
childhood cancers 92, 132–8, **134**, **135**; *see also* leukemia; retinoblastoma
childlessness **52**, **55**, 174, 198
child welfare 200–1, 203
cholestasis 69–70
chorionic villous sampling 69
chromosomal aberrations/abnormalities 21–2, 24, 61, 90, 150
chromosomal aneuploidies 98
chromosomal testing 105; *see also* comprehensive chromosome testing
chromosome segregation errors 86
cleavage stage 151, 162
cleavage-stage biopsy and fresh embryo transfer (CB-ET) 99, **101**, 102–3
clomiphene citrate 8–9, **10**, **12**, **14**, 15–16, **15**, **50**
coasting 4
cognitive development 28, **29**, 104
colorectal cancer 125
Committee of Nordic ART and Safety (CoNARTaS) 42, 44
comorbidities 88, 171, **175**
comprehensive chromosome testing (CCT) 98, **101**, 102, 105
conception: ART 24, 132, 134–7, 186, 189; mode of 35, 62, 184, 187–9; natural (NC) 20–1, **23**, 24, 28, **29–30**, 31–5, **32**, **33**, **35**, **36**, 37, 54, 62, 78, 132, 142–3, 149–50, 152, 157–8, 164, 182, 201; spontaneous 24, 42, 44–5, **51–2**, 86, 92, 99, **101**, 102–3, 149, 174, 185–6, 188–9
confounding 8, 12, 28, 69, 80, 89–90, 133, 135, 164
controlled ovarian stimulation (COS/COH) 1, 70, 81, 119, 149, 151–2, 164
corpus luteum 48–9, **50**, **51**, 53–4, **55**, 89
couples: fertile 20, 103, 137; heterosexual 188; infertile 74; male 141; same-sex 188; subfertile 20, **23**, 137
CpG islands 132, 163
craniosynostosis 89
CREATE study 137
cryopreservation methods 48, 68; slow-freezing 43, 45, 48, 68–71, 156; vitrification 21, 43, 45, 48, 68–71, 98, 105, 151–2
culdocentesis 5
cycle cancellation 4
cycle segmentation 4
cyclophosphamide 118
cytosine methylation 162–3

decidualization 81
Denmark 9, **10**, **12**, **13**, **14**, **15**, 28, **29–30**, 31, **33**, 34, **50**, **64**, 103, 111, 134–5, **134**, 137, 165
depression 170–2, **175**, 183, 185; postnatal 185; prenatal 183; *see also* postpartum depression
developmental delay 21, 28
developmental origins of health and disease (DoHaD) 161, 164, 166; hypothesis 164, 166
diabetes *see* diabetes mellitus
diabetes mellitus 14, 34, 37, **52**, 69, 74, 89–92; pregestational 89; type 1 **33**, 34, 92; type 2 3; *see also* gestational diabetes mellitus
dilation and curettage (D&C) 123
disability 91, 196, 201–2
DNA 117, 132, 162–3, 166; testing 188; *see also* DNA methylation; DNA sequence
DNA methylation 53, 92, 132, 164–5
DNA sequence 53, 132, 161, 165
DNMT 162–3
donor identity 187
donor oocytes 62, 68, 70–1, 73–81, 89
dopamine 4–5
double embryo transfer (DET) 20, **101**, 109
dystocia 54, 89

eclampsia 76; *see also* preeclampsia
Edwards, Robert 182, 197
egg donation 71, 149, 184–5
egg sharing 74
elective frozen/thawed embryo transfer (eFET) 42, 44–5, **44**, **46–7**, 53
elective single embryo transfer (eSET) 43, 45, 108–114, 118
electrolyte imbalance 1
elevated gonadotropins theory 9
embryo development 53, 98–9, 109, 150, 157, 162; *see also* in vitro embryo development
embryo grading 109
embryo implantation 102, 105, 108–9
embryonic genome activation (EGA) 162
embryonic stem cells (ESCs) 163
embryo research 195
embryos 4–5, 22, 43–5, 48, **52**, 54, **55**, 68, 70, 73, 80–1, 86, 98, 103, 108–9, *110*, 114, 119, 132, 144, 148–51, 161–5, 183, 185, 195–6, 199–200; aneuploid 22, 196; cleavage-stage 63, 98–9, 103, 109, 151; cryopreservation of 4–5, 45; cryopreserved 42–55, 70, 165; fresh **29**, 44, 70, 74, 164; frozen **29**, **36**, **52**, 70–1, 74; in vitro 166; mosaic 22; *see also* embryo development; embryo grading; embryo implantation; embryo research; embryo transfer
embryo transfer (ET) 3, 5, 20–1, 42–55, **47**, 68–71, **75**, 103, 108, 145, 164, **175**, 184; *see also* elective frozen/thawed embryo transfer; elective single embryo transfer; fresh embryo transfer; multiple embryo transfer; single embryo transfer
endocrine disorders/metabolic diseases **33**, 34, 81, 90
endometrial cancer 13–16, 123–4
endometrial development 87–8
endometrial growth 118
endometrial proliferation 88
endometrial receptivity 61, 88

Index

endometriosis 9, 12, 14, 86, 90, 111–12, **113**
endometrium preparation 49, 89
endothelial progenitor cells 49
enmeshment 186
epigenetic modifications 31, 54, 92, 163–4
epigenetic regulation 149, 161–6
epigenetics 53, 132, 162, 165–6
epilepsy **30**, 31
epithelial neoplasms 92, 136
Erb palsy 89
esophageal atresia 89
estradiol 2, 4–5, 49, 53, 63, 80, 119; valerate PO 63
estrogen 8–9, 13–14, 49, **50**, 89, 119
estrogen-only hormone replacement therapy 14
Europe 20, 43, *43*, 68, 109–10, *110*, 141, 148, 185
European Convention on Human Rights 197
European IVF Monitoring Programme (EIM) 109
European Society of Human Reproduction and Embryology (ESHRE) 73, 99, 156, 169, 176, 203n2

family(ies): ART 185–6; background 28; disclosing 188; donation 185; extended 183; heteronormative 201; heterosexual 185; history **10**, **11**, **13**, **14**; lesbian 185; meaning of 174, 182–3; non-disclosing 188–9; nuclear 183; relationships 182, 184, 188–9; SC 185–6, 188; structures 182–3, 201; surrogacy 186; two-father 185–6
femininity 174, **175**, 198
fertility drugs 8–16, 201; and cancer risk 8–16
fertility preservation 61–5, **63**, **64**, 68, 70, 118–19, **121**, 123, 125, 148, 151–2, 156, 169; embryo and oocytes cryopreservation 118–19; gonadotropin-releasing hormone analog agonists 118, 120; ovarian tissue cryopreservation 63, **64**, 118, 120, 151, 156–8; *see also* fertility sparing
fertility sparing 124
fertility treatments 8–9, 16, 123, 164, 170–1, 173, **175**, 184, 197, 200
fertilization 20, 88, 109, 114, 119, 148, 161–2, 164, 171, **175**; post- 98; *see also* in vitro fertilization
fetal arthrogryposis 158
fetal attachment 184
fetal development 69, 163, 166
financial security 183, 187
Finland **11**, **13**, **14**, **16**, 48, **64**, 109, 111, **126**
fluid resuscitation 5
fluorescent in situ hybridization (FISH) 98, **100–1**, 102–3
follicles 2, 8, 48, **52**, **55**, 118, 120, 122, 148–9, 156
follicle-stimulating hormone (FSH) 3–4, **36**, 42, **50**, **52**, **55**, 63, 120, 122, 148–9
follicular phase 49, **50**, 149
forced choice 198
fresh embryo transfer 3, 31, 43–5, **44**, **46**, 73, 89, 99, **101**, 149
frozen embryo replacements (FERs) 43, *43*
frozen/thawed embryo transfers (FETs) 21, 42–3, 89, 108; artificial/substituted 48; NC- (natural cycle) 42, **46**, 48–9, **50**, **51–2**, 53–4, **55**; tNC- (true natural cycle) 42, 48–9, **50**, **51–2**, **55**; *see also* elective frozen/thawed embryo transfer

galactosemia **63**, 156
gametes 68, 119, 132, 161, 164, 199–201; donated 183, 187–9; donor 183, 185
gametogenesis 53, 86
gastrointestinal disorders 33, **33**
gay fathers 185–6
gene editing 200–1
gene expression 53, 162–3, 166
genetic abnormalities 79
genetic imprinting 132
genomic imprinting 53, 163–4
germ cells 92, 117, 122, 124; primordial (PGCs) 162
germinal cells 118
germinal stage (GV) 119, 148
germline 163, 200, 202
gestation 69–70, 88–91, 108, 161, 165
gestational age 21–2, **23**, 31, 34, 69–70, 92, **100**, 102–3, 135, **142**, 144, 150, 158, 165, 186; *see also* large for gestational age; small for gestational age
gestational carrier 81, 141–5; *see also* surrogacy
gestational cholestasis 69
gestational diabetes mellitus (GDM) 21, 42, **52**, 68, 70, 76, **77**, 78, 87, 89–90, 99, **101**, 102, 111, **113**, **142**, 143
gestational sac **52**, **55**, 109
gestational surrogacy 62, 65, 141–5; *see also* surrogacy
GnRH analog (GnRHa) 119–20
gonadal cells 117
gonadal tissue 117
gonadotoxic damages 117
gonadotoxicity 118, 120, 125; effects 118, 123
gonadotoxic therapies 70, 156
gonadotoxic treatments 156, 158
gonadotropin hormonal stimulation 118
gonadotropin-releasing hormone (GnRH) 3–5, 42–3, **50**, 54, 118, 122, 148
gonadotropins 4, 8–9, **10**, **12**, **14**, **15**, **50**, 149
Google 171
grandparenthood 173
Greece **33**, 34, 141, 185
growth 28, 34–5, **35**, **36**, 45, 87, 114, 164–6; fetal 53–4, 88, 149, 163; follicular 3, 120, 122; of multiple follicles 8; placental 164; *see also* birth weight; endometrial growth; insulin-like growth factor; intrauterine growth restriction; vascular endothelial growth factor
Guatemala 109

heart disease 54, 81, 88, 90
Hellin's law 108
hematological cancer 123
hematopoietic stem cell transplantation (HSCT) 123, 156
hemoconcentration 1, **2**
hemolysis, elevated liver enzymes, and low platelets (HELLP syndrome) 143
hepatoblastoma 134
heterotopic transplantation 157
higher-order multiple (HOM) pregnancies 108–10, 114
histone methylation 132
Hodgkin lymphoma **64**, 118, 123, 136; *see also* non-Hodgkin lymphoma
hormone replacement therapy 9, 14

host-versus-graft rejection 143
human chorionic gonadotropin (hCG) 1–5, 42, 48, **50**, 70, 119, 148, 150
Human Fertilisation and Embryology Authority (HFEA) 70, 169, 173, 199
human genome 53
human leukocyte antigen (HLA) 74, 81
human papilloma virus 125
hypercoagulability 1
hypermethylation 132
hypertension 14, **52**, 54, 89–91, 99, **101**; chronic **52**, **55**, 76, 88, 90; pregnancy-induced 45, 69, **113**, **142**, 143; *see also* hypertensive disorders; hypertensive disorders in pregnancy
hypertensive disorders 21–2, 42, **51–2**, 61–2, 70, 73–4, **75**, 76, **77**, 80, 88–9, 99, **113**, **142**, 143; gestational hypertension 22, **23**, 76, 102, 111, **113**; preeclampsia 21–2, **23**, 24, 44–5, **44**, **46**, **51**, 53–5, **75**, 76, **77**, 80–1, 87, 89, 99, **101**, 102, **113**, **142**, 143; chronic hypertension **52**, **55**, 76, 88, 90; *see also* hypertensive disorders in pregnancy
hypertensive disorders in pregnancy (HDP) 21, 42–5, **44**, **46**, 49, **51–2**, 53–4, 68–9, 76, 88, **113**, **142**, 143
hypo-albuminemia 5
hypoestrogenism 61
hypoglycemia 54, 89, 102
hypomethylation 132
hypospadias 21, 89
hypothalamic-pituitary-adrenal (HPA) axis 184
hypothalamus 4, 8
hypothermia 102
hypovolemic hyponatremia 3
hysterectomy **10**, **11**, **13**, **14**, 123–4, **128**, 141, 144

identity 174, 182–3, 187–9; autonomy and 187; biological 189; donor 187; formation 189; gender 187; and genetic relatedness 187–8; genetic 187, 189; non-identity problem 201, 203; tracing 188
immunogenetic dissimilarity 88
immunologic oocyte theory 80
imprinting disorders 21, 53, 163–5
incessant ovulation theory 9
infancy 184–6, 189
infantilization 186
infection **64**, 102; urinary tract 69
infertility 8–9, **10**, 11–13, 15–16, 20–1, 28, 31, **32**, 33–5, 37, **52**, 53, **55**, 61, 86, 90, 103–4, 108, 110, 112, **113**, 120, 123, 125, 149, 164, 166, 169–71, 173, **175**, 176, 183, 197–8; age-related 87, 92; anovulatory 53; couple 37; iatrogenic 117; male factor 9, 37, 170; -related isolation 170; -related stress 170, **175**; -specific distress 171; treatments 28; tubal factor 31, 86; *see also* fertility treatments
informed consent 196, 202
inner cell mass (ICM) 161–2
insulin-like growth factor: I 3, 53; II 53, 163, 165
interleukin-6 3
intracytoplasmic sperm injection (ICSI) 20–2, **23**, 28, **29–30**, 31, **32**, 33–5, **33**, **35**, **36**, 37, 42, *43*, **52**, **55**, 62, 73–4, 76, **100–1**, 103, 108–9, 111, 114, 123, 137–8, 148–51, 164, 172, 200

intrauterine death **77**, 79
intrauterine growth restriction (IUGR) 81, 102–3, 118
intrauterine insemination (IUI) 20, 42, **50**, **51–2**, 123–4, 149, 169, 172
intraventricular hemorrhage 102
in vitro embryo development 161–6; *see also* in vitro maturation
in vitro fertilization (IVF) 1, 3, 20–4, **23**, 28, **29–30**, 31–5, **32**, **33**, **35**, **36**, 42, *43*, **52**, 54, **55**, 62, 73–4, **75**, 76, 78–80, 98–9, **100–1**, 102–5, 108–11, **113**, 114, 119, **121**, 123–4, 137–8, 141–5, 148–52, 157, 161, 164–5, 170–4, 182, 184–5, 195, 197, 199–200; and male factor 20–24
in vitro maturation (IVM) 20, 70, **121**, 148–52, 157
in vitro oocyte maturation 148–52; *see also* in vitro maturation
Israel **10**, **11**, **12**, **13**, **15**, **16**, 31, **32**, 33–4, **33**, **35**, 134–5, **134**, **135**, 141
IVF *see* in vitro fertilization

Japan 49, **50**
jaundice 102

labor: dystocia 89; induction 20, 89–90, 99, 144; pre- 42, **52**, 68; preterm 21, 70, 112, 122, 149
lacerations: perineal 54; vaginal/rectal 89
Langhorne histiocytosis 136
large for gestational age (LGA) 21, 42, 44–5, **47**, 53–4, **100–1**, 102–3, *104*, **113**
large offspring syndrome (LOS) 164
Latin America 109
lesbian mothers 185–6
letrozole **50**, 119
leukemia **64**, 92, 132, 134, 136–8, 156
linkage data studies 133
Locke, J. 198
low birth weight (LBW) 22, **23**, 24, 34, 42, 44, **44**, 53, 73, **75**, 78–9, 81, 91, 102, 122, **126**, **147**, 143, 164–5, 184; *see also* very low birth weight
luteal phase 2, 49, **50**, 148–9
luteinizing hormone (LH) 4, 42, 48, **52**, **55**, 149

macrosomia 21, 70, 89
malformation rates 150
masculinity 174, **175**
maternal insufficiency 81
maternal meiosis 99
maternal morbidity 20, **23**, 88, **113**
maternal outcomes 1–5, 20, 49, **51**, 87
mediators/mediating 3, 134–5
medically assisted reproduction (MAR) 68–70, 148–9, 151, 200
meiotic phase 149
melanoma 90, 92
menarche **10**, 158; early 9; post- 63
menopause 156; chemotherapy-induced 119; late 9, 14; premature 120; radiotherapy-induced 119
menstrual cycle 45, 119–23, 148, 171, **175**
messenger RNAs (mRNAs) 162
metaphase II stage 148
metformin 3, 5

Index

methylation 53, 92, 132, 163–6; *see also* cytosine methylation; DNA methylation; histone methylation; hypermethylation; hypomethylation; trimethylation
Middle East 109
Mill, J. S. 198
Millennial Cohort Study 186
miscarriage 20, 22, 48–9, 61, 74, 79, 86, **88**, 89, 98, **113**, 123–5, 141–2, **142**, 150
"missing corpus luteum" theory 54
mitochondrial dysfunction 86
mitochondrial replacement therapy 200–1
mitotic cleavage 161
mitotic cycles 161
modified natural cycle FET (mNC-FET) 42, **46**, 48–9, **50**, **51–2**
morbidity 62, 76, 89, 91, 102, 108; dermatological 34, **35**; gastrointestinal 33, **33**; ophthalmic 34, **35**; perinatal 76, 114; psychiatric 170, 172; psychological co- 175; *see also* maternal morbidity
morphogenetic event 161
morula 161–2
motherhood 125, 198
"multiple birth epidemic" 109
multiple birth outcomes 108–114
multiple embryo transfer 20, 87, 184
myomas 86
myometrial fibrosis 118

natural cycle FET (NC-FET) 42, **46**, 48–9, **51–2**, 53–4, **55**
naturally conceived children 132–5, 137–8, 151
natural reproduction 196–7, 201
neonatal hypoglycemia 54, 89
neonatal intensive care unit (NICU) 69, 99, **100–1**, 102–3, *104*, **113**, 150
neonatal mortality 20, 22
Netherlands, the 11–12, **11**, **13**, **14**, 28, **29**, 33, 34, 103, 134–6, **134**, **135**, 141, 144
neuroblastoma **64**, 134, 136–8
neurodevelopmental outcomes 28, **29–30**, 31, **36**, 186
newborns 20, 69, 91–2, 99, **100–1**, 103–4, *104*, 145, 150, 157
New Zealand 109, *110*
next-generation sequencing (NGS) 98, **101**
non-Hodgkin lymphoma 123
"non-identity problem, the" 200–1, 203
non-invasive PGT (ni-PGT) 105
nonobstructive azoospermia (NOA) 21–2
Norway 9, **10**, **11**, **12**, **13**, **14**, **15**, **16**, 35, **35**, **64**, **126**, 135, **135**
nulliparity 9, 12, 14, 74
nulliparous women 9, 15, **126**

obesity 13, **13**, 15, **16**, 34, 54, 173; non- 3
odds ratio (OR) **10**, **11**, **13**, **14**, **16**, 20, 22, **23**, 42, **44**, **52**, **55**, 69, **75**, 76, 89, 112, **127**
OD procedure 80–1
oligohydramnios 111
oligomenorrhoea 120
oligozoospermia 21, 164
oncofertility counseling 118–20
oocyte donation (OD) 55, 62, 70–1, 73, **75**, 87–8, 91–2, **113**, 141, 143–4, 149, 157; anonymous 187, 189

oocytes 1–2, 5, 20, 63, 65, 68–71, 74, 80–1, 118–19, 141, 148–52, 157, 163, 173; anonymous donation of 187, 189; autologous 62, 69–71, 74, **75**, 86–7, 89, 92, **113**; autologous vitrified 69–70; banking of 68; cryopreservation of 63, **63**, 68–71, 119, 156; fresh 69, 74; frozen 69, 71, 73–4; immature 119, 149, 151, 156–7; mature 70, 149, 156; prepubertal 156; quality of 86; retrieval of 1, 5, 43, 68, 149, 172; *see also* donor oocytes; oocyte donation
oral contraceptives 9, **10**, 14
organogenesis 164
organ transplantation 74
orthotopic auto-transplantation 157
orthotopic transplantation 158
ovarian cancer 9, 11–13, **12**, **13**, 16, 124
ovarian enlargement 1
ovarian epithelium 9
ovarian hyperstimulation syndrome (OHSS) 1–5, **2**, 42–3, 45, 54, 119, 148; iatrogenic occurrence of 1
ovarian insufficiency 55, 62–3, **63**, 73, 81, 118, 120, 148, 156
ovarian priming 148
ovarian reserve 1–2, 63, 73–4, 86, 121–2, 156, 158
ovarian stimulation 1–5, 8–9, 12–16, 20, **47**, 63, **63**, 70, 80–1, 90, 108, 118–19, 141, 148–52, 156, 164, 171
ovarian tissue cryopreservation (OTC) 63, **64**, 118, 120, 151, 156–8
ovarian tissue transplantation (OTT) **121**, 156–8
ovarian tumors 11; benign 11; borderline (BOTs) 11–13, **14**, 16, 124; epithelial 11; invasive 9, 11
ovaries 4, 8, 117–18, 122, 149; enlarged **2**, 3, **4**; prepubertal 157; *see also* ovarian cancer; ovarian enlargement; ovarian epithelium; ovarian hyperstimulation syndrome; ovarian insufficiency; ovarian priming; ovarian reserve; ovarian stimulation; ovarian tissue cryopreservation; ovarian tissue transplantation; ovarian tumors; ovulation; polycystic ovary syndrome
ovulation 8–9, 54–5, 122, 148; hormone-assisted 123; -inducing medication 134; induction 8–9, **10**, 12, **12**, **14**, **15**, 48, **50**; induction treatments 9; priming 150; suppression 3

paracentesis 5
parent-child relationships 183–9
parenthood 86, 170, 172–4, **175**, 176, 183–6, 189, 198, 201
parenting 91, 174, 182–7
parents: adoptive 185; biological 173; donor-conceiving 186; expectant 183; fertile 138; genetic 187; heterosexual 186; infertile 104; intended 141–2, 144–5, 200; lesbian 186; naturally conceiving 185; non-disclosing 188; prospective 86, 195, 198, 200–1; spontaneously conceiving 185; subfertile 20–1, 132, 135, 138
parity 9, **10**, **11**, **12**, **13**, 14, **14**, **15**, **16**, **52**, **55**, 89, 99, 103, 165
parous women 9, 11, 15
Percutaneous Epididymal Sperm Aspiration (PESA) 21–2, **23**, 24
periconception period 164, 166
perinatal complications: with donor oocytes 73–81, **77**

perinatal mortality 20–1, 44–5, 53, 74, 89, 91, **113**
perinatal outcomes 20–2, **23**, 24, 43–5, 48, 68–71, 74, 91, **100**, 102–3, **126**, 141–5, 149, 165
pituitary gland 8
pituitary suppression 4
placenta 49, 88, 99, 143, 164; manual lysis of 99; retained 20; *see also* placenta(l) abruption; placenta accrete; placenta previa; placental complications; placental disease; placentation; uterine revision
placenta(l) abruption **51**, 53, 78, 89, 99, **113**, 143
placenta accreta **51**, 99
placental complications 68, 99
placental disease **142**, 143
placenta previa 21, **51**, 53, 68, 78, 88–9, 99, **100**, 102, 111, **113**, 143
placentation 69–70, 81, 88, 112, 150
polar body biopsy 98–9, 102–3, 105
polycystic ovary syndrome (PCOS) 1, 3, *4*, 5, 14–15, 42, 45, **46–7**, **52**, 53, 111–12, **113**, 148, 150–1
postpartum depression **142**, 144–5
postpartum hemorrhage (PPH) 20, 42, **46**, **51**, 53–4, **77**, 78, 99, **101**, 102, **113**, **126**, **128**, 141, **142**, 144
preconception counseling 61–2, **128**
preeclampsia 21–2, **23**, 24, 44–5, **44**, **46**, **51**, 53–5, **75**, 76, **77**, 80–1, 87, 89, 99, **101**, 102, **113**, **142**, 143
pregnancy(ies): at advanced maternal age 86–92; AO IVF 78–9; ART 110; clinical 48, 68, 86, **88**, 102, 108, 149; complications during 61, 70–1, 73–4, 99, 111, **128**, 157; ectopic 20, 89–90; extrauterine 142, **142**; higher-order multiple 108–10, 114; IVF 74, 76, 144; IVF with AO 78–9; MAR 68; molar 86, 89; multiple 20, 31, 34, 62, 74, 76, 81, 90, 108–12, **113**, 114, 124, **142**, 143–5, 150–1, 174; natural 74, **75**, 76, **77**, 78–80, 109, 143; oocyte donation 73–4, 76, 78–80, 88, 143–4; progression of 69; singleton 20–2, **23**, 28, **29–30**, 31, 33–4, **36**, 37, 44, **46**, 53, 62, 69, 76, **77**, 78–80, 87, 91, 99, **100**, 102, 108, 110, 124, **126**, 143, 150–1, 158, 165, 185–6; spontaneous 61, 111, 122, 124–5; twin 28, 76, 91, 102–3, **113**, 114, 124, 151, 158; unwanted 86; *see also* pregnancy test
pregnancy test 171–2, **175**
preimplantation genetic diagnosis (PGD) 98, 201
preimplantation genetic screening (PGS) 98
preimplantation genetic testing (PGT) 20, 42–3, **52**, 98–105, **100–1**, *104*, 169, 196
premature ovarian insufficiency (POI) 55, **63**, 81, 118, 120, 125, 148, 156–7
prematurity 37, 81, 87, 91, **113**
prepubertal girls 117, 156
preterm birth (PTB) 20–2, **23**, 24, 28, 37, 42, 44–5, **44**, **46**, 48–9, 53–4, **55**, 69–70, 78, 89, **100**, 102–3, **113**, 122, **126**, **128**, 144, 149–50, 152, 164, 184
preterm delivery 34, 61, 73–4, **75**, **77**, 78, 81, 91, 102, 123, 125, 144
preterm prelabor rupture of membranes (PPROM) 42, **52**, 68
primordial follicle 120, 156
procreation 197
procreative liberty 197
progesterone 2, 13, 49, **50**, 53, 89; supplementation 49
pronatalism 198

prophylactic anti-coagulation 5
proteinuria 22, 90
psychosocial development 22, 24
puberty 61, 63, 65, 187

quantitative polymerase chain reaction (qPCR) 98, **101**

radiotherapy 73, 117–19, 123, 125, **128**, 156
randomized controlled trial (RCT) 3, 42, **44**, 45, **46**, 48, 53, **100–1**, 102, 104–5, 165
Rawls, J. 198
recessive disorders 79, 81
recurrent pregnancy loss (RPL) 98, 103, 105
relational autonomy 199
relative risk (RR) 8, **10**, **11**, **12**, **13**, **14**, **15**, **16**, 22, 29, 42–5, **46**, 54, 76, 78, 91, **113**, **127**, **128**, 136
relaxin 49, 89
repeated implantation failure (RIF) 98, 103, 105
reproductive autonomy 195, 198–9
reproductive choice 198, 203
reproductive liberty 196–8
reproductive medicine 195–6, 200
reproductive rights 86, 197
respiratory disorders/disease 32–3, **32**
respiratory distress syndrome **2**, 102
retinoblastoma 92, 132, 134, 136–8
rights: claim 196; liberty 196; negative 197; offspring 187–9; positive 197; vs principles 198–9; *see also* reproductive rights; right to reproduce
right to reproduce 197, 203; *see also* reproductive rights
risk reduction 5, 196

salpingo-oophorectomy 123–4, 144
Scandinavia 89, 135, **135**, 137
self-esteem **175**, 176, 183
semen quality 21
sepsis **2**, 102
severe male factor (SMF) 20, 98
sex selection 199
sex steroids 45, 54
sexual relationship 174, **175**
Silver-Russell syndrome (SRS) 21, 164
single embryo transfer (SET) 20, 43, 45, **52**, 54, **55**, 62, 81, 91, **101**, 108–14, *110*, 184
single nucleotide polymorphism array (SNP-array) 98, **100–1**
singletons 20–2, **23**, 28, **29–30**, 31, 33–4, **36**, 37, 44, **46**, 53, 62, 69, 76, **77**, 78–80, 87, 91, 99, **100**, 102, 108, 110, 124, **126**, 143, 150–1, 158, 165, 185–6; perinatal mortality rate of 91
skin disorders 34, **35**
slow-freezing 43, 45, 48, 68–71, 156
small for gestational age (SGA) 34, 42, 44–5, **47**, 53–4, **77**, 79, **113**, **126**, 149, 164
smoking **10**, **11**, **12**, **13**, **15**, **52**, **55**, 91, 173; maternal 88
social media 171
Society for Assisted Reproductive Technologies (SART) 108
Spain 86
Spanish Fertility Society 73

Index 211

sperm: cells 141; donation 74, 185; donor 22, **23**, 24, 80, 185; ejaculated 21–2; epididymal 21–2, **23**; nondonor 22; partner 22, **23**, 80; testicular 21–2; *see also* intracytoplasmic sperm injection
spermatozoa 21, 79, 164
standard deviation (SD) 42, **46**, **63**
stem cells: transplantation 123, 156; *see also* embryonic stem cells
stigmatization: and behavior problems 186
stillbirths 21–2, **36**, 44, 87, 90–1, **113**, **127**
subfertility **14**, 20–1, **23**, 33, **50**, **51**, 53, 122, 132, 135–8, **135**, 149
surrogacy 141, 185–6, 201
Sweden 9, **10**, **11**, **12**, **13**, **14**, 28, **29–30**, **32**, **33**, **35**, **36**, 37, **50**, 62–3, **64**, 109, **126**, 134–5, **134**, **135**

taxanes 122
technological imperative 195–6; imperative of demand 196; imperative of possibility and action 196
Testicular Sperm Aspiration (TESA) 21–2, **23**
Testicular Sperm Extraction (TESE) 21–2, **23**, 24
TET proteins 163
third-trimester bleeding 68–9
thromboembolic disease 5
thromboembolism **2**, 5
thrombophilia 5
thyroid-stimulating hormone (TSH) **33**, 34
toddlerhood 182, 185–6
trachelectomy 125, **128**
trimethylation 163
triple embryo transfer (TET) 109
triplets 108–10, *111*, 114, 144, 185; perinatal mortality rate 91; perinatal risks 184
trophectoderm (TE) 98–9, **101**, 102–3, *104*, 105, 161
trophectoderm biopsy 98–9, 102–5
trophectoderm cells 98
true natural cycle FET (tNC-FET) 42, 48–9, **50**, **51–2**, 55
tumor(s): borderline ovarian (BOTs) 11–13, **14**, 16, 124; brain 92, 134; cell 117; diagnosis 119; germ cell 92, 124; granulosa cell 157; hematological 157; hepatic 136–8; regression **128**; renal 136; retinoblastoma 136; solid 157; suppressor gene 132; *see also* ovarian tumors
Turner syndrome 61–65, **63**, **64**, 80, 156, 196
twins 20–1, **23**, 28, 76, 91, 102–3, 108–10, *111*, **113**, 114, 124, 132, 151, 158, 165, 184–6; dizygotic 108; monozygotic 108, 114, 132, 157; naturally conceived 91, 185; perinatal mortality rate 91; vanishing 20

ultrasound 4, 48, 90, 108, 122, 148, 151
United Arab Emirates 109
United Kingdom **10**, **11**, **12**, **13**, **14**, 15, **15**, **16**, 62, 134–5, 137, 141, 169–70, 185–6, 199, 203n1; National Health Service 199
United Nations 197; Declaration on Human Rights 197
United States **10**, **11**, **12**, **13**, **15**, **16**, 76, 86, 109, *110*, 133, 135, 141
uterine cancer **15**, **16**
uterine receptivity 87
uterine revision 99
uterine vascularization 118
uterus 9, 80, 108, 124, **128**, 141–2, 144, 196

vagina 118
vaginal deliveries 20, 90, 144
vanishing twins 20
vascular endothelial growth factor (VEGF) 3–4, 42, 49
vasoactive hormones 49
very low birth weight (VLBW) 20, 42, 69, 79, 102–3, 149, 164
very preterm birth (VPTB) 20, 42, **113**, 164
vision and hearing disorders 34, **35**
vitrification 21, 43, 45, 48, 68–71, 98, 105, 151–2

welfare standards 200–1
womanhood 198
World Health Organization (WHO) 169
"wrongful life" 200–1

zona pellucida (ZP) opening 98, 102–3
zygote 98–9, 151

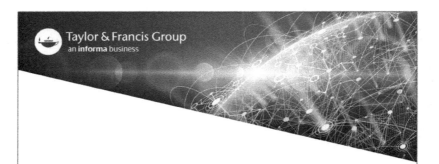

Milton Keynes UK
Ingram Content Group UK Ltd.
UKHW032302291123
433521UK00005B/53